2012
YEAR BOOK OF
PATHOLOGY
AND LABORATORY
MEDICINE®

The 2012 Year Book Series

Year Book of Anesthesiology and Pain Management™: Drs Chestnut, Abram, Black, Gravlee, Lien, Mathru, and Roizen

Year Book of Cardiology®: Drs Gersh, Cheitlin, Elliott, Gold, Graham, and Thourani

Year Book of Critical Care Medicine®: Drs Dellinger, Parrillo, Balk, Dorman, Dries, and Zanotti-Cavazzoni

Year Book of Dermatology and Dermatologic Surgery™: Dr Del Rosso

Year Book of Diagnostic Radiology®: Drs Elster, Abbara, Oestreich, Offiah, Rosado de Christenson, Stephens, and Strickland

Year Book of Emergency Medicine®: Drs Hamilton, Bruno, Handly, Minczak, Mullin, Quintana, and Ramoska

Year Book of Endocrinology®: Drs Schott, Apovian, Clarke, Eugster, Ludlam, Meikle, Oetjen, Schteingart, and Toth

Year Book of Gastroenterology™: Drs Talley, DeVault, Harnois, Murray, Pearson, Philcox, Picco, and Smith

Year Book of Hand and Upper Limb Surgery®: Drs Yao and Steinmann

Year Book of Medicine®: Drs Barker, Garrick, Gersh, Khardori, LeRoith, Panush, Talley, and Thigpen

Year Book of Neonatal and Perinatal Medicine®: Drs Fanaroff, Benitz, Donn, Neu, Papile, Polin, and Van Marter

Year Book of Neurology and Neurosurgery®: Drs Klimo, Minagar, Breningstall, Gandhi, House, Kevill, Liu, Mazia, Panagariya, Ragel, Riesenburger, Shafazand, Uhm, and Yang

Year Book of Obstetrics, Gynecology, and Women's Health®: Drs Dungan and Shulman

Year Book of Oncology®: Drs Arceci, Bauer, Chiorean, Gordon, Lawton, Murphy, Thigpen, and Tsao

Year Book of Ophthalmology®: Drs Rapuano, Cohen, Flanders, Hammersmith, Milman, Myers, Nagra, Nelson, Penne, Pyfer, Sergott, Shields, Talekar, and Vander

Year Book of Orthopedics®: Drs Morrey, Huddleston, Swiontkowski, and Trigg

Year Book of Otolaryngology-Head and Neck Surgery®: Drs Sindwani, Balough, Franco, Gapany, and Mitchell

Year Book of Pathology and Laboratory Medicine®: Drs Raab and Bissell

Year Book of Pediatrics®: Dr Stockman

Year Book of Plastic and Aesthetic Surgery™: Drs Miller, Gosman, Gurtner, Gutowski, Ruberg, Salisbury, and Smith

Year Book of Psychiatry and Applied Mental Health®: Drs Talbott, Ballenger, Buckley, Frances, Krupnick, and Mack

Year Book of Pulmonary Disease®: Drs Barker, Jones, Maurer, Spradley, Tanoue, and Willsie

Year Book of Sports Medicine®: Drs Shephard, Cantu, Feldman, Galea, Jankowski, Janssen, Lebrun, and Nieman

Year Book of Surgery®: Drs Copeland, Behrns, Daly, Eberlein, Fahey, Huber, Klodell, Mozingo, and Pruett

Year Book of Urology®: Drs Andriole and Coplen

Year Book of Vascular Surgery®: Drs Moneta, Gillespie, Starnes, and Watkins

2012

The Year Book of PATHOLOGY AND LABORATORY MEDICINE®

Editor-in-Chief
Stephen S. Raab, MD
Professor of Pathology, University of Washington, Seattle, Washington, and Memorial University of Newfoundland/Eastern Health Authority, St John's, Newfoundland, Canada

Editor-in-Chief, Laboratory Medicine
Michael G. Bissell, MD, PhD, MPH
Professor of Pathology, Ohio State University Medical Center, Columbus, Ohio

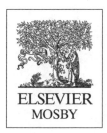

ELSEVIER
MOSBY

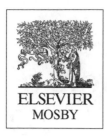

ELSEVIER
MOSBY

Vice President, Continuity: Kimberly Murphy
Editor: Katie Hartner
Supervisor, Electronic Year Books: Donna M. Skelton
Electronic Article Manager: Mike Sheets
Illustrations and Permissions Coordinator: Dawn Vohsen

Printed in the United States of America
Composition by TNQ Books and Journals Pvt Ltd, India
Printing/binding by Sheridan Books, Inc.

Editorial Office:
Elsevier
Suite 1800
1600 John F. Kennedy Blvd.
Philadelphia, PA 19103-2899

International Standard Serial Number: 1077-9108
International Standard Book Number: 978-0-323-08889-3

Contributing Editors

Reza Alaghehbandan, MD, MSc

Clinical Epidemiologist, Faculty of Medicine, Memorial University of Newfoundland; Fellow, Dr H. Bliss Murphy Cancer Care Foundation, St John's, Newfoundland, Canada

Beverley A. Carter, MD, FRCPC

Provincial Director of Pathology and Laboratory Medicine, Government of Newfoundland and Labrador, St John's, Newfoundland, Canada

S. A. Chandrakanth, MD, FRCPC

Staff Pathologist, Clinical Assistant Professor, Eastern Health, Memorial University, Newfoundland and Labrador, St John's, Newfoundland, Canada

Dana M. Grzybicki, MD, PhD

Associate Professor, Pathology, Rocky Vista University, Parker, Colorado

Miriam D. Post, MD

Assistant Professor, Department of Pathology, University of Colorado School of Medicine, Aurora, Colorado

M. Sherif Said, MD, PhD, FCAP

Associate Professor of Pathology, University of Colorado Denver; Associate Director of Pathology, Denver Health, Denver, Colorado

Maxwell L. Smith, MD

Assistant Professor, Department of Laboratory Medicine and Pathology, Mayo Clinic Arizona, Scottsdale, Arizona

Joshua Wisell, MD

Assistant Professor, Department of Pathology, University of Colorado School of Medicine, Aurora, Colorado

Table of Contents

Journals Represented   xi

ANATOMIC PATHOLOGY   1
1. Outcomes Analysis   3
2. Breast   19
3. Gastrointestinal System.   33
4. Hepatobiliary System and Pancreas   47
5. Dermatopathology   65
6. Lung and Mediastinum.   85
7. Cardiovascular   93
8. Soft Tissue and Bone   97
9. Female Genital Tract   103
10. Urinary Bladder and Male Genital Tract   129
11. Kidney   161
12. Head and Neck.   181
13. Neuropathology   219
14. Cytopathology   229
15. Hematolymphoid   245
16. Techniques/Molecular   257

LABORATORY MEDICINE   265
17. Laboratory Management and Outcomes   267
18. Clinical Chemistry   283
19. Clinical Microbiology.   297
20. Hematology and Immunology   311
21. Transfusion Medicine and Coagulation   329
22. Cytogenetics and Molecular Pathology.   343

Article Index   359
Author Index   371

Journals Represented

Journals represented in this YEAR BOOK are listed below.

Academic Emergency Medicine
AJR American Journal of Roentgenology
American Journal of Clinical Pathology
American Journal of Dermatopathology
American Journal of Gastroenterology
American Journal of Kidney Diseases
American Journal of Medicine
American Journal of Perinatology
American Journal of Surgical Pathology
American Journal of Transplantation
Archives of Pathology & Laboratory Medicine
BioMed Central Genomics
Brain Structure & Function
Breast Cancer Research and Treatment
British Journal of Surgery
British Medical Journal
Cancer
Cancer Cytopathology
Cancer Epidemiology, Biomarkers & Prevention
Cardiovascular Pathology
Chinese Medical Journals
Clinical Cancer Research
Clinical Chemistry
Clinical Infectious Diseases
Clinical Oncology
Clinical Oncology (Royal College of Radiologists)
Clinics and Research in Hepatology and Gastroenterology
Endoscopy
European Archives of Oto-rhino-laryngology
European Journal of Cancer
European Journal of Radiology
European Journal of Surgical Oncology
European Respiratory Journal
Fetal and Pediatric Pathology
Gastrointestinal Endoscopy
Gynecologic Oncology
Head & Neck Oncology
Histopathology
Human Pathology
Intensive Care Medicine
International Journal of Cancer
International Journal of Gynecology & Pathology
International Journal of Obesity
Journal of Clinical Endocrinology & Metabolism
Journal of Clinical Microbiology
Journal of Clinical Oncology
Journal of Clinical Pathology

Journal of Cutaneous Pathology
Journal of General Internal Medicine
Journal of Immunology
Journal of Infectious Diseases
Journal of Molecular Diagnostics
Journal of Neuropathology and Experimental Neurology
Journal of the American Academy of Dermatology
Journal of the American Medical Association
Journal of the American Society of Nephrology
Journal of the National Cancer Institute
Journal of Urology
Kidney International
Lancet
Modern Pathology
Molecular Cancer Therapeutics
Molecular Therapy
Nature
Nephrology Dialysis Transplantation
New England Journal of Medicine
Obstetrics & Gynecology
Oral Oncology
Pancreas
Pathology Research and Practice
Pediatric and Developmental Pathology
Placenta
Plastic and Reconstructive Surgery
Proceedings of the National Academy of Sciences of the United States of America
Public Library of Science One
Science
Thrombosis Research
Thyroid
Transfusion

STANDARD ABBREVIATIONS

The following terms are abbreviated in this edition: acquired immunodeficiency syndrome (AIDS), cardiopulmonary resuscitation (CPR), central nervous system (CNS), cerebrospinal fluid (CSF), computed tomography (CT), deoxyribonucleic acid (DNA), electrocardiography (ECG), health maintenance organization (HMO), human immunodeficiency virus (HIV), intensive care unit (ICU), intramuscular (IM), intravenous (IV), magnetic resonance (MR) imaging (MRI), ribonucleic acid (RNA), ultrasound (US), and ultraviolet (UV).

NOTE

The YEAR BOOK OF PATHOLOGY AND LABORATORY MEDICINE is a literature survey service providing abstracts of articles published in the professional literature. Every effort is made to assure the accuracy of the information presented in these pages. Neither the editors nor the publisher of the YEAR BOOK OF PATHOLOGY AND LABORATORY MEDICINE can be responsible for errors in the original materials. The editors' comments are their own opinions. Mention of specific products within this publication does not constitute endorsement.

To facilitate the use of the YEAR BOOK OF PATHOLOGY AND LABORATORY MEDICINE as a reference tool, all illustrations and tables included in this publication are now identified as they appear in the original article. This change is meant to help the reader recognize that any illustration or table appearing in the YEAR BOOK OF PATHOLOGY AND LABORATORY MEDICINE may be only one of many in the original article. For this reason, figure and table numbers will often appear to be out of sequence within the YEAR BOOK OF PATHOLOGY AND LABORATORY MEDICINE.

PART I

ANATOMIC PATHOLOGY

1 Outcomes Analysis

Resident education and quality of gross tissue examination practices of benign uteri
Ryan MS, Smith ML, Grzybicki DM, et al (Univ of Colorado, Aurora; Rocky Vista Univ, Parker, CO; et al)
J Clin Pathol 64:761-764, 2011

Introduction.—In the USA, most anatomical pathology residency training is based on an apprenticeship model in which residents learn directly by watching more senior personnel and then performing the examination. The level and the effect of the standardisation of resident trainee gross tissue examination practices have not been extensively evaluated.

Methods.—In this apprenticeship-based training programme, a retrospective report review was performed to measure the level of standardisation of gross description (for 11 mandatory descriptors) and tissue submission (for four mandatory sections) practices for uterine specimens removed for benign conditions (n=78). Practices were examined for significant relationships with error, turnaround time (TAT), resource utilisation and postgraduate year of resident (n=25) training.

Results.—Residents provided mandatory descriptors from 23.1% to 93.6% of the time and submitted mandatory sections from 82.1% to 96.2% of the time. Cases submitted by less experienced residents had a longer TAT and were associated with more errors, measured by the necessity to submit additional tissues. Less experienced residents used greater resources (submitting 9.5 tissue cassettes per case) compared with more experienced residents (7.3 cassettes per case), and a statistically significant correlation was found between the number of cassettes submitted and TAT.

Conclusions.—In this training programme, the model of apprenticeship training leads to less than optimal standardisation of gross examination practices, inefficiency, active errors and a high frequency of latent conditions leading to error.

▶ Ryan et al show that, in at least this one residency program in which residents perform gross tissue examination in an apprenticeship training model, marked variability in grossing performance was identified. Ryan et al examined the processes of the gross examination of benign uteri, and one may assume that the gross examination of larger, more complex specimens would have equal or even less standardization. Grossing performance affected overall laboratory quality metrics of turnaround time (timeliness) and efficiency, as additional work needed to be performed to improve quality. The problems in safety most likely were latent factors that could affect (although not likely with benign uteri) diagnostic or reporting error. I think the data presented by Ryan et al reveal 2 main types of problems: (1) the lack of standardized processes affects patient care, and (2) an apprenticeship training model contributes to a less-than-optimal educational environment. The necessity of changing the training paradigm (from "See one, do one, ...") is mandatory to improve patient care and education. For additional reading, please see the reference section.[1,2]

S. S. Raab, MD

References

1. Compton CC. Surgical pathology for the oncology patient in the age of standardization: of margins, micrometastasis, and molecular markers. *Semin Radiat Oncol.* 2003;13:382-388.
2. Gawande A. *The Checklist Manifesto: How to Get Things Right.* New York, NY: Metropolitan Books, LLC; 2009.

Pathology Review of Outside Material: When Does It Help and When Can It Hurt?
Smith LB (Univ of Michigan, Ann Arbor)
J Clin Oncol 29:2724-2727, 2011

Purpose.—Pathology review is performed for patients when care is transferred to a tertiary care center after diagnostic tissue has been obtained. While it has many benefits, this practice can lead to unforeseen difficulties in doctor-patient communication and patient well-being, especially if a diagnosis is overturned or modified years after treatment. The aim of this analysis is to identify clinical situations in which pathology review can result in challenging discussions between patients and oncologists.

Patients.—Representative case scenarios are presented in the subspecialty area of hematopathology. Analysis of the clinical benefits and possible harm to patients, pathologists, and treating oncologists that may ensue from pathology review is performed.

Results.—Pathology review may result in a valuable second opinion and expert subclassification. However, problematic situations may arise with pathology review, especially if the patient has already undergone definitive treatment and is referred to an academic institution in remission. Difficulties can also arise when patients do not understand the limitations of diagnosing disease on small biopsies. The patient may receive a different diagnosis or it may become apparent that the diagnosis could have been made more expeditiously. These discrepancies must be communicated to the patient and may cause confusion and distress.

Conclusion.—Pathology review can be beneficial or potentially harmful depending on the clinical situation. Preliminary recommendations are provided for selecting patients for review. Limiting pathology review to certain clinical situations and encouraging patients to get second opinions before initial treatment at local referral centers may be helpful in minimizing reassignment of diagnoses after definitive treatment.

▶ The opinions offered by Smith should be challenged by the pathology community, although they unfortunately represent not just a small minority opinion. Patient safety is 1 of the 6 domains of quality defined by the Institute of Medicine (IOM). Through the secondary review of anatomic pathology cases, we detect errors of accuracy (the diagnosis does not correspond to the actual disease process) and errors of precision (pathologists disagree on the diagnosis). The majority of medical errors do not cause patient harm, and harm may be classified by degree of severity. Patient anxiety is a form of harm. This concept of harm does not include clinical practitioner harm. Of course, when clinical practitioners are involved in a medical error, there may be consequences to those practitioners in our current health care system. However, the prevailing thought is that errors occur in a flawed system in which there are many contributing latent factors. By detecting error and performing root cause analysis, we will be able to improve the system to decrease the frequency of error. Our focus should be changing the current culture of blame and not limiting the error detection process. For additional reading, please see the reference section.[1,2]

S. S. Raab, MD

References

1. Raab SS, Grzybicki DM. Quality in cancer diagnosis. *CA Cancer J Clin.* 2010;60: 139-165.
2. McCulloch P, Catchpole K. A three-dimensional model of error and safety in surgical health care microsystems. Rationale, development and initial testing. *BMC Surg.* 2011;11:23.

Certification and maintenance of certification: updates from the American Board of Pathology
Bennett BD, Grimes MM (American Board of Pathology, Tampa, FL)
Hum Pathol 42:770-773, 2011

The American Board of Pathology continues to update the certification process to ensure that all candidates have appropriate training and credentials and meet the competency requirements of the Accreditation Council for Graduate Medical Education. The maintenance of certification process, instituted in 2006, has gone through 2 reporting cycles; and the American Board of Pathology is preparing for administration of the first maintenance of certification examination in 2014. This article updates the pathology community on these changes.

▶ Bennett and Grimes provide an update on the processes of certification and maintenance of certification (MOC) for pathologists. Since January 1, 2006, all primary and subspecialty certificates issued by the American Board of Pathology are time limited, and all pathologists certified in 2006 or later must participate in the MOC program. In the future, the MOC program may be mandated for credentialing in hospitals, so it is possible that all pathologists will need to participate. MOC is based on the 6 competency domains adopted by the Accreditation Council for Graduate Medical Education: medical knowledge, patient care, practice-based learning and improvement, professionalism, communication and interpersonal skills, and systems-based practice. There are 4 components of MOC: professional standing, lifelong learning and self assessment, cognitive expertise, and evaluation of performance in practice. The development of the assessment process is still ongoing, although our profession has a terrific opportunity to build quality improvement and education specifically into the MOC. The link between education and performance will be critical to maintain and improve professional competence. For additional reading, please see the reference section.[1,2]

S. S. Raab, MD

References

1. Bennett BD. Certification from the American Board of Pathology: getting it and keeping it. *Hum Pathol.* 2006;37:978-981.
2. Rinder HM, Grimes MM, Wagner J, Bennett BD, RISE Committee, American Society for Clinical Pathology and the American Board of Pathology. Senior pathology resident in-service examination scores correlate with outcomes of the American Board of Pathology certifying examinations. *Am J Clin Pathol.* 2011;136:499-506.

Biopsy Misidentification Identified by DNA Profiling in a Large Multicenter Trial
Marberger M, McConnell JD, Fowler I, et al (Med Univ of Vienna, Austria; Wake Forest Univ School of Medicine, Winston-Salem, NC; GlaxoSmithKline, Durham, NC; et al)
J Clin Oncol 29:1744-1749, 2011

Purpose.—The Reduction by Dutasteride of Prostate Cancer Events (REDUCE) prostate cancer risk reduction study randomly assigned 8,231 men to dutasteride or placebo for 4 years. Protocol-mandated biopsies were obtained after 2 and 4 years. After the discovery of three cases of biopsy sample misidentification in the first 2 years, all protocol-mandated biopsy samples were DNA tested to verify biopsy identity.

Methods.—Biopsy and blood DNA profiling was performed retrospectively for the year 2 scheduled biopsies and prospectively for the year 4 scheduled biopsies. Toward the end of year 2, multiple changes were made to improve sample handling and chain of custody.

Results.—Of the 6,458 year 2 and 4,777 year 4 biopsies, 26 biopsies reflecting 13 sample handling errors at year 2 (0.4%) and one biopsy reflecting one sample handling error at year 4 (0.02%) were confirmed to be mismatched to the patient for whom they were originally submitted. Of 6,733 reference blood samples profiled, 31 (0.5%) were found to be mismatched to the patient's verified identity profile. Sample identification errors occurred at local research sites and central laboratories.

Conclusion.—Biopsy misidentification is a potential problem in clinical laboratories and clinical trials. Until now, biopsy misidentification has not been studied in the setting of a large, multinational clinical trial. In the REDUCE study, process improvement initiatives halfway through the trial dramatically reduced biopsy mismatches. The potential for biopsy mismatches in clinical trials and clinical practice is an under-recognized problem that requires rigorous attention to details of chain of custody and consideration of more widespread DNA identity testing.

▶ The article by Marberger and colleagues identifies the frequency of prostate biopsy misidentification. This frequency depends on the existing organization structure of work processes. As variability in these processes among laboratories is high, the institutional frequency of this misidentification will also vary. The organizational structure depends on a number of sociotechnical factors, such as the use of technologies (eg, bar coding). A challenge in current practice is changing work processes to decrease the frequency of biopsy misidentification. Little information in this process is currently available in the published literature. In addition to technology solutions, some laboratories have achieved success in reducing misidentification errors through the use of quality improvement initiatives that focus on changing small steps in the entire process. The use of Lean tools, rules of work, and principles has been shown to drive this change, although other quality improvement systems also may be used. Rules of work stress concepts of 1-by-1 work processes that replace more traditional batch processes that are associated with higher error frequencies. The adoption of technologies or quality improvement systems reflects positive changes focused on patient safety. For additional reading, please see the reference section.[1,2]

S. S. Raab, MD

References

1. Zarbo RJ, Tuthill JM, D'Angelo R, et al. The Henry Ford Production System: reduction of surgical pathology in-process misidentification defects by bar code-specified work process standardization. *Am J Clin Pathol.* 2009;131:468-477.
2. Condel JL, Sharbaugh DT, Raab SS. Error-free pathology: applying lean production methods to anatomic pathology. *Clin Lab Med.* 2004;24:865-899.

The College of American pathologists and National Society for Histotechnology Workload Study
Kohl SK, Lewis SE, Tunnicliffe J, et al (Nebraska Methodist Hosp, Omaha; Univ of Iowa Hosp and Clinics; Royal Columbian Hosp, New Westminster, British Columbia, Canada; et al)
Arch Pathol Lab Med 135:728-736, 2011

Limited data exist in regard to productivity and staffing in the anatomic pathology laboratory. In 2004, the National Society for Histotechnology (NSH) conducted a pilot study to examine productivity and staffing in the histology laboratory. After review of the data, The College of American

TABLE 6.—Staffing Productivity (Blocks per Full-Time Equivalent per Year) by Type and Size of Laboratories Participating in College of American Pathologists/National Society for Histotechnology 2007 Survey

	n	5th Percentile	Median	95th Percentile	P Value
All institutions	792	1333	6433	13762	
Institution type					.09
Hospital laboratory	607	1456	6259	13019	
Independent laboratory	124	723	7511	16000	
Institution size					<.001
Small caseload	197	200	3169	8441	
Medium caseload	401	2618	6727	12650	
Large caseload	194	4690	9167	16649	

Pathologists (CAP)/NSH Histotechnology Committee concluded that a larger survey was required to further address and expand on the pilot study findings. In 2007, a total of 2674 surveys were sent out to North American laboratories. From the responses, comparisons of laboratory demographics and productivity were examined by institution type and workload volume. Productivity was measured as the number of paraffin-embedded tissue blocks processed per full-time equivalent per year. This manuscript presents and discusses the data collected from the CAP/NSH Workload Study (Table 6).

▶ The Institute of Medicine classifies quality into 6 domains: safety, efficiency, effectiveness, timeliness, patient centeredness, and equity. Laboratory and individual productivity is a measure of efficiency, and Table 6 shows laboratory histotechnologist staffing productivity in terms of blocks per full-time equivalent (FTE) per year. The variability in the number of blocks per FTE is pronounced; for all institutions, the mean number of blocks per FTE is 6433 with a fifth and 95th percentile of 1333 and 13762, respectively. This degree of variability reflects a lack of standardized work processes among laboratories and most likely a variable penetration of technologies that affect work flow. Although Kohl et al examined productivity in terms of several factors, such as institutional type and caseload, a large number of other factors are not assessed, which would allow individual laboratories to compare their own data with these benchmarks. At some point, future studies may yield important data that would guide assessments of histotechnologist productivity compared with other IOM metrics, such as safety and timeliness. Until then, laboratories can only compare themselves in a superficial way with these benchmarks. For additional reading, please see the reference section.[1,2]

S. S. Raab, MD

References

1. Raab SS, Grzybicki DM, Condel JL, et al. Effect of Lean method implementation in the histopathology section of an anatomical pathology laboratory. *J Clin Pathol.* 2008;61:1193-1199.
2. Buesa RJ. Staffing benchmarks for histology laboratories. *Ann Diagn Pathol.* 2010;14:182-193.

Are There Barriers to the Release of Paraffin Blocks for Clinical Research Trials? A College of American Pathologists Survey of 609 Laboratories
Fitzgibbons PL (St Jude Med Ctr, Fullerton, CA)
Arch Pathol Lab Med 135:870-873, 2011

Context.—The number of paraffin blocks submitted for patients enrolled in clinical research trials appears to be declining.

Objective.—To obtain information on laboratory policies and procedures in complying with requests to submit paraffin blocks for research.

Design.—A questionnaire was sent to members of a voluntary market research panel composed of pathologists representing a broad spectrum of experience and practice settings. The questions addressed departmental policies and the likely responses to requests to submit pathology materials for patients enrolled in clinical trials.

Results.—The survey was completed by 609 of 762 pathologists (80%) who responded to the invitation. More than 90% of respondents stated that they comply with these requests. Although 14% have a policy precluding the release of blocks for research, 84% of those will send limited tissue samples in lieu of blocks. When tumor is confined to a single block, most laboratories will not release the block but will send unstained slides. Very few laboratories require reimbursement before releasing tissues.

Conclusions.—Pathologists attempt to comply with requests for materials but usually refuse to release the only diagnostic paraffin block so that materials are retained for possible future needs. Other problems identified in this survey include difficulties in getting blocks returned when needed and poor communication between researchers and laboratories. Lack of reimbursement and inadequate consent are not significant barriers to release of materials (Table 4).

▶ Pathology departments play an important role in research by providing tissues in the form of a tissue block or unstained slide sections. Policies on the release of such tissues are not standard across laboratories, and Fitzgibbons reports the results of a survey completed by 609 pathologists. For research involving patient materials (eg, specimens), patients may have to grant consent,

TABLE 4.—Stated Reason for Policy Precluding Release of Blocks (Question 6)

	No. (%)
To ensure that material is available for future use for that patient if needed	36 (44.4)
Legal prohibition (ie, state law)	8 (9.9)
CLIA '88 regulations (eg, requirement to maintain blocks)	6 (7.4)
Risk management (medicolegal concerns)	15 (18.5)
Institutional IRB rules	7 (8.6)
Protection of intramural research studies	1 (1.2)
Other	8 (9.9)
Total	81 (100)

Abbreviations: CLIA, Clinical Laboratory Improvement Amendments of 1988; IRB, institutional review board.

which usually is obtained through institutional review boards' (IRBs) protocols and policies. In the United States, the US Food and Drug Administration and Department of Health and Human Services regulations have empowered IRBs to approve, require modifications in planned research prior to approval, or disapprove research. An IRB performs critical oversight functions for research conducted on human subjects that are scientific, ethical, and regulatory. The survey did not address the issue of IRB research study approval and how laboratories respond to this approval. In Table 4, institutional policies precluding the release of tissue blocks are listed. More information should have been provided here, because, as in many cases, the pathology laboratory is not the ultimate arbitrator in the determination of how tissues may be used. For additional reading, please see the reference section.[1,2]

S. S. Raab, MD

References

1. Leyland-Jones BR, Ambrosone CB, Bartlett J, et al. Recommendations for collection and handling of specimens from group breast cancer clinical trials. *J Clin Oncol.* 2008;26:5638-5644.
2. Hakimian R, Korn D. Ownership and use of tissue specimens for research. *JAMA.* 2004;292:2500-2505.

Pathology subspecialty fellowship application reform 2007 to 2010
Crawford JM, Hoffman RD, Black-Schaffer WS (North Shore-Long Island Jewish Health System and Hofstra North Shore-LIJ School of Medicine, Manhasset, NY; Vanderbilt Univ School of Medicine, Nashville, TN; Massachusetts General Hosp and, Harvard Medical School, Boston)
Hum Pathol 42:774-794, 2011

The specialty of Pathology and Laboratory Medicine has entered into a phase when the 4-year sequence of Anatomic Pathology and/or Clinical Pathology Residency Training is almost universally followed by 1 or more years of Subspecialty Fellowship Training. Such training may occur in one of the American Board of Pathology-recognized subspecialties or any number of "subspecialty fellowships" that, although not leading to subspecialty board certification, may nevertheless fall under the oversight of the local institutional Graduate Medical Education Committee and the Accreditation Council for Graduate Medical Education Review Committee for Pathology. Unlike the application process for first-year Pathology Residency, which is run through the National Resident Matching Program, applications for Subspecialty Pathology Fellowships are not coordinated by any consistent schedule. Competition for Subspecialty Pathology Fellowships has consistently resulted in undesirable drift of the fellowship application process to dates that are unacceptably early for many fellowship applicants. Responding to widespread dissatisfaction voiced by national pathology resident organizations, in 2007, the Association of Pathology Chairs began evaluation and potential intervention in the fellowship application process. Three years of intermittently intense discussion, surveys, and market

---

TABLE 11.—2010: The Salient Objections to a Fellowship Match

Need for the "barn door" exception: acceptance of internal Applicants
Breaking the "trust relationship" between Programs and their Internal Applicants if subject to a Match
Administrative burden for Fellowship Programs, most of which are single-position offerings
Perceived loss of control for Fellowship Program Directors Includes loss of flexibility in crafting PGY1-6/
    7 year sequence for research-track Pathology Residents
Concern that Programs that comply with a Match will be at a disadvantage to those that do not
Lack of clear paradigm for 2- (or 3-) fellowship sequences
Joint jurisdictional issues (Dermatopathology, Molecular Genetic Pathology)
Joint specialty entry points (Blood Banking/Transfusion Medicine; Dermatopathology, Molecular Genetics
    Pathology)

---

analysis, have led the Council of the Association of Pathology Chairs to recommend implementation of a Pathology Subspecialty Fellowship Matching program starting in the 2011 to 2012 recruiting year, for those Applicants matriculating in fellowship programs July 2013. We report on the data that informed this decision and discuss the pros and cons that are so keenly felt by the stakeholders in this as-yet-incomplete reform process (Table 11).

▶ The old adage that some things change and some things stay the same applies to pathology residency education. Educational methods for residents generally involve apprenticeship training models in which residents learn from experts and others at higher educational levels by watching and then doing. Other specialties are attempting to change this paradigm by alternative training methods such as simulation. The increasing complexity of clinical and diagnostic services has led to the evolution of team-centered care (resulting in clinicians and pathologists working more closely together) and subspecialty training for clinicians and pathologists. Crawford et al discuss the process of pathology subspecialty fellowship application reform, which, in my opinion, is necessary to further the development of pathology subspecialty training. Crawford et al report that the number of trainees enrolling in fellowship programs has increased dramatically and that the number of traditional and nontraditional training programs also has increased. In Table 11, Crawford and colleagues list some of the objections to a fellowship matching program, and these objections partly represent internal program control and autonomy issues and programmatic remnants of the traditional old system of trainee education. The pathology fellowship application system needs to change to benefit the trainees, rather than maintain the status quo of the existing system. For additional reading, please see the reference section.[1,2]

S. S. Raab, MD

References

1. Roth AE. The origins, history, and design of the resident match. *JAMA*. 2003;289:909-912.
2. Alexander CB. Pathology graduate medical education (overview from 2006-2010). *Hum Pathol*. 2011;42:763-769.

Mislabeling of Cases, Specimens, Blocks, and Slides: A College of American Pathologists Study of 136 Institutions

Nakhleh RE, Idowu MO, Souers RJ, et al (Mayo Clinic Florida, Jacksonville; Virginia Commonwealth Univ Health System, Richmond; College of American Pathologists, Northfield, IL; et al)
Arch Pathol Lab Med 135:969-974, 2011

Context.—Accurate specimen labeling is a major patient-safety initiative by the Joint Commission and the College of American Pathologists. Inadequate specimen labels have led to patient injury from wrong patient diagnosis, wrong side treatment, and delay in diagnosis.

Objectives.—To quantify the rates of mislabeled cases, specimens, blocks, and slides and to identify the sources of error and the ways in which errors are detected.

Design.—In this voluntary-subscription Q-Probes study, participants prospectively reviewed surgical pathology cases for 8 weeks or until 30 errors (mislabeled cases, specimens, blocks, and slides) were identified. Information collected on each labeling error included the work location where the defect occurred, what was mislabeled, the number of items affected, the point of detection, and the consequences of the mislabeling error, along with institutional demographics and practice. The rates of mislabeled cases, specimens, blocks, and slides were tested for association with institutional demographics and practice variables.

Results.—Of the 136 institutions providing information on a total of 1811 mislabeling occurrences, the overall mislabeling rates per 1000 were 1.1 cases, 1.0 specimen, 1.7 blocks, and 1.1 slides. Of all mislabeling events, 27.1% were cases, 19.8% specimens, 25.5% blocks, and 27.7% slides. The work locations at which the errors occurred were 20.9% before accessioning, 12.4% at accessioning, 21.7% at block labeling, 10.2% during gross pathology, and 30.4% at tissue cutting. Errors were typically detected in the first or second steps immediately following the error. Lower mislabeled slide rates were associated with continuous individual case accessioning and use of formal checks at accessioning. Routinely including a statement in the gross description that the specimen is labeled with the patient's name and is properly identified was also associated with lower rates of specimen mislabeling. The errors were corrected before reports were issued 96.7% of the time; for 3.2% of errors, a corrected report was issued. In 1.3% of error occurrences, participants gauged that patient care was affected.

Conclusions.—This study quantified mislabeling rates across 136 institutions of cases (0.11%), specimens (0.1%), blocks (0.17%), and slides (0.11%). Errors in labeling appear nearly equally throughout the system of accessioning, gross pathology processing, and tissue cutting. Errors are typically detected in the immediate steps after the errors occurred, reinforcing the need for quality checks throughout the system (Table 9).

▶ The frequency of specimen mislabeling depends on the detection method, and in the article by Nakhleh et al, cases were prospectively reviewed. The

TABLE 9.—Statistically Significant Correlations Between Mislabeling Rates and Various Practice Variables

Characteristic (No. of Laboratories Responding), N = 136	Institutions, No.	Median Mislabeling Rate (per 1000)
A. Relationship between *slide* mislabeling rate and practice variable		
Surgical pathology cases are typically processed by		
Batch accessioning	55	2.1
Continuous individual case accessioning	72	0.5
Institutions have a formal (documented) check for accessioning/labeling errors at accessioning		
Yes	67	0.6
No	32	2.3
B. Relationship between *specimen* mislabeling rate and practice variables		
The gross description routinely includes a statement indicating that the specimen is labeled with the patient's name and is properly identified		
Yes	75	0.6
No	53	1.3
C. Relationship between *block* mislabeling rate and practice variables		
Institution has a committee specifically designated for patient safety/quality assurance		
Yes	92	1.2
No	38	0.5

manner of how cases were reviewed is not explicitly stated, and other authors have shown that the harder one looks, the higher the frequency of detected error. I find the statistically significant correlation between mislabeling frequency and practice variable (Table 9) useful in determining factors that pathology practices could change to decrease mislabeling. These practices include redundancy checks, redesign of work flow (ie, continuous individual case accessioning compared with batching), and establishment of protocols. The factor of an institutional committee designated for patient safety and quality assurance is a component of culture, which many investigators consider to be highly influential on error frequency. Patient safety cultures show variable levels of maturity reflecting their engagement on factors such as error disclosure and quality improvement. A culture that establishes committees and conferences on patient safety have a higher maturity level than cultures that do not. For additional reading, please see the reference section.[1,2]

S. S. Raab, MD

References

1. Grimm EE, Schmidt RA. Reengineered workflow in the anatomic pathology laboratory: costs and benefits. *Arch Pathol Lab Med.* 2009;133:601-604.
2. Meier FA, Zarbo RJ, Varney RC, et al. Amended reports: development and validation of a taxonomy of defects. *Am J Clin Pathol.* 2008;130:238-246.

Current experience and attitudes to biomedical scientist cut-up: results of an online survey of UK consultant histopathologists

Simmons EJV, Sanders DSA, Carr RA (Coventry and Warwickshire Pathology Service, UK)
J Clin Pathol 64:363-366, 2011

Aims.—To assess the current utilisation of biomedical scientist (BMS) surgical specimen cut-up in the UK and attitudes of consultant histopathologists to the practice.

Methods.—Email invitations were sent to all UK consultant histopathologists to participate in an online survey (SurveyMonkey) assessing attitudes to and utilisation of BMS surgical specimen cut-up.

Results.—463 individual replies were received (35% response rate) from 1320 invitations to participate, covering 181 UK histopathology departments. A majority of the respondents were either fully in favour of BMS cut-up (52.7%), or in favour but with some reservation (46.2%). Only five respondents (1.1%) were completely opposed to BMS cut-up. 267 (57.7%) respondents reported that their BMS staff loaded biopsies only. 148 (32%) reported BMS cut-up of more complex benign specimens, and 83 (17.9%) reported BMS handling of orientated skin specimens. Only 39 (8.4%) reported that BMS staff in their departments currently cut-up larger cancer resections.

Conclusions.—This survey is representative of current BMS cut-up practice in the UK. The majority of UK consultant histopathologists replying to this survey support BMS cut-up to some degree, but utilisation of BMS cut-up is rather limited and patchy at present. Cost, staffing constraints, perceived quality issues and individual consultant preferences are cited as reasons for limited uptake currently. Recognised benefits of promoting BMS cut-up include better use of consultant time, enhanced team working, BMS job satisfaction and career progression, and better adherence to standard operating procedures.

▶ Simmons et al present the results of a survey of United Kingdom pathologists on their opinions regarding issues in "cut-up," known as gross tissue examination in North America. My impression is that the biomedical scientist is similar to a North American pathologists' assistant in scope of activities. Formalized training and a proposed examination are underway in the United Kingdom. Although biomedical scientists appear to be prevalent, pathologists' opinions regarding their tasks are variable, similar to what pathologists in the United States once thought. Only a small percentage reported that biomedical scientists could "cut-up" large specimens. The development of pathologist extenders is occurring on a global basis. For additional reading, please see reference list.[1]

S. S. Raab, MD

Reference

1. Duthie FR, Nairn ER, Milne AW, McTaggart V, Topping D. The impact of involvement of biomedical scientists in specimen dissection and selection of blocks for histopathology: a study of time benefits and specimen handling quality in Ayrshire and Arran area laboratory. *J Clin Pathol.* 2004;57:27-32.

Inappropriate calibration and optimisation of pan-keratin (pan-CK) and low molecular weight keratin (LMWCK) immunohistochemistry tests: Canadian Immunohistochemistry Quality Control (CIQC) experience

Copete M, Garratt J, Gilks B, et al (Univ of Saskatchewan, Saskatoon, Canada; Lions Gate Hosp, Vancouver, British Columbia, Canada; Univ of British Columbia, Vancouver, Canada; et al)
J Clin Pathol 64:220-225, 2011

Aims.—Pan-cytokeratin (pan-CK) and low molecular weight cytokeratin (LMWCK) tests are the most common immunohistochemistry (IHC) tests used to support evidence of epithelial differentiation. Canadian Immunohistochemistry Quality Control (CIQC), a new provider of proficiency testing for Canadian clinical IHC laboratories, has evaluated the performance of Canadian IHC laboratories in two proficiency testing challenges for both pan-CK and LMWCK.

Methods.—CIQC has designed a 70-sample tissue microarray (TMA) for challenge 1 and a 30-sample TMA for challenge 2. There were 13 participants in challenge 1, and 62 in challenge 2. All results were evaluated and scored by CIQC assessors and compared with reference laboratory results.

Results.—Participating laboratories often produced false-negative results that ranged from 20% to 80%. False-positive results were also detected. About half of participating clinical laboratories have inappropriately calibrated IHC tests for pan-CK and LMWCK, which are the most commonly used markers for demonstration of epithelial differentiation. The great majority of laboratories were not aware of the problem with calibration of pan-CK and LMWCK tests because of inappropriate selection of external positive controls and samples for optimisation of these tests. Benign liver and kidney are the most important tissues to include as positive controls for both pan-CK and LMWCK.

Conclusions.—Participation in external quality assurance is important for peer comparison and proper calibration of IHC tests, which is also helpful for appropriate selection of positive control material and material for optimisation of the tests (Fig 4).

▶ Copete and colleagues report on the challenges in the calibration of immunohistochemical tests in laboratories and the benefits of participating in external quality control programs. In this article, the authors evaluated low-molecular-weight cytokeratin and pan-cytokeratin, which are used in most laboratories in North America. The take home messages include: (1) for the antibody cocktail AE1/AE3, appropriate controls must be selected to show

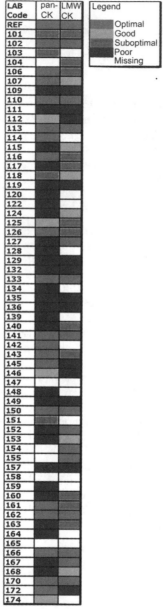

FIGURE 4.—Garrattogram of challenge 2. An overview of results is also shown in a tabular summary of test results. Red designates poor results or an immediate need for test optimisation. This type of presentation of results gives immediate insight into the level of national concordance as well as the extent of a problem with a specific test. For interpretation of the references to color in this figure legend, the reader is referred to web version of this article. (Reprinted from Copete M, Garratt J, Gilks B, et al. Inappropriate calibration and optimisation of pan-keratin (pan-CK) and low molecular weight keratin (LMWCK) immunohistochemistry tests: Canadian Immunohistochemistry Quality Control (CIQC) experience. *J Clin Pathol.* 2011;64:220-225.)

that both clones are optimized, (2) tissues with low expression levels may be useful for optimal calibration, and (3) benign tissues with predictable levels of expression could be better external controls than tumor tissues. Fig 4 shows a Garrattogram showing laboratory performance and identifying the laboratories with poor performance in a sample of Canadian laboratories. For additional reading, please see reference list.[1,2]

S. S. Raab, MD

References

1. Canadian Association of Pathologists-Association canadienne des pathologistes National Standards Committee, Torlakovic EE, Riddell R, Banerjee D, et al. Canadian Association of Pathologists-Association canadienne des pathologistes National Standards Committee/Immunohistochemistry: best practice recommendations for standardization of immunohistochemistry tests. *Am J Clin Pathol.* 2010;133:354-365.
2. Rüdiger T, Höfler H, Kreipe HH, et al. Quality assurance in immunohistochemistry: results of an interlaboratory trial involving 172 pathologists. *Am J Surg Pathol.* 2002;26:873-882.

Error rates in reporting prostatic core biopsies
Oxley JD, Sen C (North Bristol NHS Trust, Bristol, UK)
Histopathology 58:759-765, 2011

Aims.—To evaluate the false-negative and false-positive error rates both in a screening and a non-screening population.

Methods and Results.—A total of 4192 prostatic biopsies were reported in a 6-year period by 15 consultant histopathologists, two of whom had an interest in uropathology and were deemed to be specialists (J.O. and C.S.). All biopsies were reviewed prior to the multidisciplinary team (MDT) meeting. The overall false-negative rate was 1.7% (screening 2.1%, non-screening 1.5%). The overall false-positive rate was 0.5% (screening 0.9%, non-screening 0.4%). These error rates varied among pathologists, with the false-negative rate ranging from 0% to 9.3%, and the false-positive rate ranging from 0% to 3.8%.

Conclusion.—The false-negative rate was three times greater than the false-positive rate, showing that detection of significant pathology is far greater in the negative biopsies. More errors occurred in the screening population than in the non-screening population. The consultants making the most errors were non-specialists, but the specialists also made false-negative errors, suggesting that just using specialist reporting alone would not have eradicated errors (Table 3).

▶ Oxley and Sen report on the diagnostic precision in prostate needle core biopsies. Important points in this article are: (1) subspecialists make fewer errors than nonsubspecialists, but they still make errors, and (2) individual pathologists have a variable error frequency, with some pathologists making more false-negative and others making more false-positive errors (Table 3).

TABLE 3.—Number of Biopsies Reported by Each Pathologist and Error Rate per Pathologist and for the Group Overall; Also Shown are Data for the Screening and Non-Screening Patients

| | | | False-Negative | | | False-Positive | | |
Consultant	Total Number	Number per Month	Number of Biopsies Originally Reported as Benign, Atypia or HGPIN	Number of Errors	Rate (%)	Number of Biopsies Originally Reported as Cancer	Number of Errors	Rate (%)
1	1403	19.8	791	2	0.3	575	0	0.0
2	645	10.4	357	12	**3.4**	271	4	**1.5**
3	499	7.8	277	4	1.4	198	0	0.0
4	399	5.6	222	3	1.4	165	1	**0.6**
5	285	8.1	161	8	**5.0**	105	4	**3.8**
6	221	7.6	133	3	**2.3**	86	0	0.0
7	180	6.9	95	1	1.1	74	0	0.0
8	139	5.4	84	0	0.0	53	0	0.0
9	137	9.1	69	0	0.0	59	0	0.0
10	135	2.2	86	8	**9.3**	44	0	0.0
11	57	5.7	35	0	0.0	22	0	0.0
12	49	24.5	29	0	0.0	16	0	0.0
13	28	9.3	16	0	0.0	9	0	0.0
14	13	6.5	10	0	0.0	3	0	0.0
15	2	2	2	0	0.0	0	0	0.0
Overall	4192	58.2	2367	41	1.7	1680	9	0.5
Screened	1141	15.8	747	16	**2.1**	344	3	**0.9**
Non-screened	3051	42.4	1620	25	1.5	1336	6	0.4

Rates in bold type are greater than the overall rate; consultants 1 and 3 had a special interest in uropathology.
HGPIN, High-grade prostatic intraepithelial neoplasia. False-negative % error rate = biopsies detected as cancer or suspicious for cancer/biopsies originally reported as benign, atypia, HGPIN × 100.
False-positive % error rate = biopsies detected as not cancer/biopsies originally reported as cancer × 100.

These are really difficult problems to fix and involve education and pathology cultural issues. A large portion of fixing this problem involves consensus building and teamwork. For additional reading, please see reference list.[1,2]

S. S. Raab, MD

References

1. Berney DM, Fisher G, Kattan MW, et al. Trans-Atlantic prostate group. Pitfalls in the diagnosis of prostatic cancer: retrospective review of 1791 cases with clinical outcome. *Histopathology.* 2007;51:452-457.
2. Wolters T, van der Kwast TH, Vissers CJ, et al. False-negative prostate needle biopsies: frequency, histopathologic features, and follow-up. *Am J Surg Pathol.* 2010;34:35-43.

2 Breast

Effect of Occult Metastases on Survival in Node-Negative Breast Cancer

Weaver DL, Ashikaga T, Krag DN, et al (Univ of Vermont College of Medicine and Vermont Cancer Ctr, Burlington; et al)
N Engl J Med 364:412-421, 2011

Background.—Retrospective and observational analyses suggest that occult lymph-node metastases are an important prognostic factor for disease recurrence or survival among patients with breast cancer. Prospective data on clinical outcomes from randomized trials according to sentinel-node involvement have been lacking.

Methods.—We randomly assigned women with breast cancer to sentinel-lymph-node biopsy plus axillary dissection or sentinel-lymph-node biopsy alone. Paraffin-embedded tissue blocks of sentinel lymph nodes obtained from patients with pathologically negative sentinel lymph nodes were centrally evaluated for occult metastases deeper in the blocks. Both routine staining and immunohistochemical staining for cytokeratin were used at two widely spaced additional tissue levels. Treating physicians were unaware of the findings, which were not used for clinical treatment decisions. The initial evaluation at participating sites was designed to detect all macrometastases larger than 2 mm in the greatest dimension.

Results.—Occult metastases were detected in 15.9% (95% confidence interval [CI], 14.7 to 17.1) of 3887 patients. Log-rank tests indicated a significant difference between patients in whom occult metastases were detected and those in whom no occult metastases were detected with respect to overall survival (P = 0.03), disease-free survival (P = 0.02), and distant-disease–free interval (P = 0.04). The corresponding adjusted hazard ratios for death, any outcome event, and distant disease were 1.40 (95% CI, 1.05 to 1.86), 1.31 (95% CI, 1.07 to 1.60), and 1.30 (95% CI, 1.02 to 1.66), respectively. Five-year Kaplan-Meier estimates of overall survival among patients in whom occult metastases were detected and those without detectable metastases were 94.6% and 95.8%, respectively.

Conclusions.—Occult metastases were an independent prognostic variable in patients with sentinel nodes that were negative on initial examination; however, the magnitude of the difference in outcome at 5 years was small (1.2 percentage points). These data do not indicate a clinical benefit of additional evaluation, including immunohistochemical analysis, of initially negative sentinel nodes in patients with breast cancer. (Funded by the National Cancer Institute; ClinicalTrials.gov number, NCT00003830.)

▶ Considerable research and debate have taken place regarding the significance of occult metastases (metastases not found on initial examination of lymph nodes) for disease recurrence or survival in breast cancer patients. The onus is on the anatomic pathologist to provide accurate information regarding the lymph node status of the patient to the oncologist for optimal treatment planning. Anatomic pathologists have not yet reached consensus on how to best examine sentinel lymph nodes for tumor deposits. Significant variability exists within and between laboratories. Although National Surgical Adjuvant Breast and Bowel Project trial B-32 was designed to compare sentinel node resection to conventional axillary dissection in clinically node-negative breast cancer patients, Weaver et al were able to perform a prospective study of a subset of registered patients. While the group found that there was clinical significance to the finding of occult metastases with respect to overall survival, disease-free survival, and distant disease-free survival, the magnitude of this impact was small. The identification of occult metastases was not needed for clinical decision making, and their findings argue against any additional examination of a sentinel lymph node, other than a single hematoxylin and eosin of each 2-mm slice of lymph node blocked in initially node-negative patients. They did support continuing to divide lymph node metastases into isolated tumor cells, micrometastases, and macrometastases.

This article will aid pathologists in developing protocols for the examination of sentinel lymph nodes of breast cancer patients, which should lead to uniformity of staging and care for breast cancer patients.

B. A. Carter, MD, FRCPC

Prognostic Value of a Combined Estrogen Receptor, Progesterone Receptor, Ki-67, and Human Epidermal Growth Factor Receptor 2 Immunohistochemical Score and Comparison With the Genomic Health Recurrence Score in Early Breast Cancer
Cuzick J, Dowsett M, Pineda S, et al (Queen Mary Univ of London, UK; Royal Marsden Hosp, London, UK; et al)
J Clin Oncol 29:4273-4278, 2011

Purpose.—We recently reported that the mRNA-based, 21-gene Genomic Health recurrence score (GHI-RS) provided additional prognostic information regarding distant recurrence beyond that obtained from classical clinicopathologic factors (age, nodal status, tumor size, grade, endocrine treatment) in women with early breast cancer, confirming earlier reports. The aim of this article is to determine how much of this information is contained in standard immunohistochemical (IHC) markers.

Patients and Methods.—The primary cohort comprised 1,125 estrogen receptor—positive (ER-positive) patients from the Arimidex, Tamoxifen, Alone or in Combination (ATAC) trial who did not receive adjuvant chemotherapy, had the GHI-RS computed, and had adequate tissue for the four IHC measurements: ER, progesterone receptor (PgR), human epidermal growth factor receptor 2 (HER2), and Ki-67. Distant recurrence was the primary end point, and proportional hazards models were used with sample splitting to control for overfitting. A prognostic model that used classical variables and the four IHC markers (IHC4 score) was created and assessed in a separate cohort of 786 patients.

Results.—All four IHC markers provided independent prognostic information in the presence of classical variables. In sample-splitting analyses, the information in the IHC4 score was found to be similar to that in the GHI-RS, and little additional prognostic value was seen in the combined use of both scores. The prognostic value of the IHC4 score was further validated in the second separate cohort.

Conclusion.—This study suggests that the amount of prognostic information contained in four widely performed IHC assays is similar to that in the GHI-RS. Additional studies are needed to determine the general applicability of the IHC4 score.

▶ Molecular profiling of breast cancer is significantly more costly than histologic examination and/or immunohistochemical staining. Furthermore, the superior predictive and prognostic value of molecular profiling compared with current practice is controversial. Most agree that the pathologic nodal status, tumor grade, tumor size, and estrogen receptor (ER) status are the most clinically important factors for consideration when selecting women with early breast cancer for adjuvant systemic therapy. Nonetheless, there is pressure to have all breast cancers undergo genetic assessment.

In this study from the United Kingdom, the United States, and Australia, the authors examine 1125 ER-positive patients from the Arimidex, Tamoxifen, Alone or in Combination (ATAC) trial who had not received adjuvant chemotherapy. Immunohistochemical analysis of ER, progesterone receptor, Her2/neu, and Ki-67 was carried out. The results were compared with the mRNA-based 21-gene genomic health recurrence score, which had been shown in a previous study to be superior to histologic examination alone.

The study concludes that the amount of predictive and prognostic information found in 4 routine immunohistochemical assays was similar to that of the molecular profile.

The market for molecular profiling of breast cancer is currently being flooded with new kits and technologies. Many institutions are adapting this testing in a routine fashion with little evidence-based medicine to support the decision. This study raises doubts about this costly addition to breast cancer diagnosis and treatment.

B. A. Carter, MD, FRCPC

The effect of delay in fixation, different fixatives, and duration of fixation in estrogen and progesterone receptor results in breast carcinoma

Apple S, Pucci R, Lowe AC, et al (UCLA Ctr for the Health Sciences)
Am J Clin Pathol 135:592-598, 2011

Accurate determination of estrogen receptor (ER) and progesterone receptor (PR) status in breast carcinoma is essential. Preanalytic variation may contribute to discordant results. Recently, American Society of Clinical Oncology (ASCO)/College of American Pathologists (CAP) made recommendations to normalize fixation for breast biomarkers. To evaluate this, a 4-cm invasive lobular carcinoma was processed according to ASCO/CAP guidelines. The remainder was stored fresh at 4°C for 4 days and cut into biopsy-sized pieces. Each was fixed in 10% formalin, Pen-Fix (Richard-Allan Scientific, Kalamazoo, MI), Bouin solution, Sakura Molecular Fixative (Sakura Tissue-Tek Xpress, Torrance, CA), zinc formalin, or 15% formaldehyde for times ranging between 1 and 168 hours. Immunohistochemical studies for ER and PR were performed and interpreted. After 4 days at 4°C, all samples showed no degradation or ER/PR staining differences, except 2 Bouin-fixed samples, in comparison with the patient's sample processed according to ASCO/CAP guidelines. In our study, the preanalytic variables of fixative type, fixation time, and 4 days of ischemic time did not affect immunohistochemical accuracy for ER/PR.

▶ Recent recommendations from the American Society of Clinical Oncology (ASCO)/College of American Pathologists (CAP), National Comprehensive Cancer Network,[1] and multiple international guidelines groups have focused on the effects of preanalytical variations in routine immunohistochemical staining for hormone receptor status in breast cancer. These guidelines often contain impositions that are not necessarily in sync with the standard activities of operating suites and anatomic pathology laboratories.

Apple et al compared stain quality in cancers limited to ASCO/CAP preanalytic guidelines to cancer subjected to variable fixatives, prolonged ischemic time, and fixation time. The study found no significant difference.

This study, although not without limitations, serves here as a representative of the many articles published in the past few years regarding handling of breast cancer tissue specimens in the anatomic pathology laboratory. It provides evidence that acting outside the guidelines is not necessarily harmful to the patient. This article and multiple similar ones offer laboratories some wiggle room outside the strict impositions of guidelines. It serves as a reminder that guidelines are just that and not standard of practice.

B. A. Carter, MD, FRCPC

Reference

1. Tong LC, Nelson N, Tsourigiannis J, Mulligan AM. The effect of prolonged fixation on the immunohistochemical evaluation of estrogen receptor, progesterone receptor, and HER2 expression in invasive breast cancer: a prospective study. *Am J Surg Pathol.* 2011;35:545-552.

Assessment of Ki67 in Breast Cancer: Recommendations from the International Ki67 in Breast Cancer Working Group

Dowsett M, Nielsen TO, A'Hern R, et al (Royal Marsden Hosp and Breakthrough Breast Cancer Centre, London, UK; Univ of British Columbia, Vancouver, Canada; The Inst of Cancer Res, Sutton, Surrey, UK; et al)

J Natl Cancer Inst 103:1-9, 2011

Uncontrolled proliferation is a hallmark of cancer. In breast cancer, immunohistochemical assessment of the proportion of cells staining for the nuclear antigen Ki67 has become the most widely used method for comparing proliferation between tumor samples. Potential uses include prognosis, prediction of relative responsiveness or resistance to chemotherapy or endocrine therapy, estimation of residual risk in patients on standard therapy and as a dynamic biomarker of treatment efficacy in samples taken before, during, and after neoadjuvant therapy, particularly neoadjuvant endocrine therapy. Increasingly, Ki67 is measured in these scenarios for clinical research, including as a primary efficacy endpoint for clinical trials, and sometimes for clinical management. At present, the enormous variation in analytical practice markedly limits the value of Ki67 in each of these contexts. On March 12, 2010, an international panel of investigators with substantial expertise in the assessment of Ki67 and in the development of biomarker guidelines was convened in London by the cochairs of the Breast International Group and North American Breast Cancer Group Biomarker Working Party to consider evidence for potential applications. Comprehensive recommendations on preanalytical and analytical assessment, and interpretation and scoring of Ki67 were formulated based on current evidence. These recommendations are geared toward achieving a harmonized methodology, create greater between-laboratory and between-study comparability, and allow earlier valid applications of this marker in clinical practice (Table 1).

▶ St Gallen 2011[1] delivered firm support for the use of Ki67 in early breast cancer. Subsequently, many pathologists have been asked to include this information in their pathology report for breast cancer patients.

This commentary article provides insights and advice on this topic. Paramount was the admission that many cutoffs have been used, and in the absence of standardization of methodology, they provide little value outside the studies and the centers that performed them. Thresholds used for prognosis are not the same as those used for eligibility for neoadjuvant trials or for use as a pharmacodynamic marker. The International Ki67 in Breast Cancer Working Group was unable to come to consensus regarding the cut point(s) that might be used in clinical practice.

The group noted that no established quality assurance schemes are in place to ensure that the procedures for Ki67 analysis in one laboratory lead to scores comparable to those in others. They also confirmed the biological heterogeneity of Ki67 staining across specimens and agreed that scoring systems remain controversial.

TABLE 1.—Factors that May Affect Ki67 Immunohistochemistry*

Setting	Factor	Variables	Important?	Comments
Preanalytical	Type of biopsy	Core vs whole section	No	Both are suitable. Some data suggest that whole section may give higher scores than core biopsy.
	Type of fixative	Previously frozen, or EtOH or EDTA fixative, or previous acid decalcification vs neutral buffered formalin	Yes	Avoid all but neutral buffered formalin. Others reduce Ki67 staining compared with neutral buffered formalin.
	Time to fixation	Integrity of nuclei	Yes	For visual analysis, has little impact unless extreme. Important for image analysis.
	Means of storage	Tissue in paraffin block vs cut section	Yes	Prolonged storage of formalin-fixed paraffin-embedded tissue block at room temperature has little effect on Ki67. Avoid prolonged exposure to air of cut sections on glass slides.
Analytical	Antigen retrieval	Yes vs no	Yes	Required. Microwave processing recommended.
	Specific antibody	MIB1 vs other antibodies against Ki67 antigen	Yes	MIB1 is the most widely validated antibody. SP6 antibody against Ki67 appears promising but insufficient data to support routine use at this time.
	Colorimetric detection system	Avidin–biotin immunoperoxidase vs polymer detection†	No	Both suitable.
Interpretation and scoring	Counterstain	Completeness and intensity of stain	Yes	Important that all negative nuclei are counterstained.
	Method of reading	Cellular component, staining intensity	Yes	1) Count all positive cells within region in which all nuclei have been stained. 2) Scoring requires determination of percentage cells positive. 3) No interpretation of intensity.
	Area of slide read	Edge vs central; hot spots vs area without hot spots vs all areas	Yes	Controversial: currently recommend average score across the section.
Data analysis	Image	Visual vs automated analysis	Unknown	Unknown whether either method is superior.
	Cut point	Any vs no staining; arbitrary vs data-derived cut point; or continuous variable	Controversial	It is controversial because there is no recommended consensus cut point at this time. Select cut point based on context (prognosis, prediction of specific therapy, selection of patients for trial, use as pharmacodynamic or endpoint biomarker). Endpoint must be validated in separate independent study of similar design with same endpoints.

*EtOH = ethanol.
†The polymer detection method uses polymeric antibodies and increases the number of available enzymes or ligands binding at the antigenic site, thus increasing their reactivity to chromogen.

The members of this group are involved in a number of initiatives that may lead to clarification for their recommendations. But right now, routine Ki67 staining in pathology laboratories is not ready for prime time.

On a separate note, their assertion that the most widely practiced measurement of breast cancer proliferation index involves the immunohistochemical (IHC) assessment of Ki67 antigen is premature because there have been no studies comparing it to the well-studied and standardized Modified Bloom-Richardson (Nottigham) method of mitotic count.

B. A. Carter, MD, FRCPC

Reference

1. Gnant M, Harbeck N, Thomssen C. St. Gallen 2011: summary of the consensus discussion. *Breast Care (Basel)*. 2011;6:136-141.

Accuracy and Completeness of Pathology Reporting - Impact on Partial Breast Irradiation Eligibility

Pignol JP, Rakovitch E, Zeppieri J, et al (Univ of Toronto, Ontario, Canada)
Clin Oncol (R Coll Radiol) 2011 [Epub ahead of print]

Aims.—Accelerated partial breast irradiation (APBI) is an alternative to whole breast irradiation that is delivered over a shorter period of time with less toxicity. Appropriate patient selection is critical to its success and the American Society for Radiation Oncology (ASTRO) has published detailed selection criteria for 'suitable' patients. This study evaluated the effect of those selection criteria on APBI eligibility based on pathology reports.

Materials and Methods.—From March 2004 to March 2007 all patients referred to a single cancer centre for breast radiotherapy were screened for participation in a phase I/II trial of permanent breast seed implant brachytherapy. Eligible patients underwent a computed tomography simulation and those referred from an outside institution had a secondary expert breast pathology assessment. Initial and expert pathology reports were compared regarding completeness and accuracy.

Results.—In total, 143 patients were eligible for the trial; 79 patients had surgery carried out outside our institution. In the initial pathology report, the most frequently missing critical information was the resection margin width (29.1%) and the presence of extensive *in situ* carcinoma (11.4%). Comparing initial and reviewed pathology, the agreement was higher than 90% for most features. The main source of disagreement was the width of the negative resection margin, with 34.4% disagreement ($P = 0.016$), although it changed eligibility in only 3.6%. There was major disagreement in the evaluation of lymphovascular invasion. Overall, pathology review changed the eligibility for a patient from 'suitable' for APBI to 'cautionary' in 18.6% of the cases.

Conclusion.—Using stringent eligibility criteria has a direct effect on patient screening for APBI. The use of synoptic pathology reporting and a quality assurance programme with secondary expert assessments are recommended.

▶ This study is important as a reminder of the importance of using synoptic or checklist-type reporting in breast cancer pathology. The surgical pathology report remains the primary source of information to guide treatment. Failure to report critical elements is an increasing problem in pathology, owing to the heightened complexity of these reports and the number of elements that are important for patient care.

This study highlights just that at a radiotherapy center. The American Society for Radiation Oncology has published detailed selection criteria for patients suitable for accelerated partial breast irradiation (APBI), a less toxic treatment choice for patients with breast cancer. This study of pathology reports found that the use of synoptic pathology reporting ensured detailed communication of important prognostic features and proper eligibility for trial inclusion. In the authors' hands, almost 20% of patients initially included in a trial were suspect after completion of all criteria in the checklist pathology report.

The College of American Pathologists (CAP) has developed checklists that contain all of the scientifically validated data elements that are to be reported for cancer specimens. These high-quality pathology reports contain information that is critical for patient management as well as for cancer surveillance, resource planning, and quality purposes, responsibilities that fit into the duties of 21st-century anatomic pathologists.

Pathology reports represent a rich data source for cancer registries, assuring adequate report content with the use of synoptic checklist reports and using report formatting suggestions that aid report comprehension. Using stringent eligibility criteria has a direct effect on patient screening for APBI.

B. A. Carter, MD, FRCPC

ER, HER2, and TOP2A expression in primary tumor, synchronous axillary nodes, and asynchronous metastases in breast cancer
Jensen JD, Knoop A, Ewertz M, et al (Odense Univ Hosp, Denmark)
Breast Cancer Res Treat 2011 [Epub ahead of print]

At recurrence of breast cancer, the therapeutic target is the metastases. However, it is current practice to base the choice of systemic treatment on the biomarker profile of the primary tumor. In the present study, confirmatory biopsies were obtained from suspected metastatic lesions and compared with the primary tumors with respect to ER, HER2, and *TOP2A*. In the prospective tissue-collection study, 81 patients had biopsy from a suspected relapse. Additional archived paired material was included, leaving a total of 119 patients with paired primary tumor, synchronous axillary nodes (available in 52 patients) and asyncronous metastases available for analysis. ER, HER2, and *TOP2A* expression of primary tumors, axillary nodes and metastases were re-analysed and determined centrally by immunohistochemistry, chromogenic in situ hybridization, and fluorescence in situ hybridization. Of the 81 patients with a biopsy from a suspected relapse, 65 (80%) were diagnosed with recurrent breast carcinoma, 3 (4%) were diagnosed with other malignancies, 6 (7%) had benign conditions, and in 7 (9%) patients the biopsy was non-representative. Discordance in ER, HER2, and *TOP2A* (aberration vs. normal) status between primary tumor and corresponding asynchronous metastasis was 12% (14/118), 9% (10/114), and 23% (17/75), respectively. There were no significant associations with biomarker discordance and prior adjuvant therapy, or location of biopsy. Expression of ER, HER2, and *TOP2A* displayed discordance with a sufficient frequency to emphasize the role of confirmatory biopsies from metastatic lesions in future management of recurrent breast cancer.

▶ In most institutions, current systemic treatment options for breast cancer patients at the time of metastases are based on the biomarker profile of the primary breast excision specimen. However, the therapeutic targets are the metastases. It has long been thought that the biomarker status of the primary tumor is equal to that of any future metastases. This thinking is being questioned. Many think that there may be a change in the biology of the cancer at the time of metastasis. Tumor heterogeneity must also be taken into account when thinking of clonal metastatic capability. Increasing use of targeted therapy in breast cancer makes this issue vitally important.

In this prospective study, Jensen et al looked at 119 patients with biopsies from metastatic lesions and primary tumors and compared them regarding estrogen receptor (ER), Her2, and Top2 immunohistochemical expression. Discordance status between primary tumor and corresponding asynchronous metastases was significant. Coupling this with the fact that recent genetic studies have suggested that there can be changes in molecular phenotype between the primary and relapsed breast cancer, one can estimate that up to 20% of breast cancer patients may have a complete change in management if the metastases are biopsied.

Expression of ER and Her2/neu in this study and others shows a discordance rate of sufficient frequency to recommend biopsy of metastatic sites after considering the difficulty, cost, and side effects of the clinical management of recurrent breast cancer. Practicing pathologists as part of the multidisciplinary treatment team should encourage biopsies of metastatic deposits over the entire course of disease progression.

B. A. Carter, MD, FRCPC

All atypia diagnosed at stereotactic vacuum-assisted breast biopsy do not need surgical excision
de Mascarel I, Brouste V, Asad-Syed M, et al (Comprehensive Cancer Ctr, Bordeaux, France)
Mod Pathol 24:1198-1206, 2011

The necessity of excision is debatable when atypia are diagnosed at stereotactic vacuum-assisted breast biopsy (microbiopsy). Among the 287 surgical excisions performed at Institut Bergonié from 1999 to 2009, we selected a case—control study group of 151 excisions; 52 involving all the diagnosed cancers and 99 randomly selected among the 235 excisions without cancer, following atypical microbiopsy (24 flat epithelial atypia; 50 atypical ductal hyperplasia; 14 lobular neoplasia; 63 mixed lesions). Mammographical calcification (type, extension, complete removal) and histological criteria of epithelial atypia (type, number of foci, size/extension), topography and microcalcification extension at microbiopsy were compared according to the presence or absence of cancer at excision. Factors associated with cancer at excision were Breast Imaging Reporting and Data System (BI-RADS5) lesions, large and/or multiple foci of mammographical calcifications, histological type, number, size and extension of atypical foci. Flat epithelial atypia alone was never associated with cancer at excision. BI-RADS5, atypical ductal hyperplasia (alone or predominant) and >3 foci of atypia were identified as independent pejorative factors. There was never any cancer at excision when these pejorative factors were absent ($n = 31$). Presence of one ($n = 59$), two ($n = 23$) or three ($n = 14$) factors was associated with cancer in 24, 15 and 13 cases with an odds ratio = 5.8 (95% CI: 3—11.2) for each additional factor. We recommend that mammographical data and histological characteristics be taken into account in the decision-making process after diagnosis of atypia on microbiopsy. With experienced senologists and strict histological criteria, some patients could be spared surgery resulting in significant patient, financial and time advantages.

▶ Stereotactic breast biopsies are increasingly being performed in routine practice and the diagnosis of epithelial aytpia more often being made. There are still no clear guidelines for the management of patients when any type of epithelial atypia is diagnosed. This is largely due to the fact that the interobserver reproducibility in the classification of radiologic lesions at present remains low to moderate, and distinguishing between columnar cell change, flat epithelial atypia, and atypical ductal hyperplasia is sometimes very difficult for the practicing pathologist. There have been confounding results published in the past few years; this study should help put the issue to rest.

The study by de Mascarel et al strictly defines criteria on which to base the decision of whether or not to excise when atypias are diagnosed. They compared mammographic findings with histologic characteristics on minimal sampling techniques according to the presence or absence of cancer in a very large case-control group of surgical excisions.

They conclude that with mammographic criteria and strict histologic criteria, one can place patients into 3 generally reliable groups: those requiring no surgery, those who should be excised, and a small group for whom discussion at a multidisciplinary meeting is necessary. Adoption of the criteria is straightforward for pathologists.

Of special interest, they found that flat epithelial atypia was never associated with cancer at excision and that differentiating columnar cell lesions from pure flat epithelial atypia on needle cores does not change patient management. De Mascarel et al recommend no excision, but close follow-up.

B. A. Carter, MD, FRCPC

A multisite performance study comparing the reading of immunohistochemical slides on a computer monitor with conventional manual microscopy for estrogen and progesterone receptor analysis
Nassar A, Cohen C, Agersborg SS, et al (Mayo Clinic, Rochester, MN)
Am J Clin Pathol 135:461-467, 2011

A multisite study was conducted to assess the performance of the Aperio digital pathology system (Aperio Technologies, Vista, CA) for reading estrogen receptor (ER) and progesterone receptor (PR) slides on a computer monitor. A total of 520 formalin-fixed breast tissue specimens were assayed at 3 clinical sites for ER and PR (260 each). Percentage and average staining intensity of positive nuclei were assessed. At each site, 3 pathologists performed a blinded reading of the glass slides using their microscopes initially and later using digital images on a computer monitor. Comparable percentages of agreements were obtained for manual microscopy (MM) and manual digital slide reading (MDR) (ER, percentage of positive nuclei with cutoffs: MM, 91.3%-99.0%/MDR, 91.3%-100.0%; PR, percentage of positive nuclei with cutoffs: MM, 83.8%-99.0%/MDR, 76.3%-100.0%). Reading ER and PR slides on a computer monitor using the Aperio digital pathology system is equivalent to reading the slides with a conventional light microscope.

▶ Digital images can be used for a variety of applications, including rapid interpretations, primary diagnosis, and second opinions. Digital slide scanners for scanning glass slides are becoming increasingly popular because current scanners are fast enough and produce good enough images for diagnostic purposes.

The authors of this report conducted a 3-site study of over 500 samples that assessed the performance of the Aperio digital pathology system for reading estrogen receptor and progesterone receptor (PR) slides on a computer monitor. They found that reading estrogen receptor and PR slides on a computer monitor using the Aperio digital pathology system is equivalent to reading the slides with a conventional light microscope. It is inevitable that this technology will be paired with Image Analysis in the very near future. Image Analysis has been shown to improve accuracy in quantification of biomarkers.

In 2011, the atmosphere around immunohistochemical staining for hormone receptor status in breast cancer is filled with many strict guideline impositions. They cover all phases of the test cycle, but the analytic and postanalytic portions have daunting requirements. Many pathologists are choosing to send their samples to a central laboratory for biomarker status. Digital approaches can partially alleviate the time consumed with slide shipping, improve standardization, and provide a digital archive for referring pathologists. For central laboratories performing immunohistochemistry for peripheral or low-volume laboratories, this new(ish) technology will be a time and money saver without compromising the quality of patient care.

B. A. Carter, MD, FRCPC

Benign epithelial inclusions in axillary lymph nodes: report of 18 cases and review of the literature
Fellegara G, Carcangiu ML, Rosai J (Natl Cancer Inst, Milan, Italy)
Am J Surg Pathol 35:1123-1133, 2011

The occurrence of various types of heterotopic epithelial structures in lymph nodes is a well-documented phenomenon. Here, we report on the presence of such inclusions in axillary lymph nodes. A total of 18 cases were identified. All patients were women, their ages ranging from 32 to 79 years (median, 57 y). Thirteen patients had concomitant or antecedent breast abnormalities, and 12 of them had undergone nodal sampling for staging purposes. The other 5 patients had noted enlarging axillary masses, with no clinical evidence of previous or concomitant breast or genital tract pathology. We classified the nodal inclusions on morphologic grounds into 3 main categories: those composed exclusively of glandular structures (glandular-type inclusions; 10 cases, 56%); those made up only of squamous cysts (squamous-type inclusions; 2 cases, 11%); and those containing both glandular and squamous epithelia (mixed glandular-squamous-type inclusions; 6 cases, 33%). We speculate about the possible mechanism for the migration of the epithelial cells into the lymph nodes, discuss the modifications that they may later undergo as a result of local and systemic factors, and consider the differential diagnosis with other conditions, particularly with metastatic well-differentiated breast carcinoma.

▶ With so much new breast cancer—staging literature regarding isolated tumor cells, micrometastases, and macrometastases in axillary lymph nodes,[1,2] this paper serves as a reminder that not everything found in a lymph node of a breast cancer patient need be regarded as a poor prognostic sign. With the rising number of women who are undergoing presurgical minimal sampling biopsies of the breast and the inherently friable nature of some breast lesions, an approach to epithelial inclusions in the lymph node is needed.

Dr Rosai's group reports on the presence of heterotopic epithelial inclusions in 18 patients with axillary lymph node sampling. Twelve of these patients had undergone nodal sampling for breast cancer staging. Like many authors before them, they agree that these inclusions are likely of no metastatic importance for the patient. Many of us in practice think that these findings are increased after instrumentation of the tumor site, and are approximately proportionate to the degree of manipulation.

Clear concise language is used in this article to differentiate benign inclusions from cancer. Prudence should be used to avoid the overtreatment of epithelium without native metastatic capability.

This paper should be required reading for the many pathologists who are faced with this dilemma.

B. A. Carter, MD, FRCPC

References

1. Carter BA, Jensen RA, Simpson JF, Page DL. Benign transport of breast epithelium into axillary lymph nodes after biopsy. *Am J Clin Pathol.* 2000;113:259-265.
2. Diaz NM, Vrcel V, Centeno BA, Muro-Cacho C. Modes of benign mechanical transport of breast epithelial cells to axillary lymph nodes. *Adv Anat Pathol.* 2005;12:7-9.

Anaplastic large cell lymphoma and breast implants: results from a structured expert consultation process
Kim B, Roth C, Young VL, et al (RAND Health and Pardee RAND Graduate School, Boston, MA)
Plast Reconstr Surg 128:629-639, 2011

Background.—There are increasing concerns about a possible association between anaplastic large cell lymphoma (ALCL) and breast implants. The authors conducted a structured expert consultation process to evaluate the evidence for the association, its clinical significance, and a potential biological model based on their interpretation of the published evidence.

Methods.—A multidisciplinary panel of 10 experts was selected based on nominations from national specialty societies, academic department heads, and recognized researchers in the United States.

Results.—Panelists agreed that (1) there is a positive association between breast implants and ALCL development but likely underrecognition of the true number of cases; (2) a recurrent, clinically evident seroma occurring 6 months or more after breast implantation should be aspirated and sent for cytologic analysis; (3) anaplastic lymphoma kinase-negative ALCL that develops around breast implants is a clinically indolent disease with a favorable prognosis that is distinct from systemic anaplastic lymphoma kinase-negative ALCL; (4) management should consist of removal of the involved implant and capsule, which is likely to prevent recurrence, and evaluation for other sites of disease; and (5) adjuvant radiation or chemotherapy should not be offered to women with capsule-confined disease. Little agreement, however, was found regarding etiologic risk factors for implant-associated ALCL.

Conclusion.—The authors' assessment yielded consistent results on a number of key issues regarding ALCL in women with breast implants, but substantial further research is needed to improve our understanding of the epidemiology, clinical aspects, and biology of this disease.

Clinical Question/Level of Evidence.—Risk, V.

▶ The importance of this article lies largely in its ability to affect practice in the anatomic pathology gross room.

This expert evaluation of evidence suggests that anaplastic large cell lymphoma (ALCL) may be found more often in women with silicone or saline implants than expected. Of late, many articles on this topic, with diametrically opposing results, have been published. This article puts to rest any doubts about association. I would expect that as access to cosmetic and reconstructive procedures widens, the numbers of cases seen in the pathology laboratory will increase.

Most cases of ALCL of the breast have been diagnosed in symptomatic women with revisions of late-onset persistent lymphoma. The recommendations from the article state that tissue should be submitted for histologic examination in symptomatic women with late-onset persistent lymphoma. However, the authors note that the disease is also found in asymptomatic women with implants and in those with capsular contractures or masses adjacent to the implant. I think that this article may change practice in that all tissues submitted from breast implant patients should be examined carefully and strong consideration should be given for submission of tissue for pathologist assessment and diagnosis.

This article also contributes to pathologists' knowledge base and offers a differential diagnosis for a complex clinical preparation. The tissues collected from seromas and capsules in this scenario often show bizarre cells with the diagnosis of breast carcinoma at the top of the differential list. If one is not cognizant of the association between ALCL and implants, it could be left off of the diagnostic list altogether.

B. A. Carter, MD, FRCPC

3   Gastrointestinal System

A quantitative assessment of the risks and cost savings of forgoing histologic examination of diminutive polyps
Kessler WR, Imperiale TF, Klein RW, et al (Indiana Univ School of Medicine, Indianapolis; Med Decision Modeling, Inc, Indianapolis, IN)
Endoscopy 43:683-691, 2011

Background and Aims.—Endoscopic prediction of polyp histology is rapidly improving to the point where it may not be necessary to submit all polyps for formal histologic assessment. This study aimed to quantify the expected costs and outcomes of removing diminutive polyps without subsequent pathologic assessment.

Methods.—Cross-sectional analysis of a colonoscopy database for polyp histology; decision models that quantify effects on guideline-recommended surveillance and subsequent costs and consequences. The database was composed of consecutive colonoscopies from 1999 to 2004 at a single-institution tertiary care center. Patients were those found to have at least one diminutive polyp removed during colonoscopy, irrespective of indication. The main outcome measurements include up-front cost savings resulting from forgoing pathologic assessment; frequency and cost of incorrect surveillance intervals based on errors in histologic assessment; number needed to harm (NNH) for perforation and/or interval cancer.

Results.—Incorrect surveillance intervals were recommended in 1.9% of cases when tissue was submitted for pathologic assessment and 11.8% of cases when it was not. Based on the annual volume of colonoscopy in the US, the annual up-front cost savings of forgoing the pathologic assessment would exceed a billion dollars. An upper estimate on the downstream costs and consequences of forgoing pathology suggests that less than 10% of the up-front savings would be offset and the NNH exceeds 11 000.

Conclusion.—Endoscopic diagnosis of polyp histology during colonoscopy and forgoing pathologic examination would result in substantial up-front cost savings. Downstream consequences of the resulting incorrect surveillance intervals appear to be negligible.

▶ Cost analyses, such as the one performed by Kessler et al, are meant to guide clinical practice protocols, not necessarily definitively determine a new practice guideline. The performance of colonoscopy with biopsy is invaluable in

33

colorectal screening, and the authors reach the conclusion that not performing histologic examination of diminutive polyps may result in considerable cost savings at little increased risk. The utility and accuracy of such analyses depend on a number of factors, such as framing and assumptions performed in the analysis. In this article, the authors examine whether tissue should be sent to pathology and not whether tissue should be biopsied at all (for a diminutive polyp). In the current environment, tissue discarding (without histologic examination) is determined by institutional decision-making practices (eg, hospital or clinic policies), and it is unclear if cost analyses guide their decisions. The assumptions include a number of factors (Fig 3 in the original article) that are evaluated in 1-way sensitivity analyses. For some factors, relatively wide variability in outcome (additional incorrect surveillance) is observed. The factors evaluated in the sensitivity analyses depend on several factors themselves, such as endoscopist skill and experience, which, in turn, raises the question of the quality of the skill of practitioners who perform endoscopy. Nonetheless, the findings are intriguing and suggest that overbiopsy is the general problem, similar to overtesting for many laboratory tests. A major issue, outlined by this article, is the challenge in preanalytic decision making, which is a major cause of higher costs in the health care system. For additional reading, please see the reference section.[1,2]

S. S. Raab, MD

References

1. Rex DK. Narrow-band imaging without optical magnification for histologic analysis of colorectal polyps. *Gastroenterology.* 2009;136:1174-1181.
2. Ignjatovic A, East JE, Suzuki N, Vance M, Guenther T, Saunders BP. Optical diagnosis of small colorectal polyps at routine colonoscopy (Detect InSpect ChAracterise Resect and Discard; DISCARD trial): a prospective cohort study. *Lancet Oncol.* 2009;10:1171-1178.

How to Classify Adenocarcinomas of the Esophagogastric Junction: As Esophageal or Gastric Cancer?
Gertler R, Stein HJ, Loos M, et al (Technische Universität München, Munich, Germany; et al)
Am J Surg Pathol 35:1512-1522, 2011

Background.—To evaluate whether so-called cardiac adenocarcinomas (adenocarcinomas of the esophagogastric junction type II and III, ie AEG II and III) are better staged as cancers of the esophagus or as cancers of the stomach.

Methods.—A single-center cohort of 1141 patients operated for AEG II and III is staged according to the seventh edition of the TNM classification for cancers of the esophagus and cancers of the stomach. Kaplan-Meier and Cox regression analyses are used to evaluate the prognostic performance of these 2 staging schemes.

Results.—For so-called cardiac adenocarcinomas, the esophageal T classification is monotone. That is, it defines subgroups with continuous decreasing survival with increasing T stage. And it is distinct. That is, survival of these monotonic subgroups differs significantly. The gastric T classification is monotone but not distinct for pT2 versus pT3 ($P = 0.641$) and for pT4a versus pT4b tumors ($P = 0.130$). The type of infiltrated adjacent structure matters with significant differences in prognosis between the esophageal subgroups T4a and T4b ($P < 0.001$). For the N classification, both the esophageal and gastric schemes are monotone and distinct, with decreasing prognosis with increasing number of lymph node metastases. The subclassification of N3a and N3b disease according to the gastric scheme defines 2 subgroups with significant differences in prognosis ($P < 0.01$). Both the gastric and esophageal schemes include heterogeneous stage groups (2 and 1, respectively) and are not distinctive between several stage groups (4 and 3, respectively).

Conclusions.—Neither the esophageal nor the gastric scheme proves to be clearly superior over the other, and neither is perfect for AEG II and III. Our analysis includes further hints that so-called cardiac adenocarcinomas have different biological properties compared with genuine gastric and genuine esophageal cancers.

▶ A very important aspect of pathology practice lies in the correct classification and staging of malignancies. To a large extent, the correct classification and staging of tumors depends on following specific rules, and for gastrointestinal tract malignancies, we now follow the rules of the seventh edition of the TNM classification system. In this system, a tumor within 5 cm of the esophagogastric junction that extends into the esophagus is classified and staged with the esophageal scheme. All other tumors are staged with the gastric scheme. The importance of a thorough gross examination is absolutely necessary for correct classification. Based on these rules, the staging system determines patient prognosis and stage-specific treatments. Gertler et al examined whether adenocarcinomas of the esophagogastric junction II (true carcinomas of the cardia - AEG II) and AEG III (subcardial gastric carcinomas) are better staged as cancers of the esophagus or of the stomach and found that neither scheme was superior. The authors also found other important aspects of the TNM classification system that affect prognosis. These findings indicate that practicing pathologists need to be up to date with the current TNM system and be aware that patients will have differences in prognosis based on subclassifications of different schemes. For additional reading, please see the reference section.[1,2]

S. S. Raab, MD

References

1. Siewert JR, Stein HJ. Classification of adenocarcinoma of the oesophagogastric junction. *Br J Surg.* 1998;85:1457-1459.
2. von Rahden BH, Feith M, Stein HJ. Carcinoma of the cardia: classification as esophageal or gastric cancer? *Int J Colorectal Dis.* 2005;20:89-93.

Gastric Hyperplastic Polyps: A Heterogeneous Clinicopathologic Group Including a Distinct Subset Best Categorized as Mucosal Prolapse Polyp

Gonzalez-Obeso E, Fujita H, Deshpande V, et al (Hosp General de Ciudad Real, Spain; Kagoshima Univ Graduate School of Med and Dental Sciences, Japan; Massachusetts General Hosp and Harvard Med School, Boston; et al)
Am J Surg Pathol 35:670-677, 2011

Background.—Gastric hyperplastic polyps are the second most common subtype of gastric polyps. There has been an ongoing debate about their precise diagnostic criteria and etiological associations.

Materials and Methods.—A total of 208 gastric polyps that were originally diagnosed as hyperplastic polyps in our department during an 8-year period were reviewed using recently emphasized diagnostic criteria, and their clinicopathologic associations were explored.

Results.—Only 41 cases were confirmed as hyperplastic polyps, whereas 103 cases (49%) were reclassified as polypoid foveolar hyperplasia, and 64 cases (31%) were diagnosed as gastric mucosal prolapse polyps. Gastric mucosal prolapse polyps were distinguished by basal glandular elements, hypertrophic muscle fibers ascending perpendicularly from the muscularis mucosae, and by thick-walled blood vessels. This hitherto undescribed polyp is more commonly sessile than hyperplastic polyps ($P=0.0452$) and is found more often in the antropyloric region (P: 0.0053). Only 20.6% of hyperplastic polyps were associated with *Helicobacter pylori* infection.

Conclusions.—Our findings highlight that gastric polypoid lesions that have morphologic similarities may be related to various mechanisms, including inflammatory and prolapse processes. The predominantly antral location of gastric mucosal prolapse polyps, a zone of pronounced peristalsis, suggests that mucosal prolapse plays a role in the development of these common polyps. Evaluation of the prevalence and clinical associations of these distinctive polyps awaits further studies (Fig 3).

▶ It's the battle of the gastric polyps. The most common type of gastric polyp is the fundic gland polyp. The second most common polyp is the hyperplastic polyp, with a prevalence of approximately 14%. A publication by Abraham et al[1] spurred the debate that some small hyperplastic polyps were examples of polypoid foveolar hyperplasia (PFH), which display foveolar elongation and hyperplasia and lack cyst formation and stromal changes. Some pathologists believe that PFH is simply a precursor of hyperplastic polyps and do not make the separation. Others believe that the separation is important for several reasons, one being that large hyperplastic polyps are associated with a low risk of malignant transformation. The article by Gonzalez-Obeso and colleagues suggest that there is yet another subtype of the hyperplastic polyp that they term the *mucosal prolapse polyp* (MPP). The MPP has thick-walled vessels, thick bundles of smooth muscle, and a prominent basal glandular component. Fig 3 depicts these 3 polyp types. By reviewing 208 cases originally diagnosed as hyperplastic polyp, Gonzalez-Obeso et al separated their cases into 3 polyp

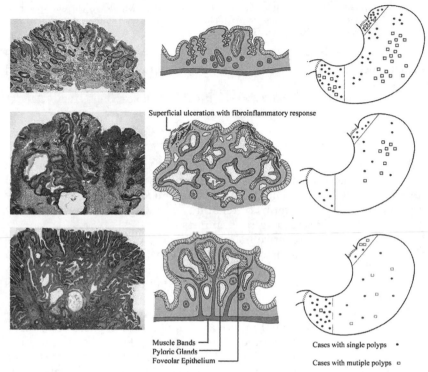

FIGURE 3.—The panels show the characteristic histologic features of 3 types of mucosal polyps with foveolar hyperplasia and their schematic representation. The top row shows the characteristic features of PFH; the middle row, gastric hyperplastic polyp; and the lower row, gastric mucosal prolapse polyp. The column on the right shows the distribution of polyps in the 3 gastric regions. Squares characterize multiple polyps, and the circle indicates cases with single polyps (blue: foveolar epithelium; gold: pyloric glands; red: fibroblasts; pink: smooth muscle). For interpretation of the references to color in this figure legend, the reader is referred to web version of this article. (Reprinted from Gonzalez-Obeso E, Fujita H, Deshpande V, et al. Gastric hyperplastic polyps: a heterogeneous clinicopathologic group including a distinct subset best categorized as mucosal prolapse polyp. *Am J Surg Pathol.* 2011;35:670-677, with permission from Lippincott Williams & Wilkins.)

types, although their data show a degree of overlap in histologic features. The importance for the practicing pathologist is whether the diagnosis of these 3 entities is reproducible (are we precise?) and does this separation have clinical implications (are we accurate in the sense that we describe different diseases that are associated with different management strategies or risks?). Currently, we do not seem to know the answers to these 2 questions, and studies such as the one by Gonzalez-Obeso put us on the right course of knowledge seeking. For additional reading, please see the reference section.[2]

S. S. Raab, MD

References

1. Abraham SC, Singh VK, Yardley JH, Wu TT. Hyperplastic polyps of the stomach: associations with histologic patterns of gastritis and gastric atrophy. *Am J Surg Pathol.* 2001;25:500-507.

2. Carmack SW, Genta RM, Schuler CM, Saboorian MH. The current spectrum of gastric polyps: a 1-year national study of over 120,000 patients. *Am J Gastroenterol.* 2009;104:1524-1532.

Virtual microscopy for histology quality assurance of screen-detected polyps

Risio M, Bussolati G, Senore C, et al (IRCC, Candiolo-Torino, Italy; Univ of Torino, Italy; CPO Piemonte, Torino, Italy)
J Clin Pathol 63:916-920, 2010

Aim.—Histology quality assurance is crucial for screening programmes and can be performed by circulating glass slides, which has certain intrinsic disadvantages. The present study aimed to assess the accuracy of virtual microscopy in terms of reliability and diagnostic reproducibility in colorectal cancer screening programmes.

Methods.—457 consecutive lesions detected in people undergoing colonoscopy were examined histologically in two pathology units, using both traditional optical microscopy and virtual microscopy (6–12 months later). Intra- and inter-observer agreement using the two approaches was determined using κ statistics.

Results.—Intra- and inter-observer agreements were substantially unmodified by the use of the virtual microscopy approach compared with traditional optical microscopy; moreover, for some histological features critical for patient management in colorectal cancer screening programmes (such as the presence of a villous component within the adenoma), virtual microscopy increased interobserver agreement (κ statistics 0.66 versus 0.52).

Conclusions.—This study shows that virtual microscopy can be an effective tool for diagnostic quality assurance in colorectal cancer screening programmes, and its accuracy is equivalent to or higher than that of optical microscopy in the validation of histological criteria (eg, advanced adenoma) crucial for patient management in screening programmes.

▶ Risio et al examine virtual microscopy compared with light microscopy in external quality assessment scheme. The interobserver agreement data would suggest that cases (at least for colon polyps) could be sent to reviewers through electronic format rather than as glass slides. For additional reading, please see the reference section.[1,2]

S. S. Raab, MD

References

1. Cross SS, Burton JL, Dubé AK, et al. Offline telepathology diagnosis of colorectal polyps: a study of interobserver agreement and comparison with glass slide diagnoses. *J Clin Pathol.* 2002;55:305-308.
2. Cross SS, Betmouni S, Burton JL, et al. What levels of agreement can be expected between histopathologists assigning cases to discrete nominal categories? A study of the diagnosis of hyperplastic and adenomatous colorectal polyps. *Mod Pathol.* 2000;13:941-944.

Adenoma detection rate increases with each decade of life after 50 years of age

Diamond SJ, Enestvedt BK, Jiang Z, et al (Oregon Health and Sciences Univ, Portland)
Gastrointest Endosc 74:135-140, 2011

Background.—The adenoma detection rate (ADR) has recently been used as a quality measure for screening colonoscopy. We hypothesize that the ADR will increase with each decade of life after 50 years of age.

Objective.—The aim of this study was to define age-based goals for the ADR and advanced neoplasia to improve the quality of colonoscopy.

Methods.—Using the Clinical Outcomes Research Initiative database, we identified patients who underwent screening colonoscopy between 2005 and 2006. Pathology of polyp findings was reviewed, and the ADR and the prevalence of advanced neoplasia were calculated based on age and sex.

Results.—A total of 7756 polypectomies (44.9%) were performed on 17,275 patients between 2005 and 2006. Of these polyps, 56.3% (4363) were adenomas or more advanced lesions. The ADR was higher in men than women and increased with age. The ADR in men younger than age 50 was 24.7 (95% CI, 18.2-31.2); for those 50 to 59 years of age, it was 27.8 (95% CI, 26.5-29.1); for those 60 to 69 years of age, it was 33.6 (95% CI, 31.7-35.4); for those 70 to 79 years of age, it was 34.3 (95% CI, 31.5-37.1); and for those older than 80 years of age, it was 40.0 (95% CI, 32.9-47.1). The ADR in women younger than 50 years old was 12.6 (95% CI, 6.8-18.4); in those 50 to 59 years of age, it was 17.0 (85% CI, 15.9-18.1); for those 60 to 69 years of age, it was 22.4 (95% CI, 20.8-24.0); for those 70 to 79 years of age, it was 26.1 (95% CI, 23.7-28.5); and for those older than 80 years of age, it was 26.9 (95% CI, 21.4-32.5).

Limitations.—The Clinical Outcomes Research Initiative database offers access to demographic information as well as endoscopy and pathology data, but there is limited clinical information about patients in the database.

Conclusion.—The ADR, and, importantly, the rate of advanced neoplasia increased with each decade of life after the age of 50 and are higher in men than women in each decade of life (Table 2).

▶ Pathologists play an important role in evaluating the quality of clinical services. In the article by Diamond et al, colon biopsy pathologic diagnoses are used to evaluate the quality of colonoscopy screening services through the adenoma detection rate (ADR, which is defined as the number of adenomas identified per 100 screened patients) and the advanced neoplasia (including cancer and high-grade dysplasia) frequency. The authors concluded that the ADR (Table 2) and advanced neoplasia frequency increased by decade of life. This metric could be used to evaluate the quality of entire programmatic screening services, hospitals, clinicians, and pathologists. The role of databases, depending on pathology data, is becoming increasingly important in guiding care through quality improvement initiatives. Consequently, pathologist inclusion in the construction of these databases and the appropriate use of pathology data sets are critical. A major

TABLE 2.—Adenoma Detection rate for Men and Women

Age, y	ADR	95% CI	P value	Trend
Men				
<50	24.7	18.4-1.9	.378	<.0001
50-59	27.8	26.5-9.1	Reference	
60-69	33.6	31.7-5.5	<.0001	
70-79	34.3	31.5-7.2	<.0001	
>80	40	32.9-7.4	<.0001	
Women				
<50	12.6	7.4-19.7	.191	<.0001
50-59	17	15.9-18.1	Reference	
60-69	22.4	20.8-24.1	<.0001	
70-79	26.1	23.7-28.6	<.0001	
>80	26.9	21.5-32.9	<.0001	

ADR, Adenoma detection rate; CI, confidence interval.

role of pathologists is in information transfer and management, and clinical teams that include pathologists are important to health care organizations. For additional reading, please see the reference section.[1,2]

S. S. Raab, MD

References

1. Lieberman DA, Weiss DG, Bond JH, Ahnen DJ, Garewal H, Chejfec G. Use of colonoscopy to screen asymptomatic adults for colorectal cancer. Veterans Affairs Cooperative Study Group 380. *N Engl J Med*. 2000;343:162-168.
2. Kaminski MF, Regula J, Kraszewska E, et al. Quality indicators for colonoscopy and the risk of interval cancer. *N Engl J Med*. 2010;362:1795-1803.

A Prospective Study of Duodenal Bulb Biopsy in Newly Diagnosed and Established Adult Celiac Disease

Evans KE, Aziz I, Cross SS, et al (Sheffield Teaching Hosp Trust, UK; Royal Hallamshire Hosp, Sheffield, UK)

Am J Gastroenterol 106:1837-1842, 2011

Objectives.—Recent reports suggest that the duodenal bulb may be the only site to demonstrate villous atrophy (VA) in celiac disease. However, there is a paucity of data from newly diagnosed adult celiac patients and no data from those patients with established celiac disease. The objective of this study was to compare the histological findings in the duodenal bulb and distal duodenum of patients with adult celiac disease (newly diagnosed or established) against controls.

Methods.—A total of 461 patients were prospectively recruited. Biopsies were graded using the Marsh criteria.

Results.—In all, 461 patients (300 females and 161 males) with median age 51 years were analyzed. In all, 126 had newly diagnosed celiac disease, 85 established celiac disease, and 250 controls. New diagnosis celiac disease

TABLE 2.—The Modified Marsh Criteria Used to Classify Duodenal Mucosal Damage in Celiac Disease

Marsh Grade	Histological Findings
0	Normal
1	Raised IELs (>25 per 100 enterocytes)
2	Raised IELs with crypt hyperplasia
3a	Raised IELs, crypt hyperplasia and partial villous atrophy
3b	Raised IELs, crypt hyperplasia and subtotal villous atrophy
3c	Raised IELs, crypt hyperplasia and total villous atrophy

IELs, intraepithelial lymphocytes.

(9%, P < 0.0001) and established celiac disease (14%, P < 0.0001) were more likely than controls to have VA in the bulb alone. Overall, when comparing the histological lesion of the bulb against the distal duodenum, 31/85 with established celiac disease (P < 0.0001) and 21/126 newly diagnosed (P = 0.0067) had a discrepancy in the severity of the lesion between the two sites compared with 18/250 controls. In all, 24/31 with established celiac disease and 16/21 newly diagnosed had the more severe lesion in the bulb.

Conclusions.—VA may be present only in the duodenal bulb. This study suggests that the optimal assessment of patients in whom celiac disease is suspected (with positive serology) and those with established celiac disease requires a duodenal bulb biopsy in addition to distal duodenal biopsies (Table 2).

▶ Clinical sampling in all areas of pathology is one of the most important factors in correctly establishing a disease (or nondisease) process. The quality of clinical sampling includes technical performance skills and cognitive decision making, such as selecting the correct area for sampling. In the study by Evans et al, the data indicate that sampling the duodenal bulb is important in correctly diagnosing celiac disease. Pathologists have an important role in the process by both histologically diagnosing the disease (Table 2) and checking to see if the duodenal bulb has been sampled. Because communication among health care professionals has been established as a critical component in patient safety (and diagnostic accuracy!), pathologists may assist in improving patient care in gastrointestinal pathology through several methods. The most important method in this scenario is by directing communication with endoscopists that the duodenal bulb has been sampled. In this manner, the pathologist is the quality check of a complex process of testing and evaluation. For additional reading, please see the reference section.[1,2]

S. S. Raab, MD

References

1. Oberhuber G, Granditsch G, Vogelsang H. The histopathology of coeliac disease: time for a standardized report scheme for pathologists. *Eur J Gastroenterol Hepatol.* 1999;11:1185-1194.

2. Rostom A, Murray JA, Kagnoff MF. American Gastroenterological Association (AGA) Institute technical review on the diagnosis and management of celiac disease. *Gastroenterology.* 2006;131:1981-2002.

Inter-observer variation in the histological diagnosis of polyps in colorectal cancer screening

van Putten PG, Hol L, van Dekken H, et al (Erasmus Univ Med Centre, Rotterdam, The Netherlands; St Lucas Andreas Hosp, Amsterdam, The Netherlands; et al)
Histopathology 58:974-981, 2011

Aim.—To determine the inter-observer variation in the histological diagnosis of colorectal polyps.

Methods and Results.—Four hundred and forty polyps were randomly selected from a colorectal cancer screening programme. Polyps were first evaluated by a general (324 polyps) or expert (116 polyps) pathologist, and subsequently re-evaluated by an expert pathologist. Conditional agreement was reported, and inter-observer agreement was determined using kappa statistics. In 421/440 polyps (96%), agreement for their non-adenomatous or adenomatous nature was obtained, corresponding to a very good kappa value of 0.88. For differentiation of adenomas as non-advanced and advanced, consensus was obtained in 266/322 adenomas (83%), with a moderate kappa value of 0.58. For the non-adenomatous or adenomatous nature, both general and expert pathologists, and expert pathologists between each other, showed very good agreement {kappa values of 0.89 [95% confidence interval (CI) 0.83—0.95] and 0.86 (95% CI 0.73—0.98), respectively}. For categorization of adenomas as non-advanced and advanced, moderate agreement was found between general and expert pathologists, and between expert pathologists [kappa values of 0.56 (95% CI 0.44—0.67) and 0.64 (95% CI 0.43—0.85), respectively].

Conclusions.—General and expert pathologists demonstrate very good inter-observer agreement for differentiating non-adenomas from adenomas, but only moderate agreement for non-advanced and advanced adenomas. The considerable variation in differentiating non-advanced and advanced adenomas suggests that more objective criteria are required for risk stratification in screening and surveillance guidelines.

▶ In this study, advanced adenomas are defined as adenomas of ≥10 mm in size, with ≥25% villous histology, or with high-grade dysplasia. Van Putten and colleagues found that pathologists have a lack of precision in separating adenomas from advanced adenomas (Table 3 in the original article shows inter-observer kappa values), and this lack of precision results in pathologists disagreeing about which patients should have more or less aggressive follow-up screening (surveillance colonoscopy 3 years after removal of an advanced adenoma versus 5-10 years after removal of 1 to 2 nonadvanced adenomas). Pathologists will need to reach consensus on distinguishing adenomas and advanced adenomas, and this will require a great deal of hard work. Reaching consensus ultimately requires a great deal of teamwork and working together to determine when specific criteria are present. For additional reading, please see the reference section.[1,2]

S. S. Raab, MD

References

1. Costantini M, Sciallero S, Giannini A, et al. SMAC Workgroup. Interobserver agreement in the histologic diagnosis of colorectal polyps. the experience of the multicenter adenoma colorectal study (SMAC). *J Clin Epidemiol.* 2003;56: 209-214.
2. Yoon H, Martin A, Benamouzig R, Longchampt E, Deyra J, Chaussade S, Groupe d'étude APACC. Inter-observer agreement on histological diagnosis of colorectal polyps: the APACC study. *Gastroenterol Clin Biol.* 2002;26:220-224.

Current practice patterns among pathologists in the assessment of venous invasion in colorectal cancer

Messenger DE, Driman DK, McLeod RS, et al (Mount Sinai Hosp, Toronto, Ontario, Canada; London Health Sciences Centre, Ontario, Canada; et al)
J Clin Pathol 64:983-989, 2011

Aims.—Venous invasion (VI) is a known independent prognostic indicator of recurrence and survival in colorectal cancer. The guidelines of the Royal College of Pathologists (RCPath) state that, in a series of resections, extramural VI should be detected in at least 25% of specimens. However, there is widespread variability in the reported incidence, and this may affect patient access to adjuvant therapy. This study aims to clarify the current practice patterns of pathologists regarding the assessment of VI and to identify factors associated with an increased self-reported VI detection rate.

Methods.—A population-based survey was mailed to 361 pathologists in the province of Ontario, Canada.

Results.—The overall response rate was 64.9%. Most pathologists were practicing in community-based centres (66.2%) and approximately half had been in practice for over 15 years (53.5%). A subspecialist interest in gastrointestinal (GI) pathology was declared by 27.3% of pathologists. The majority of pathologists (70.2%) reported that they detected VI in less than 10% of resection specimens, with only 9.1% reporting VI detection rates above 20%. Standardised reporting criteria were applied by 62.1%. Special stains were employed by 57.6% if VI was suspected on H&E-stained sections. Practice in a university-affiliated centre, a subspecialist interest in GI pathology and the acceptance of the 'orphan arteriole' sign were all independently associated with a self-reported VI detection rate above 10% on multivariate analysis.

Conclusions.—Self-reported VI detection rates are low among most pathologists. Even among specialist GI pathologists practicing in university-affiliated centres, few reported a detection rate close to that recommended

TABLE 3.—Factors Predictive of a Self-Reported Venous Invasion Detection Rate Above 10% on Logistic Regression

Factor	OR (95% CI)	p Value
Tumour within an endothelium lined space surrounded by a rim of smooth muscle		
No	1.00	0.228
Yes	3.74 (0.44 to 31.9)	
Tumour nodule adjacent to an artery where smooth muscle can be identified (orphan arteriole sign)		
No	1.00	0.025
Yes	3.74 (1.18 to 11.8)	
Routine use of special stain if fail to detect VI on standard H&E stain		
No	1.00	0.132
Yes	2.21 (0.79 to 6.22)	
Type of hospital practice		
Community	1.00	0.024
University	2.44 (1.13 to 5.31)	
Subspecialist interest		
Non-gastrointestinal	1.00	0.048
Gastrointestinal	2.24 (1.01 to 4.99)	

Factors entered into model if p<0.10 on univariate analysis.
VI, venous invasion.

by the RCPath. Strategies to increase the detection of VI may be required (Table 3).

▶ Messenger and colleagues found that the reporting of venous invasion in colorectal cancer cases is low in both subspecialists and even lower nonsubspecialists. These data were measured using a self-reporting survey tool and reflect, at least in this group of pathologists, that there is significant underreporting. Specific practice and pathologist characteristics are associated with higher reporting frequencies (Table 3), and these may serve as a basis for improving the quality of venous invasion reporting. These include the adoption of standardized criteria, use of histochemical studies (ie, elastic staining), and implementing forms of redundancy (eg, secondary review) in practice. For additional reading, please see reference list.[1,2]

S. S. Raab, MD

References

1. Abdulkader M, Abdulla K, Rakha E, Kaye P. Routine elastic staining assists detection of vascular invasion in colorectal cancer. *Histopathology.* 2006;49:487-492.
2. Sternberg A, Mizrahi A, Amar M, Groisman G. Detection of venous invasion in surgical specimens of colorectal carcinoma: the efficacy of various types of tissue blocks. *J Clin Pathol.* 2006;59:207-210.

What Impact Has the Introduction of a Synoptic Report for Rectal Cancer Had on Reporting Outcomes for Specialist Gastrointestinal and Nongastrointestinal Pathologists?

Messenger DE, McLeod RS, Kirsch R (Mount Sinai Hosp, Toronto, Ontario, Canada)
Arch Pathol Lab Med 135:1471-1475, 2011

Context.—Synoptic pathology reports increase the completeness of reporting for colorectal cancer. Despite the perceived superiority of specialist reporting, service demands dictate that general pathologists report colorectal cancer specimens in many centers.

Objective.—To determine differences in the completeness of rectal cancer reporting between specialist gastrointestinal and nongastrointestinal pathologists in both the narrative and synoptic formats.

Design.—Pathology reports from rectal cancer resections performed between 1997 and 2008 were reviewed. A standardized, synoptic report was formally introduced in 2001. Reports were assessed for completeness according to 10 mandatory elements from the College of American Pathologists checklist.

Results.—Overall, synoptic reports (n = 315) were more complete than narrative reports (n = 183) for TNM stage, distance to the circumferential radial margin, tumor grade, lymphovascular invasion, extramural venous invasion, perineural invasion, and regional deposits (all $P < .01$). Compared with those by nonspecialist pathologists, narrative reports by gastrointestinal pathologists were more complete for lymphovascular invasion (59.3% versus 35.9%, $P = .02$) and extramural venous invasion (70.4% versus 35.9%, $P = .001$), but there was no difference in completeness once a synoptic report was adopted. Gastrointestinal pathologists tended to report the presence of extramural venous invasion more frequently in both the narrative (18.5% versus 5.1%, $P = .01$) and synoptic formats (25.5% versus 14.6%, $P = .02$).

Conclusions.—Completeness of reporting, irrespective of subspecialist interest, was dramatically increased by the use of a synoptic report. Improvements in completeness were most pronounced among nongastrointestinal pathologists, enabling them to attain a level of report completeness comparable to that of gastrointestinal pathologists. Further studies are required to determine whether there are actual discrepancies in the detection of prognostic features between specialist gastrointestinal and nongastrointestinal pathologists.

▶ Messenger et al show that synoptic reporting improves report completeness and essentially decreases reporting hand-off errors of omission. Synoptic reporting most likely also improves the efficiency of care because clinicians do not need to call for additional details necessary for patient management. In the end, synoptic reporting also improves the efficiency of pathologists because they do not need to reexamine cases to assess histologic parameters that were omitted from the original report. The authors stress the point that gastrointestinal subspecialists use synoptic reports more frequently than non-subspecialists, although I think that finding is just a by-product of features such as familiarity and ease of use. The key point here is the importance of report standardization for all pathologists, regardless of practice type, diagnostic acumen, experience, and other factors. For additional reading, please see reference list.[1,2]

S. S. Raab, MD

References

1. Rigby K, Brown SR, Lakin G, Balsitis M, Hosie KB. The use of a proforma improves colorectal cancer pathology reporting. *Ann R Coll Surg Engl.* 1999;81:401-403.
2. Beattie GC, McAdam TK, Elliott S, Sloan JM, Irwin ST. Improvement in quality of colorectal cancer pathology reporting with a standardized proforma—a comparative study. *Colorectal Dis.* 2003;5:558-562.

4 Hepatobiliary System and Pancreas

Fibrolamellar carcinomas are positive for CD68
Ross HM, Daniel HDJ, Vivekanandan P, et al (The Johns Hopkins Univ School of Medicine, Baltimore, MD; et al)
Mod Pathol 24:390-395, 2011

Fibrolamellar carcinomas are a unique type of liver carcinoma that arise in non-cirrhotic livers of young individuals. Despite their distinctive appearance, recent studies have demonstrated a lack of consistency in how fibrolamellar carcinomas are diagnosed by pathologists. As a potential aide in diagnosis, we investigated the staining properties of CD68. The CD68 gene encodes for a transmembrane glycoprotein located within lysosomes and endosomes. Macrophages as well as other cell types rich in lysosomes/endosomes are CD68 positive. Cases of fibrolamellar carcinoma were collected from four academic centers. Control groups included hepatocellular carcinomas arising in both non-cirrhotic livers and cirrhotic livers. A group of cholangiocarcinomas were also stained. CD68 immunostaining was scored for both intensity and distribution on a scale of 0 to 3+. Twenty-three primary fibrolamellar carcinomas and 9 metastases (total of 24 individuals) were immunostained and showed a distinctive granular, dot-like or stippled pattern of cytoplasmic staining in nearly all cases (31/32), with a median distribution and intensity score of 3+. In control hepatocellular carcinomas that arose in non-cirrhotic livers, 10/39 showed CD68 staining with a median distribution and intensity score of 2+. In hepatocellular carcinomas arising in cirrhotic livers, 3/27 cases showed CD68 positivity, all with stippled dot-like cytoplasmic staining similar to that of fibrolamellar carcinomas. All five cholangiocarcinomas were negative. Overall, CD68 positivity was strongly associated with fibrolamellar carcinomas, $P<0.001$ and had a sensitivity of 96%, a specificity of 80%, and a negative predictive value of 98%. In sum, tumor positivity for CD68 staining was highly sensitive for fibrolamellar carcinoma and a lack of CD68 staining should suggest caution in making a diagnosis of fibrolamellar carcinoma (Fig 1).

▶ Hepatocellular neoplasms with fibrosis can be challenging to diagnose, and additional widely available immunohistochemical markers to assist in the

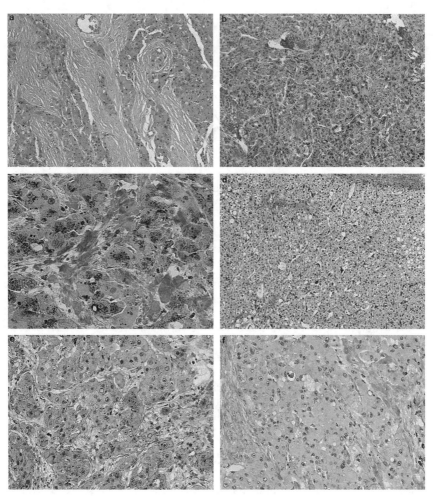

FIGURE 1.—Fibrolamellar carcinomas are CD68 positive. (a) H&E, original magnification, ×40. The typical morphology of fibrolamellar carcinoma can be seen. (b) CD68, original magnification, ×40: fibrolamellar carcinomas show a distinctive granular or stippled cytoplasmic staining pattern. (c) CD68, original magnification, ×160: High-power image of CD68 staining in fibrolamellar carcinoma. (d) CD68, original magnification, ×40: the background liver (same case as b, c) shows CD68 staining in Kupffer cells, but not the hepatocytes. (e) CD68, original magnification, ×100: another case of fibrolamellar carcinoma showing weaker but still positive CD68 staining. (f) CD68, original magnification, ×100: in some cases of fibrolamellar carcinoma, the tumor showed a larger circumscribed dotlike staining pattern of CD68. (Reprinted from Ross HM, Daniel HDJ, Vivekanandan P, et al. Fibrolamellar carcinomas are positive for CD68. *Mod Pathol.* 2011;24:390-395, Copyright 2011, with permission from Macmillan Publishers Ltd.)

classification would be useful. Although fibrolamellar carcinoma of the liver has a "classic" histologic appearance (large polygonal cells, abundant eosinophilic cytoplasm, vesiculated nuclei, prominent nucleoli, and lamellar fibrosis) and clinical presentation, it is not consistently diagnosed. On the basis of these findings, the authors suggest the combined use of classic histologic features and reactivity for CK7 and CD68 to make the diagnosis of fibrolamellar carcinoma. The granular or dot-like pattern of CD68 staining is important to recognize (Fig 1). Strengths of this study include the use of internal controls (Kupffer cells) to be sure the staining worked, the use of metastatic samples, and the use of full tissue sections to understand the pattern of staining. Unfortunately, biopsy specimens were not included in the study, so the applicability to biopsy specimens may not be appropriate. In addition, pathologist interpretation was used as the gold standard for classification into fibrolamellar and control hepatocellular carcinoma. These findings require confirmation from other investigators before the method receives widespread clinical use.

M. L. Smith, MD

The steatohepatitic variant of hepatocellular carcinoma and its association with underlying steatohepatitis

Salomao M, Remotti H, Vaughan R, et al (Columbia Univ College of Physicians and Surgeons, NY; Columbia Univ, NY)
Hum Pathol 2011 [Epub ahead of print]

Steatohepatitis and metabolic syndrome are increasingly recognized as important risk factors for development of hepatocellular carcinoma. We have recently described a histologic subtype of hepatocellular carcinoma termed *steatohepatitic hepatocellular carcinoma*, which shows features resembling stcatohepatitis in the nonneoplastic liver. The present study is undertaken to assess the association between the steatohepatitic hepatocellular carcinoma variant and underlying steatohepatitis and features of metabolic syndrome. We examined all hepatocellular carcinomas diagnosed on resections and explant specimens over a 3.5-year period at our institution. Tumors were classified as either conventional hepatocellular carcinoma or steatohepatitic hepatocellular carcinoma variant based on their predominant histopathologic pattern. The underlying chronic liver disease in each case was determined. The steatohepatitic hepatocellular carcinoma variant represented 13.5% (16/118) of cases. All but one case of steatohepatitic hepatocellular carcinoma occurred in patients with underlying steatohepatitis. Steatohepatitic hepatocellular carcinoma was diagnosed in 35.7% of patients with either nonalcoholic steatohepatitis or alcoholic liver disease compared with 1.3% of patient with other chronic liver diseases ($P < .0001$). The steatohepatitic hepatocellular carcinoma group had a significantly higher number of metabolic syndrome risk factors (2.44 versus 1.48, $P = .01$) and a higher percentage of patients with at least 3 metabolic syndrome components (50% versus 22.5%, $P = .02$). Immunohistochemically, there were diffuse loss of cytoplasmic CK8/18 and increased numbers of activated hepatic stellate cells within steatohepatitic hepatocellular carcinoma, in a pattern identical to that seen in steatohepatitis in nonneoplastic liver. Hepatocellular carcinomas showing a "steatohepatitic" histologic phenotype are strongly associated with underlying steatohepatitis and metabolic syndrome. This association further supports a possible role of steatohepatitis in human hepatocarcinogenesis.

▶ This article raises 2 important points for discussion. First, the authors show a correlation between a variant of hepatocellular carcinoma (HCC), namely, the steatohepatitic hepatocellular carcinoma (SH-HCC), and a diagnosis of steatohepatitis in the nonneoplastic liver. This is the first example of a specific variant of HCC having clinical significance. Three of the following 5 criteria were required in greater than 50% of the tumor for a diagnosis of SH-HCC: 1) steatosis, 2) hepatocyte ballooning, 3) Mallory bodies, 4) inflammation, and 5) pericellular fibrosis. Secondly, does the presence of steatohepatitis features histologically increase risk for the development of HCC, regardless of the degree of fibrosis? Can fat alone act to promote malignant transformation? These are topics for future study and consideration. Based on these changes it may be appropriate to report SH-HCC in needle biopsies of liver tumors and suggest the possibility of underlying steatohepatitis. Although there was a trend toward better survival in the SH-HCC group, it was not statistically significant.

M. L. Smith, MD

Telangiectatic Variant of Hepatic Adenoma: Clinicopathologic Features and Correlation Between Liver Needle Biopsy and Resection
Mounajjed T, Wu T-T (Mayo Clinic, Rochester, MN)
Am J Surg Pathol 35:1356-1363, 2011

Telangiectatic hepatic adenoma (THA) is a benign neoplasm treated by resection. The role of liver needle biopsy in identifying THA before resection has not been evaluated. We identified 55 patients who have undergone resection for hepatic adenoma (HA), THA, or focal nodular hyperplasia (FNH) after needle biopsy. Needle biopsies and resections were evaluated for the following: (1) abortive portal tracts; (2) sinusoidal dilatation; (3) ductular reaction; (4) inflammation; (5) aberrant naked vessels; (6) nodules, fibrous septa, and/or central stellate scar. THA diagnosis was made if the lesion had the first 4 criteria and lacked criterion 6. Most patients (36 of 55), including patients with THA (12 of 16), had multiple lesions (0.2 to 14.4 cm). Patients with THA showed no difference in age, body mass index, prevalence of diabetes or glucose intolerance, or presence of oral contraceptive (OCP) use from patients with HA or FNH, but patients with THA had longer periods of OCP use than patients with HA. Thirty-one percent of THAs had tumor hemorrhage. Of sampled THAs, 27% showed steatosis compared with 76% of sampled HAs ($P < 0.05$). All resected HAs and FNHs were correctly diagnosed on needle biopsy. Of 14 patients with resected THA, 3 histologic patterns were noted on needle biopsy: (1) All THA criteria and naked vessels were present in 6 patients (43%). (2) Consistent with HA: naked vessels only were present in 4 patients (29%). (3) Suggestive of THA: some but not all THA criteria were present in 4 patients (29%). No needle biopsy of a THA was

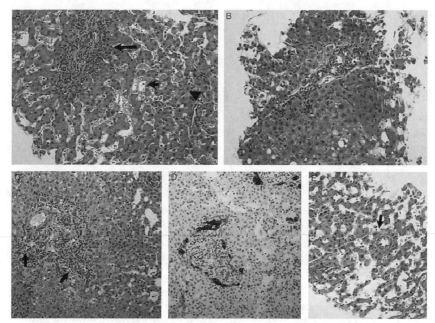

FIGURE 3.—Histologic findings in liver needle biopsy specimens from THA. A, All histologic features were present in some needle biopsy specimens. Abortive portal tracts with inflammation (long arrow) and sinusoidal dilatation (short arrow) and small aberrant naked vessels (arrowhead) were noted in this biopsy (case 1). B, Abortive portal tracts containing multiple sections of small, thick-walled arteries were also present (case 1). C, In this case, ductular reaction was difficult to discern on H&E (arrows). D, CK7 immunostain highlights ill-formed cholangioles. A diagnosis of THA was rendered on needle biopsy in this case (case 1). E, Only aberrant naked vessels and sinusoidal dilatation were present in this biopsy leading to a misdiagnosis of HA (case 8). (Reprinted from Mounajjed T, Wu T-T. Telangiectatic variant of hepatic adenoma: clinicopathologic features and correlation between liver needle biopsy and resection. *Am J Surg Pathol.* 2011;35:1356-1363, with permission from Lippincott Williams & Wilkins.)

TABLE 4.—Summary of Liver Needle Biopsy Findings in Lesions Consequently Diagnosed as THA at Resection

	Abortive Portal Tracts	Ductular Proliferation	Inflammation	Sinusoidal Dilatation	Aberrant Naked Vessels
Diagnostic of THA (n = 6)	6	6	5	6	6
Suggestive of THA (n = 4)	4	0	0	2	4
Consistent with HA (n = 4)	0	0	0	1	4
Total	10/14	6/14	5/15	9/14	14/14

HA, hepatic adenoma; THA, teleangiectatic hepatic adenoma.

misdiagnosed as FNH. Although evaluation of resection specimens is the gold standard for diagnosis of THA, liver needle biopsy is a useful diagnostic tool that leads to adequate treatment (Fig 3, Table 4).

▶ Based on the impressive work by Bioulac-Sage et al,[1] telangiectatic hepatic adenoma (THA) is increasingly being recognized as a benign liver lesion distinct from traditional hepatic adenoma (HA) and focal nodular adenoma (FNH). This article reviews an institution's experience with the needle biopsy diagnosis of these benign lesions and comparisons with resection specimens. An interesting finding not discussed in the abstract was the finding of multiple lesion types in 20% of patients. A combination of HA and FNH was most common. This underscores the similarities these lesions have in their presentation and possible biology. Fig 3 shows the histologic features required for a diagnosis of THA on needle biopsy. THA was most often misdiagnosed as HA primarily because of the presence of unpaired arteries and the lack of other findings of typical THA (Table 4). Fortunately HA and THA have similar patient management and risk of hemorrhage and are thus similarly treated.

For additional reading on THA, I suggest the article by Bioulac-Sage et al.[1]

M. L. Smith, MD

Reference

1. Bioulac-Sage P, Rebouissou S, Cunha AS, et al. Clinical, morphologic, and molecular features defining so-called telangiectatic focal nodular hyperplasias of the liver. *Gastroenterology.* 2005;128:1211-1218.

Identification of Malignant Cytologic Criteria in Pancreatobiliary Brushings With Corresponding Positive Fluorescence In Situ Hybridization Results
Barr Fritcher EG, Caudill JL, Blue JE, et al (Mayo Clinic and Foundation, Rochester, MN)
Am J Clin Pathol 136:442-449, 2011

Cytologic evaluation of pancreatobiliary brushings is specific but poorly sensitive for malignancy. Detection of polysomic cells by fluorescence in situ hybridization (FISH) is significantly more sensitive than routine cytology with similar specificity. The purpose of this study was to identify cytologic criteria most associated with malignancy in specimens unaffected by sample failure. Endoscopic brushings were split equally for routine cytologic and FISH analyses per clinical practice. We retrospectively evaluated 16 cytologic criteria on Papanicolaou-stained slides. We assumed that the presence of polysomic cells by FISH indicated successful tumor sampling in specimens from patients with pathologic evidence of malignancy on follow-up. We compared cytologic criteria of malignant brushings with corresponding positive FISH results (positive control, n = 39) with those without evidence of malignancy and corresponding negative FISH results (negative control, n = 30). The presence of single abnormal cells, irregular nuclear membranes, and enlarged nuclei were independent predictors of malignancy by logistic regression ($P < .05$) (Table 1).

▶ Polysomy in ductal epithelial cells as measured by florescence in situ hybridization (FISH) using probes for chromosomes 3, 7, 17, and 9p21 (Urovysion) is increasingly being used in the diagnosis and management of pancreatobiliary neoplasms. Table 1 highlights the main results in this study. Many cytologic

TABLE 1.—Frequency and Performance Characteristics of Cytologic Criteria Evaluated in 69 Pancreatobiliary Brushings Using Corresponding FISH Results to Identify Specimens Likely to Contain Tumor Cells

Cytologic Criteria	Positive Control* (n = 39)	Negative Control† (n = 30)	P‡	Sensitivity (%)	Specificity (%)
Architectural features					
Architectural disarray	31	11	<.001	79.5	63.3
3-dimensional depth of focus	10	1	<.05	25.6	96.7
Cell within cell	1	0	.37	2.6	100.0
Anisonucleosis	21	3	<.001	53.8	90.0
Abnormal groups (≥10 cells) present	37	21	<.01	94.9	30.0
Abnormal clusters (2-9 cells) present	34	11	<.0001	87.2	63.3
Abnormal single cells present	30	3	<.0001	76.9	90.0
Nuclear features					
Increased nuclear/cytoplasmic ratio	35	14	<.0001	89.7	53.3
Enlarged nuclei	23	3	<.0001	59.0	90.0
Irregular nuclear membranes	36	11	<.0001	92.3	53.3
Prominent nucleoli	27	10	<.01	69.2	66.7
Coarse chromatin	21	12	.25	53.8	60.0
Irregular chromatin distribution	10	3	.10	25.6	90.0
Overall cellularity					
>20 groups (≥10 cells) present	26	21	.77	66.7	30.0
>20 clusters (2-9 cells) present	23	12	.12	59.0	60.0
>20 single cells present	30	15	.05	76.9	50.0

FISH, fluorescence in situ hybridization.
*Corresponding positive FISH result and pathologic evidence of malignancy on follow-up.
†Corresponding negative FISH result without clinicopathologic evidence of malignancy on follow-up.
‡Comparison of positive control with negative control.

criteria were associated with tumor in the positive control group (higher sensitivities) but were also found in the negative control group (lower sensitivity). The findings suggest that extra attention be given to single abnormal cells (single cell with at least 1 abnormal nuclear feature), nuclear membrane abnormalities, and nuclear enlargement (3 times normal cell size) when examining pancreatobiliary brushings. A definitive definition of nuclear membrane abnormalities was not given. A major assumption in this study was that a positive FISH result indicated the presence of tumor on the Pap-stained slide. Further investigation of the usefulness of these specific cytologic findings is required in a prospective study.

M. L. Smith, MD

Diagnostic Utility of CD10 in Benign and Malignant Extrahepatic Bile Duct Lesions

Tretiakova M, Antic T, Westerhoff M, et al (Univ of Chicago Med Ctr, IL; et al)
Am J Surg Pathol 2011 [Epub ahead of print]

CD10, a cell surface enzyme with neutral metalloendopeptidase activity, is a marker for intestinal epithelial brush border. It is also present in normal bile ducts and gallbladder epithelia but is absent in cholangiocarcinomas.

However, the expression profile of CD10 in benign and malignant extrahepatic biliary lesions has not been studied. In this study, 69 biopsies, 9 resections, and 9 cell blocks prepared from fine-needle aspirations of the extrahepatic bile ducts from 86 patients were studied immunohistochemically for CD10 expression. The majority of cases contained normal biliary epithelium (NL, n = 64), along with foci of benign or malignant lesions in various combinations. Benign lesions included reactive atypia (n = 35), low-grade dysplasia of unknown significance (n = 21), and bile duct adenoma (BDA, n = 1). Malignant lesions included high-grade dysplasia (HGD, n = 45) and invasive adenocarcinoma (IC, n = 30). As expected, the NL showed strong continuous staining at the apical surface in all cases. Benign lesions were also CD10 positive in all but 3 cases; however, the staining pattern was discontinuous, with positive cells varying from 20% to 80%. None of the malignant lesions showed CD10 immunoreactivity, except for 2 HGD cases and 1 IC case, which exhibited focal staining. The Pearson χ^2 and Fisher exact tests showed significant statistical difference in CD10 expression among the study groups ($P < 0.001$). Our findings suggest that absence of CD10 expression in strips of atypical biliary epithelial cells may be a phenotype associated with malignant transformation and may serve as a useful marker to aid in the evaluation of bile duct biopsies, in which distinction between benign and malignant lesions on biopsies or cytology specimens can be extremely challenging because of limited sampling, crush artifact, and frequent inflammatory/reactive changes (Table 1).

▶ This is another study investigating the usefulness of ancillary testing to aid in the diagnosis of extrahepatic biliary lesions that are notoriously difficult to classify. Classification into study groups was based on consensus diagnosis among 3 study pathologists. No follow-up resection data were available to confirm initial pathologic classification. This leads to the possibility that some cases may have been misclassified initially. Strengths of the study include the large study size and the use of a variety of specimens, including fine-needle aspiration cell blocks, biopsies, and resection cases. A large number of cases in the low-grade dysplasia group (86.4%, Table 1) showed discontinuous staining,

TABLE 1.—Demographic Data of Studied Patients and CD10 Expression in Different Types of Lesions

Histologic Lesion	No. Cases	Mean Age	M:F Ratio	CD10 (+) Continuous*	CD10 (+) Discontinuous*	CD10 (−)
Normal biliary mucosa	64	67.1	1:1	60 (93.75%)	4 (6.25%)	0
R A	35	59.2	1.2:1	0	33 (94.3%)	2 (5.7%)
LGD and BDA	22	69.5	1.5:1	2 (9%)	19 (86.4%)	1 (4.6%)
HGD	45	69.1	0.7:1	0	2 (4%)	43 (96%)
Invasive carcinoma	30	68.7	1:1		1 (3%)	29 (97%)

F indicates female; M, male.
*All CD10-positive cases with both continuous and discontinuous staining patterns showed moderate-to-strong immunoreactivity. The difference in CD10 expression was strongly statistically significant between all studied lesions ($P < 0.001$).

which was not helpful diagnostically, as both benign and malignant lesions also showed a percentage of discontinuous staining. One may argue that these indeterminate-/low-grade cases are the more difficult ones to classify, and thus CD10 may not add much to these categories. Florescence in situ hybridization for chromosomes 3, 7, 17, and 9p21 (UroVysion) has also been used in pancreatobiliary lesions as a marker of malignant transformation. An interesting follow-up study would be to compare the use of combined CD10 immunohistochemistry, UroVysion, and cell black cytology for the diagnosis of these lesions prospectively.

M. L. Smith, MD

Costaining for keratins 8/18 plus ubiquitin improves detection of hepatocyte injury in nonalcoholic fatty liver disease
Guy CD, Nonalcoholic Steatohepatitis Clinical Research Network (Duke Univ Med Ctr, Durham, NC; et al)
Hum Pathol 2011 [Epub ahead of print]

Nonalcoholic fatty liver disease is a global health dilemma. The gold standard for diagnosis is liver biopsy. Ballooned hepatocytes are histologic manifestations of hepatocellular injury and are characteristic of steatohepatitis, the more severe form of nonalcoholic fatty liver disease. Definitive histologic identification of ballooned hepatocytes on routine stains, however, can be difficult. Immunohistochemical evidence for loss of the normal hepatocytic keratin 8/18 can serve as an objective marker of ballooned hepatocytes. We sought to explore the utility of a keratin 8/18 plus ubiquitin double immunohistochemical stain for the histologic evaluation of adult nonalcoholic fatty liver disease. Double immunohistochemical staining for keratin 8/18 and ubiquitin was analyzed using 40 adult human nonalcoholic fatty liver disease core liver biopsies. Ballooned hepatocytes lack keratin 8/18 staining as previously shown by others, but normal-size hepatocytes with keratin loss are approximately 5 times greater in number than keratin-negative ballooned hepatocytes. Keratin-negative ballooned hepatocytes, normal-size hepatocytes with keratin loss, and ubiquitin deposits show a zonal distribution, are positively associated with each other, and are frequently found adjacent to or intermixed with fibrous matrix. All 3 lesions correlate with fibrosis stage and the hematoxylin and eosin diagnosis of steatohepatitis (all $P < .05$). Compared with hematoxylin and eosin staining, immunohistochemical staining improves the receiver operating characteristics curve for advanced fibrosis (0.77 versus 0.83, 0.89, and 0.89 for keratin-negative ballooned hepatocytes, normal-size hepatocytes with keratin loss, and ubiquitin, respectively) because immunohistochemistry is more sensitive and specific for fibrogenic hepatocellular injury than hematoxylin and eosin staining. Keratin 8/18 plus ubiquitin double immunohistochemical stain improves detection of hepatocyte injury in nonalcoholic fatty liver disease. Thus,

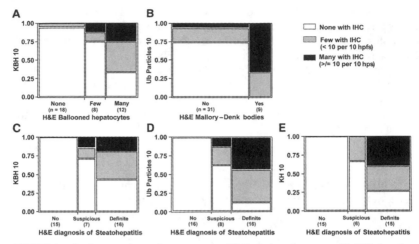

FIGURE 2.—Contingency plot analyses comparing H&E scoring parameters with IHC detection of hepatocellular injury. A, The H&E scoring of BH is compared with the IHC analysis of KBH. B, The H&E scoring of MDB is compared with the IHC analysis of Ub deposits. C, The H&E diagnosis of SH is compared with the IHC analysis of KBH. D, The H&E diagnosis of SH is compared with the IHC analysis of Ub deposits. E, The H&E diagnosis of SH is compared with the IHC analysis of KH. (Reprinted from Guy CD, Nonalcoholic Steatohepatitis Clinical Research Network. Costaining for keratins 8/18 plus ubiquitin improves detection of hepatocyte injury in nonalcoholic fatty liver disease. *Hum Pathol.* 2011;[Epub ahead of print], Copyright 2011, with permission from Elsevier.)

it may help differentiate nonalcoholic steatohepatitis from nonalcoholic fatty liver (Fig 2).

▶ Pathologists pore over fatty liver disease biopsies very carefully searching for definitively ballooned hepatocytes to justify a diagnosis of steatohepatitis. Unfortunately, these crucial cells are often not identified with certainty. The lack of pathologist reproducibility on the identification of ballooned hepatocytes and, thus, a diagnosis of steatohepatitis has been documented. This retrospective immunohistochemical staining article was designed to see if there are stains that may help pathologists in the identification of injured hepatocytes in cases of fatty liver disease. Fig 2 shows the main results of the study. It is interesting that some cases classified histologically as definite for steatohepatitis did not show immunohistochemical evidence of hepatocyte injury, raising questions of sensitivity. Hepatopathology experts performed the histologic analysis in this study, and it would be interesting to see how generalizable the results are to a general pathology practice. Furthermore, many of the example images supplied in the study show hepatocyte injury morphology that is very consistent with ballooning degeneration. Only 7 cases in the study were classified based on histology as suspicious for steatohepatitis. In these cases, the presence or absence of immunohistochemical evidence of hepatocyte damage may be used to support a more definitive classification. A follow-up study may be to evaluate the use of immunohistochemistry in cases that are borderline or indeterminate for hepatocyte injury.

M. L. Smith, MD

The Liver in Celiac Disease: Clinical Manifestations, Histologic Features, and Response to Gluten-Free Diet in 30 Patients

Mounajjed T, Oxentenko A, Shmidt E, et al (Mayo Clinic, Rochester, MN)
Am J Clin Pathol 136:128-137, 2011

Descriptive reports of liver histologic features in celiac disease (CD) are sparse, and the effect of a gluten-free diet (GFD) on the course of liver injury is poorly understood. We reviewed liver biopsy specimens in 30 patients with CD and performed immunostains for IgG, IgG4, IgM, and IgA. Subsequent liver biochemical tests and compliance with the GFD were recorded. Of the patients, 19 had autoimmune-mediated liver disease (AILD; autoimmune hepatitis, 9; primary sclerosing cholangitis, 7; and primary biliary cirrhosis, 3). The remaining 11 patients had cryptogenic hepatitis (5), hepatitis C (2), steatohepatitis (2), sarcoidosis (1), and T-cell lymphoma (1). The liver disease diagnosis preceded the CD diagnosis in all groups except steatohepatitis. Although 82% of patients without AILD had symptomatic CD, only 26% of patients with AILD had such symptoms. The pathology of the specific liver disease was not atypical in histologic features or IgG/IgM ratios. While GFD improved cryptogenic hepatitis, it did not seem to affect AILD. We propose that AILD and cryptogenic hepatitis in patients with CD represent distinct clinical, histologic, and immunohistochemical entities rather than 2 ends of a spectrum of liver injury.

▶ Celiac disease is associated with a large number of hepatic abnormalities that have been poorly defined. This article strictly defines patients with celiac disease and then describes the liver pathology in this patient group. An expected number of autoimmune-associated diseases were documented. Five cases were defined as cryptogenic liver disease and deserve further discussion. These patients had relatively mild elevations of aspartate aminotransferase and alanine aminotransferase and largely nonspecific changes on liver biopsy, including Kuppfer cell hyperplasia, macrovesicular steatosis, and ductular proliferation. These findings are important to note because it is not uncommon to receive liver biopsies from patients with celiac disease with mild elevations of transaminases. Careful study of the biopsies for these subtle changes and suggestions to their etiology and possible response to gluten-free diets is warranted. Weaknesses of this study include the relatively small sample size and the retrospective histologic review of liver biopsies that may have led to more detailed histologic scrutiny.

M. L. Smith, MD

The role of the pathologist in diagnosing and grading biliary diseases

Nakanuma Y, Harada K (Kanazawa Univ Graduate School of Medicine, Japan)
Clin Res Hepatol Gastroenterol 35:347-352, 2011

Pathological features of primary biliary cirrhosis (PBC) are reviewed. Immune-mediated, non-suppurative cholangitis is the initial lesion and is followed by the gradual and extensive destruction of bile ducts and

TABLE 1.—Scoring for Staging of Primary Biliary Cirrhosis

A. *Scoring of fibrosis*

Score 0	No portal fibrosis, or fibrosis limited to portal tracts
Score 1	Portal fibrosis with periportal fibrosis or incomplete septal fibrosis
Score 2	Bridging fibrosis with variable lobular disarray
Score 3	Liver cirrhosis with regenerative nodules and extensive fibrosis

B. *Scoring of bile duct loss*

Score 0	No bile duct loss
Score 1	Bile duct loss in < 1/3 of portal tracts
Score 2	Bile duct loss in 1/3−2/3 of portal tracts
Score 3	Bile duct loss in > 2/3 of portal tracts

C. *Scoring of deposition of copper granules or orcein-positive granules*

Score 0	No deposition of granules
Score 1	Deposition of granules in several periportal hepatocytes in <1/3 of portal tracts
Score 2	Deposition of granules in variable periportal hepatocytes in 1/3−2/3 of portal tracts
Score 3	Deposition of granules in many hepatocytes in >2/3 of portal tracts

TABLE 2.—Staging by Summing for Scores of Three and Two Items

	Sum of score	
Stage	3 items	2 items
Stage 1 (no progression)	0	0
Stage 2 (mild progression)	1−3	1−2
Stage 3 (moderate progression)	4−6	3−4
Stage 4 (advanced progression)	7−9	5−6

Three items; fibrosis, bile duct loss and deposition of copper granules on orcein-positive granules. Two items; fibrosis and bile duct loss.

development of chronic cholestasis. Simultaneously, necro-inflammatory activities of the hepatic parenchyma and limiting plates of milder form develop not infrequently. Eventually, liver fibrosis and cirrhosis develop. A new system applicable to needle liver biopsies in which staging is evaluated using a combination of three factors (fibrosis, cholestasis, and bile duct loss) and necro-inflammatory activities of the bile duct and hepatic parenchyma are graded, is proposed. The clinical and therapeutic evaluation of PBC using this system is warranted (Tables 1-3).

▶ Although widely used in clinical practice, traditional grading and staging systems were initially developed for the assessment of chronic hepatitis, and, therefore, the terminology and features are geared to histologic changes of chronic hepatitis, including viral hepatitis and autoimmune hepatitis. The lack of a system tailored to the specific histologic findings seen in steatohepatitis led to the introduction of the nonalcoholic fatty liver disease activity score and the Brunt fibrosis staging system for steatohepatitis. The benefits of a specific system led to more precise classification of disease and more standardization of reporting, both important aspects for pathologists. The biliary system proposed by Nakanuma

TABLE 3.—Grading of Activities of Cholangitis and Hepatitis of Primary Biliary Cirrhosis

A. Activities of cholangitis (CA)

CA 0 (no activities)	No cholangitis, but mild duct epithelial damage may be present
CA 1 (mild activities)	One evident chronic cholangitis in the specimen, with or without other duct injuries in less than 1/3 of portal tracts or fibrous septa
CA 2 (moderate activities)	Chronic cholangitis in between CA1 and CA3
CA 3 (marked activities)	At least one CNSDC in the specimen, with or without other duct injuries in 2/3 of portal tracts of fibrous septa

B. Activities of hepatitis (HA)

HA 0 (no activities)	No interface hepatitis, and no or minimum lobular hepatitis
HA 1 (mild activities)	Interface hepatitis affecting 10 continuous hepatocytes in less than 1/3 of portal tracts, and mild to moderate lobular hepatitis
HA 2 (moderate activities)	Interface hepatitis affecting 10 continuous hepatocytes in more than 2/3 of portal tracts, and mild to moderate lobular hepatitis
HA 3 (marked activities)	Interface hepatitis affecting 20 continuous hepatocytes in over half portal tracts, and moderate lobular hepatitis, or bridging or zonal necrosis

CNSDC: chronic non suppurative destructive cholangitis.

follows in a similar fashion by incorporating changes specific to primary biliary cirrhosis (PBC). The activity of PBC (Table 3) takes into account both cholangitis lesions and the activity of hepatitis. The staging system involves fibrosis, bile duct loss, and periportal copper deposition (Tables 1 and 2). Because of the fundamental differences in pathophysiology, different disease processes need specific grading systems. This system should be evaluated prospectively clinically and would be a strong foundation for clinical research in PBC.

For further reading on the proposed staging system, I recommend the article by Nakanuma et al.[1]

M. L. Smith, MD

Reference

1. Nakanuma Y, Zen Y, Harada K, Sasaki M, Nonomura A, Uehara T, et al. Application of a new histological staging and grading system for primary biliary cirrhosis to liver biopsy specimens: interobserver agreement. *Pathol Int.* 2010; 60:167-174.

Hepatic granulomas: A clinicopathologic analysis of 86 cases

Turhan N, Kurt M, Ozderin YO, et al (Turkiye Yuksek Ihtisas Teaching and Res Hosp, Ankara, Turkey; et al)
Pathol Res Pract 207:359-365, 2011

The aim of this study was to determine the prevalence and histopathological characteristics of hepatic granulomas.

All records of liver biopsies/resections evaluated in our pathology department between 2002 and 2009 were retrospectively reviewed. Specimens with hepatic granulomas were reexamined by a designated pathologist. Type and localization of granulomas, size of granulomas and epithelioid histiocytes, and the morphological findings of surrounding liver tissue were recorded in an attempt to establish a correlation with relevant clinical, laboratory and radiological findings.

Out of 1420 liver biopsy/resected specimens evaluated at our institution during the study period, 86 cases of epithelioid cell granulomas (6.05%) were observed. Of the 86 cases, 23 were men and 63 were women. The most common underlying etiology was PBC in 38 patients, infections in 34, malignancies in five, sarcoidosis in four, and foreign bodies in three patients. One case (1.2%) of a drug-induced hepatic granuloma was encountered, while another case was deemed idiopathic (of unknown etiology). Contrary to common belief, granulomas were observed not only in early stage PBC but also in cases with stage 3 disease. Out of all the PBC cases with granulomas, 55.6% had stage 3 disease, and besides periductal granulomas, intraacinar granulomas were also seen. For sarcoidosis, intra- and peri-granulomatous fibrosis was observed in as many as 75% of cases. A large majority of granulomas (82.4%) associated with infections were of the necrotizing type.

Extensive evaluation of the morphological characteristics of hepatic granulomas and surrounding liver tissue along with clinical, radiological, and other laboratory findings may help arrive at an accurate diagnosis in a majority of cases. Rather than being a final diagnosis, the presence of hepatic granulomas entails the need for further investigations towards identifying the underlying etiology, with a pathologist being at the center of the diagnostic process.

▶ Hepatic granulomas can be a frustrating finding for a pathologist in that it may be difficult to establish a definitive diagnosis that will be helpful to the clinical team. This article offers some interesting observations from a retrospective review. One important finding was the presence of granulomas in the liver parenchyma in cases of primary biliary cirrhosis (PBC). This is in contrast to current concepts and suggests PBC should be included in the differential diagnosis in any cases of hepatic granulomas, either portal or lobular based. I was surprised to see how few cases were drug induced or idiopathic. In my practice, these categories seem to be the most frequent. Perhaps the retrospective nature of these case reviews allowed the investigators the follow-up time needed to establish a more definitive diagnosis in the majority of cases. Granulomas with necrosis should be assumed to be infectious until proven otherwise. Weaknesses of this article include selection bias and review bias because all cases were from the same institution and were retrospectively reviewed by a single pathologist.

M. L. Smith, MD

Autoimmune Pancreatitis (AIP) Type 1 and Type 2: An International Consensus Study on Histopathologic Diagnostic Criteria

Zhang L, Chari S, Smyrk TC, et al (Mayo Clinic, Rochester, MN; et al)
Pancreas 40:1172-1179, 2011

Objectives.—To develop and validate histologic diagnostic criteria for autoimmune pancreatitis (AIP) and its types.

Methods.—Thirteen pathologists participated in this 2-phase study to develop diagnostic criteria for AIP types 1 and 2 (phase 1) and validate them (phase 2). A virtual library of 40 resected pancreata with AIP and other forms of chronic pancreatitis (CP) was constructed. Readers reviewed the slides online and filled out a questionnaire for histopathologic findings and diagnosis.

Results.—Diagnostic criteria for AIP and its types were proposed according to the results from the top 5 reviewers in phase 1. The interobserver agreement was significantly improved in phase 2 by applying the proposed diagnostic criteria. Features distinguishing AIP from alcoholic and obstructive forms of CP were periductal lymphoplasmacytic infiltrate, inflamed cellular stroma with storiform fibrosis, obliterative phlebitis, and granulocytic epithelial lesions. Although there was overlap, 2 types of AIP were recognized. Type 1 had dense lymphoplasmacytic infiltrate with storiform fibrosis and obliterative phlebitis, whereas type 2 was distinguished from type 1 by the presence of granulocytic epithelial lesions.

Conclusions.—Autoimmune pancreatitis can be distinguished from other forms of CP with substantial interobserver agreement. The 2 types of AIP can be distinguished by the proposed consensus histopathologic diagnostic criteria (Table 4).

▶ This is an excellent article that provides a data-driven consensus opinion on the diagnostic criteria and terminology for autoimmune pancreatitis. Over the last decade, several articles have described 2 unique forms of autoimmune pancreatitis (AIP) with different clinical and histologic features. One of the difficulties in this area has been the use of a variety of diagnostic terms for

TABLE 4.—Diagnostic Pathologic Features of Type 1 and Type 2 AIP

	Pathologic Features	Type 1	Type 2
Common features of AIP	Periductal lymphoplasmacytic infiltrate	Yes	Yes
	Inflammatory cellular stroma	Yes	Yes
Diagnostic features of AIP type 1	Storiform fibrosis	Prominent	Occasional
	Obliterative phlebitis	Yes	Occasional
	Lymphoid follicles	Prominent	Occasional
	IgG4+ plasma cell infiltration*	Marked	Less prominent
Diagnostic features of AIP type 2	GEL	No	Yes
	Acinar neutrophilic infiltrate	No	Very common

*IgG4 immunostain was not included in this study. This criterion was proposed based on the literature and agreement among all reviewers.

the different patterns of AIP. This is an important addition because it can serve to standardize the reporting of AIP and facilitate future collections of cases for study. Among pathologists with gastroenterology expertise, the use of the consensus diagnostic features improved the interobserver agreement. Table 4 outlines the important diagnostic features of AIP, AIP type 1, and AIP type 2. It is worth highlighting that this study was done on resected pancreata rather than needle core biopsies. The use of resected specimens, small study size (both number of pathologists and number of cases), and use of pathologists with gastroenterology expertise raise questions about the applicability of the criteria in the hands of general surgical pathologists on needle core biopsy specimens. Nevertheless, the criteria give a standardized framework for future studies.

M. L. Smith, MD

The Concept of Hepatic Artery-Bile Duct Parallelism in the Diagnosis of Ductopenia in Liver Biopsy Samples

Moreira RK, Chopp W, Washington MK (Columbia Univ College of Physicians and Surgeons, NY; Vanderbilt Univ, Nashville, TN)
Am J Surg Pathol 35:392-403, 2011

Absence of bile ducts (BDs) in > 50% of portal tracts is currently the most widely accepted criterion for the diagnosis of ductopenia. In this study, we describe an alternative method for the quantitative assessment of BDs based on the percentage of portal tracts containing unpaired hepatic arteries (HAs). Diagnostic criteria for ductopenia were defined as follows: 1. presence of at least 1 unpaired HA in > 10% of all portal tracts; 2. at least 2 unpaired HAs present in different portal tracts in a given sample. In liver biopsies from patients with primary biliary cirrhosis and suspected chronic allograft rejection (n = 32), loss of BD was detected in 59.4% of patients using the unpaired HA method compared with 43.7% ($P = 0.31$), 21.9% ($P = 0.005$), and 12.5% ($P = 0.001$) by the traditional method, depending on specific adequacy criteria used (no adequacy criteria, > 10 portal tracts, or > 5 complete portal tracts per biopsy, respectively). The percentage of portal tracts containing BD(s) was significantly affected by the degree of portal inflammation, fibrosis stage, percentage of complete portal tracts, and biopsy width, whereas none of these factors influenced the prevalence of unpaired arteries. The unpaired HA method showed higher sensitivity for the detection of mild degrees of loss of BD compared with the traditional method, and was not influenced by factors that affected the percentage of portal tracts containing BDs (Table 5).

▶ Over the years, radiologists are increasingly performing liver biopsies using smaller-gauge needles and often via a transjugular route. This often results in thinner needle core biopsies of hepatic tissue for histologic evaluation. Most of the time, this does not pose a significant problem. However, ductopenia is classically defined as a portal tract without a bile duct in more than 50% of

TABLE 5.—Proposed Diagnostic Criteria for Ductopenia in Liver Needle Biopsy Samples

(1) Unpaired HA present in at least 10% of portal tracts
(2) At least 2 unpaired hepatic arteries present (in different portal tracts) in a given sample, regardless of
the total number of portal tracts

*A hepatic artery branch of any size within a complete portal tract not accompanied by a bile duct; or, in an incomplete portal tract, a hepatic artery branch measuring >20 μm with no bile duct present within a radius of 10 hepatic artery diameters.

portal areas. In thin-needle core biopsy specimens, many portal tracts may be incomplete, making it more difficult to establish a diagnosis of ductopenia with certainty. This interesting study provides a morphologic baseline for the hepatic artery-bile duct microscopic anatomy and suggests other criteria for the diagnosis of ductopenia (Table 5). The concept relies on an unpaired hepatic artery rather than a ductless portal tract. The proposed criteria make the diagnosis of ductopenia more frequent with the use of less-stringent definitions. This study broadens the radius in which to look for a bile duct from 3 to 10 hepatic artery diameters based on morphometry data of normal liver specimens. Deficiencies of the study include the use of only 10 normal liver specimens for the establishment of baseline morphometric data and a relatively small number of nonductopenic cases subject to analysis (n = 30). Nevertheless, these data are intriguing and should be investigated further with correlations to laboratory testing and outcomes.

M. L. Smith, MD

Histologic characteristics of pancreatic intraepithelial neoplasia associated with different pancreatic lesions
Recavarren C, Labow DM, Liang J, et al (The Mount Sinai Med Ctr, NY; Penn State Hershey Med Ctr, PA; et al)
Hum Pathol 42:18-24, 2011

Pancreatic intraepithelial neoplasia (PanIN) has been found in association with pancreatic ductal adenocarcinoma, intraductal papillary-mucinous neoplasm (IPMN), mucinous cystic neoplasm, and other pancreatic lesions, but the characteristics of PanINs associated with these lesions are not well characterized. In this study, 185 partial or total pancreatectomy specimens were collected, and 173 had complete slides for review, which included 74 pancreatic ductal adenocarcinomas, 28 IPMNs, 7 mucinous cystic neoplasms, 44 other nonductal tumors, and 20 nontumorous lesions. Differences in grade, extent, and duct involvement among PanINs associated with different lesions were analyzed. Patients with PanINs were older than those without, regardless of associated tumor or lesions. No sex predilection was noted. PanINs were found in 89%, 96%, 86%, 64%, and 55% pancreata with ductal adenocarcinomas, IPMNs, mucinous cystic neoplasm, other nonductal tumors, and nontumorous lesions, respectively. PanIN 1 and 2

TABLE 5.—The Grade of PanINs Differs Among Pancreas With Ductal Tumors, Nonductal Tumors, and Nontumorous Lesions

Positive Cases	PanIN 1 + 2, n (%)	Grade PanIN 3, n (%)	P
PDA (66)	59 (89)	38 (58)	
IPMN (27)	25 (93)	4 (15)	<.05
MCN (6)	6 (100)	0	<.01
NDT (28)	27 (96)	1 (4)	<.01
NTL (11)	10 (91)	1 (9)	<.01

NDT includes neuroendocrine tumors, solid pseudopapillary tumors, serous, ampullary tumors, granular cell tumor, acinar cell carcinoma, metastatic carcinoma. NTL includes chronic pancreatitis, incidental pancreatectomy specimen, and rejected allograft.

were commonly associated with all types of lesions, but high-grade PanIN 3 was more frequently associated with ductal adenocarcinomas. Ductal involvement of PanINs was more extensive in association with ductal adenocarcinomas than in any other types of pancreatic tumors or lesions. PanINs associated with pancreatic ductal adenocarcinomas affected both the main and branched ducts, whereas PanINs associated with other types of pancreatic tumors or lesions were mainly present in the branch ducts. No statistical differences were observed in distribution, extent, and grade of PanINs among IPMNs, mucinous cystic neoplasms, other nonductal tumors, and nontumorous lesions. Our study demonstrated a high concurrence between PanINs and other precancerous lesions and histologic features of PanINs associated with different pancreatic diseases (Table 5).

▶ This retrospective study investigated the prevalence and distribution of pancreatic intraepithelial neoplasia (PanIN) in 173 pancreatectomy specimens. Table 5 highlights an important point with respect to PanIN in that only PanIN 3, which can be conceptualized as high-grade dysplasia or carcinoma in situ, is strongly correlated with pancreatic ductal carcinoma. Strengths of this article are the large number of cases available for review and the broad array of etiologies ranging from invasive ductal carcinoma to noncancerous lesions. The biggest weakness is the retrospective nature of the data collection. I was surprised at the high prevalence of PanIN, not only in neoplastic conditions but also in nonneoplastic conditions. Fifty-five percent of nontumorous lesions showed at least PanIN 1. The retrospective review may have resulted in a bias toward a decreased threshold for PanIN. Based on this high prevalence and lack of correlation with malignancy, one may argue that the presence of PanIN 1 and 2 does not add clinically significant information and should not be reported.

M. L. Smith, MD

5 Dermatopathology

Assessment of Copy Number Status of Chromosomes 6 and 11 by FISH Provides Independent Prognostic Information in Primary Melanoma
North JP, Vetto JT, Murali R, et al (Oregon Health and Science Univ, Portland; et al)
Am J Surg Pathol 35:1146-1150, 2011

Melanoma incidence has been rising steadily for decades, whereas mortality rates have remained flat. This type of discordant pattern between incidence and mortality has been linked to diagnostic drift in cancers of the thyroid, breast, and prostate. Ancillary tests, such as fluorescent in situ hybridization (FISH), are now being used to help differentiate melanomas from melanocytic nevi. Multicolor FISH has been shown to distinguish between these 2 with 86.7% sensitivity and 95.4% specificity. To assess the ability of FISH to differentiate melanomas with metastatic or lethal potential from those with an indolent disease course, we performed FISH with probes targeting 6p25, centromere 6, 6q23, and 11q13 on 144 primary melanomas with a minimal tumor thickness of 2 mm and compared the development of metastatic disease and melanoma-specific mortality as well as relapse-free and disease-specific survival between FISH-positive and FISH-negative cases. Of the melanomas, 82% were positive by FISH according to previously defined criteria. The percentage was significantly higher (93%) in cases that developed systemic metastases (n=43) than in patients that did not (77%, n=101). FISH-positive primaries had a significantly increased risk of metastasis or melanoma-related death compared with FISH-negative cases odds ratio 4.11; confidence interval, 1.14-22.7 and odds ratio 7.0, confidence interval 1.03-300.4, respectively. FISH status remained an independent parameter when controlling for known prognostic factors. These data indicate that the group of melanomas diagnosed with routine histopathology that lack aberrations detected by FISH is enriched for melanomas with a more indolent disease course. This suggests that molecular techniques can assist in a more accurate identification of tumors with metastatic potential.

▶ Fluorescence in situ hybridization (FISH) studies to detect chromosomal abnormalities known to occur in melanoma have been gaining acceptance as an ancillary diagnostic tool. This study uses a panel of 4 previously described FISH probes on a cohort of melanoma lesions. Those patients identified to have a chromosomal abnormality in their tumor by FISH fared worse. Surprisingly, in predicting which lesions would produce a metastasis, the FISH findings were independent of standard contemporary prognostic indicators, including the tumor thickness and sentinel lymph node status. These cases were all unequivocal melanoma cases; as opposed to previous FISH studies, which attempted to separate benign from malignant lesions, this study evaluated a potential role in melanoma patient stratification. These findings also indicate that FISH-negative lesions are less likely to metastasize, indirectly hinting at a role in histologically difficult cases; although, this has been directly addressed by others.[1] The melanomas in the study were all at least 2 mm thick, a feature that collected patients with more serious disease and, accordingly, more patients with subsequent metastases. This approach likely helped to "maximize the number of end points reached," as the authors explain, but does not address the value in thinner melanomas, which account for the large majority of cases.[2] The study had an average follow-up of less than 3 years, leaving open the possibility that the FISH studies identify quickly progressive tumors and not necessarily overall lethality. In addition, the FISH studies fell short of statistical significance for independently predicating disease-specific survival.

J. Wisell, MD

References

1. Vergier B, Prochazkova-Carlotti M, de la Fouchardière A, et al. Fluorescence in situ hybridization, a diagnostic aid in ambiguous melanocytic tumors: European study of 113 cases. *Mod Pathol.* 2011;24:613-623.
2. Criscione VD, Weinstock MA. Melanoma thickness trends in the United States, 1988-2006. *J Invest Dermatol.* 2010;130:793-797.

Fluorescence *in situ* hybridization, a diagnostic aid in ambiguous melanocytic tumors: European study of 113 cases
Vergier B, Prochazkova-Carlotti M, de la Fouchardière A, et al (CHU Bordeaux-Université Victor Segalen Bordeaux 2, France; Centre Léon Bérard (CLCC), Lyon, France; et al)
Mod Pathol 24:613-623, 2011

Some melanocytic tumors are ambiguous, so the reproducible histopathological diagnosis of benign or malignant lesion is difficult. This study evaluated the contribution of fluorescence *in situ* hybridization (FISH) first in 43 non-equivocal melanomas and nevi, and then in 113 ambiguous melanocytic tumors selected by expert pathologists from six different European institutions. We included two groups of ambiguous tumors: patients without recurrence (5-year minimal follow-up) and with metastases. An independent triple-blind histopathological review was performed to classify tumors as 'favor benign' (A−) or 'favor malignant' (A+). A four-color probe set targeting 6p25, 6q23, 11q13 and CEP6 was used for FISH. In the 43 non-equivocal melanomas and nevi, sensitivity was 85% and specificity 90%. Ninety out of 95 ambiguous melanocytic tumors included were FISH interpretable (67 FISH negative and 23 FISH positive). Of the 90 patients, 69 presented no recurrence and 21/90 exhibited metastases. These ambiguous tumors were mostly spitzoid tumors (45/90). Histopathological reviewers classified these tumors as favor malignant (49/90) and favor benign (32/90), whereas nine cases had a discordant diagnosis. By comparison with outcome, the sensitivity and specificity of histopathological review were 95 and 52%, and the sensitivity and specificity of FISH were 43 and 80%. Compared with histopathological review, the sensitivity and specificity of FISH were 34.5 and 91%. Interestingly, by combining the histopathological diagnosis with FISH results, the diagnosis was optimized, especially by increasing specificity (76% instead of 52% for expert diagnosis alone) and by improving sensitivity compared with FISH alone (90 *vs* 43% for FISH result alone). The value of this FISH test is to add a reproducible demonstration of malignancy to the histopathological diagnosis, especially in doubtful/ambiguous melanocytic tumors. A positive FISH test reinforces the diagnosis of melanoma, allowing such tumors (particularly thick tumors) to be managed as melanomas.

▶ This report adds to the growing interest in using fluorescence in situ hybridization (FISH) studies to help differentiate benign from malignant melanocytic lesions. Three chromosomal targets at 6p25, 6p23, and 11q13 have received the most attention. Some of the previous studies utilizing probes for these loci have performed quite well, with some studies achieving sensitivities and specificities of 90% and higher.[1] This latter study and similar larger series, however, have used unequivocal cases of nevi, primary melanoma, and metastatic melanoma to evaluate the performance of FISH testing. If a pathologist firmly believes that a case represents melanoma, there is little utility for an additional diagnostic test, even one with high sensitivity and specificity. While cases that have confidently been signed out as benign in time have proven erroneous, no test has yet proven to be more valuable than histopathology for the diagnosis of melanocytic lesions, and it is not practical to subject every benign histopathologic diagnosis to an additional test. It is for the difficult cases that pathologists have been asking for help. This current study evaluates the performance of FISH studies on cases that were more likely to have been signed out with tentative diagnoses, the "ambiguous melanocytic tumors." This series included many of the perennially challenging "Spitzoid" lesions, which comprised half of the ambiguous tumors. The performance characteristics of the FISH studies as a solitary test compared with patient outcome in this large collection of ambiguous tumors are much less impressive (sensitivity of 43% and specificity of 80%) than in the studies with confidently classified cases. It is important to remember that this is the subset of cases in which any increase in our ability to accurately classify lesions as benign or malignant would be welcome. Indeed, the authors note modest overall improvement in the ability to classify melanomas when the FISH studies and the histologic diagnosis are combined, but concede that multivariate analysis found only the "expert diagnoses" correlated with the presence of metastases. Another smaller, but similar study found better performance in a group of difficult melanocytic lesions, demonstrating a degree of variability in using FISH studies.[2] Several variables could be proposed to explain this difference, not the least of which being the inherently subjective practice of deciding what constitutes a difficult case. Nevertheless, both of these reports do indicate a limited role for the use of these FISH probes in the diagnosis of melanoma, but more importantly demonstrate that molecular-based testing is likely to continue to improve our ability to comfortably classify melanocytic lesions.

J. Wisell, MD

References

1. Morey AL, Murali R, McCarthy SW, Mann GJ, Scolyer RA. Diagnosis of cutaneous melanocytic tumours by four-colour fluorescence in situ hybridisation. *Pathology.* 2009;41:383-387.
2. Gerami P, Jewell SS, Morrison LE, et al. Fluorescence in situ hybridization (FISH) as an ancillary diagnostic tool in the diagnosis of melanoma. *Am J Surg Pathol.* 2009;33:1146-1156.

Atypical Intradermal Smooth Muscle Neoplasms: Clinicopathologic Analysis of 84 Cases and a Reappraisal of Cutaneous "Leiomyosarcoma"
Kraft S, Fletcher CDM (Brigham and Women's Hosp, Boston, MA)
Am J Surg Pathol 35:599-607, 2011

Atypical or mitotically active dermal smooth muscle neoplasms are uncommon lesions, which are most often termed "cutaneous leiomyosarcoma," although preexisting—mostly small—series suggest a low risk of aggressive behavior. To further investigate these tumors, 84 cases from consultation and institutional files were analyzed for pathologic and clinical characteristics. There was a striking male-to-female preponderance (4.3:1), with a mean age of 56 years (range, 6 to 82y). Nine patients had a history of malignancies (6 of the skin). Tumors measured 1.3 cm on average and were predominantly located on the trunk (32) and lower extremities (30). Histologically, all tumors were confined to the dermis or showed only very superficial, focal subcutaneous extension. The majority showed an infiltrative growth pattern with fascicles of atypical eosinophilic spindle cells ramifying between dermal collagen fibers. Primary tumors showed a mean mitotic rate of 4.7/10 high-power fields. By the Fédération Nationale des Centres de Lutte Contre le Cancer grading system, 97% of primary tumors were grade I lesions, with only 3% showing necrosis. All tumors were immunopositive for smooth muscle actin; 98% expressed desmin, 90% caldesmon, and 45% pankeratin (usually focal). Follow-up in 52 cases (mean, 51 mo) showed no metastases or tumor-related deaths. Eighteen tumors showed local recurrence at a mean interval of 43 months; 12 of the recurrent lesions showed positive margins in the primary excision and 1 showed margins <0.2 cm. Margin status was not available for the other 5 cases, which recurred locally. Recurrent tumors showed, on average, 13.7 mitoses/10 high-power fields. Of recurrences, 47% were grade I lesions, 35% were grade II, and 18% were grade III, and 28% showed necrosis. The primary excision of tumors, which later recurred, showed no difference in grade, presence of necrosis, or mitotic rate, compared with those that did not recur; there were no discernible clinical differences either. In summary, these tumors, when confined to the dermis or showing only minimal subcutaneous involvement, seem to carry no evident risk of metastasis; hence, the designation "sarcoma" is inappropriate. Margin status is the most important predictor of recurrence. On excision with clear margins, the risk of local recurrence is very low. Hence, we propose the term "atypical intradermal smooth muscle neoplasm" as being more appropriate.

▶ Leiomyosarcomas occurring in superficial tissues are uncommon lesions. Previously reported series of these tumors have included both cutaneous and subcutaneous lesions. This current series focuses solely on tumors based in the dermis, but includes lesions with extension into the subcutis. This is an important distinction, as tumors arising within the subcutis may have a different pathogenesis and behave more aggressively. The authors of this study found that these dermal-based tumors had a nonaggressive course. All of the lesions that initially recurred had positive margins, and once the recurrent tumors had been completely excised, no further recurrences were documented. None of the tumors in this series were associated with metastases, though, a similar series from 2010[1] showed that one such tumor with subcutaneous extension metastasized 15 years after the initial excision, indicating that metastatic potential may still exist. In this latter study, none of the tumors confined to the dermis showed evidence of metastasis. Given this less-aggressive pattern of progression, the authors of the more recent study avoid the designation of "sarcoma," instead preferring to classify these lesions as "atypical intradermal smooth muscle neoplasms." While not everyone may concur with this nosologic dissent, it is becoming clear that these lesions should be separated from their subcutaneous and deep soft tissue counterparts.

J. Wisell, MD

Reference

1. Massi D, Franchi A, Alos L, et al. Primary cutaneous leiomyosarcoma: clinicopathological analysis of 36 cases. *Histopathology.* 2010;56:251-262.

Sebaceous Carcinoma: An Immunohistochemical Reappraisal
Ansai S-I, Takeichi H, Arase S, et al (Nippon Med School, Tokyo, Japan; Univ of Tokushima Graduate School, Japan; et al)
Am J Dermatopathol 33:579-587, 2011

The rates of distant metastases and tumor death in sebaceous carcinoma (SC) have been reported to be higher than those of other cutaneous carcinomas, such as squamous cell carcinoma (SCC) and basal cell carcinoma (BCC), regardless of whether they occur in ocular or extraocular regions. Therefore, strict differentiation of SC from SCC and BCC is required. In this article, we report immunohistochemical findings of SC and compare these data to those of SCC, BCC, and sebaceoma. An immunohistochemical study was performed using 7 antibodies [anti-carcinoembryonic antigen (CEA), anti-epithelial membrane antigen (EMA), anti–CA15-3, anti–CA19-9, anti–androgen receptor (AR), anti-epithelial antigen (Ber-EP4), and anti-adipophilin (ADP)] on 35 cases of SC (16 cases in ocular and 19 cases in extraocular regions) and 10 cases of each SCC (5 cases in ocular and 5 cases in extraocular regions), BCC (5 cases in ocular and 5 cases in extraocular regions), and sebaceoma (no cases arose on the eyelids). In summary, the typical immunophenotypes of SC were EMA+, CA15-3+, AR+, Ber-EP4−, and ADP+; those of sebaceoma were CEA−, EMA+, Ber-EP4−, and ADP+; those of SCC were CEA−, EMA+, CA19-9−, AR−, Ber-EP4−, and ADP−; and those of BCC were CEA−, EMA−, CA15-3−, Ber-EP4+, and ADP−. Other antibody tests for each neoplasm were positive in about half of the cases. The detection of AR and ADP was useful for differentiating SC from SCC, whereas the determination of EMA, CA15-3, Ber-EP4, and ADP was valuable in differentiating SC from BCC.

▶ Sebaceous carcinoma (SC) has been regarded by some as "high-risk" epithelial tumors in an effort to set them apart from the much more common and usually less aggressive basal cell (BCC) and squamous cell (SCC) carcinomas. Although posing significant differences in behavior from these latter tumors, the rare SC has long been known to histologically mimic its more common superficial epithelial counterparts[1] posing a potential hazard for pathologists. The cagey histopathologist, when faced with an SC, may realize that he or she is not dealing with a mundane BCC or SCC but may find a variety of other uncommon tumors have also entered the differential diagnosis, including balloon cell melanoma and other adnexal tumors. Enter the role of immunohistochemical (IHC) studies that have been used to help confirm or refute the occasionally tricky diagnosis of SC. This current report details the behavior of 7 of the antibodies purported to indicate sebaceous differentiation in 65 tumors, with more than half being SC. The most promising single marker put forth by this investigation is adipophilin, a protein involved in adipocyte fatty acid uptake. Antibodies to this protein labeled nearly all SCs, no BCCs, and a single SCC (out of 10). Other markers were shown to be useful in either BCCs or SCCs within this group of tumors, but not in both. As with most forays into an IHC evaluation of an individual case, having a panel is helpful. This panel approach has been particularly valid for evaluating sebaceous neoplasia because no single marker has stood out as diagnostic. The approach taken by the authors of this study has added utility compared with more limited studies because they performed the entire 7-marker panel on each case, allowing for direct comparison of the markers in this set of tumors. This lessens the degree of indirect comparisons often made across different studies, with different patients in different laboratories.

J. Wisell, MD

Reference

1. Doxanas MT, Green WR. Sebaceous gland carcinoma. Review of 40 cases. *Arch Ophthalmol.* 1984;102:245-249.

A two-antibody mismatch repair protein immunohistochemistry screening approach for colorectal carcinomas, skin sebaceous tumors, and gynecologic tract carcinomas
Mojtahed A, Schrijver I, Ford JM, et al (Stanford Univ, CA)
Mod Pathol 24:1004-1014, 2011

Mismatch repair protein immunohistochemistry is a widely used method for detecting patients at risk for Lynch syndrome. Recent data suggest that a two-antibody panel approach using PMS2 and MSH6 is an effective screening protocol for colorectal carcinoma, but there are limited data concerning this approach for extraintestinal tumors. The purpose of this study was to review the utility of a two-antibody panel approach in colorectal carcinoma and extraintestinal tumors. We evaluated mismatch repair protein expression in two cohorts: (1) a retrospective analysis of intestinal and extraintestinal tumors ($n = 334$) tested for mismatch repair protein immunohistochemistry and (2) a prospectively accrued series of intestinal, gynecologic tract, and skin sebaceous neoplasms ($n = 98$). A total of 432 cases were analyzed, including 323 colorectal, 50 gynecologic tract, 49 skin sebaceous, and 10 other neoplasms. Overall, 102/432 tumors (24%) demonstrated loss of at least one mismatch repair protein. Concurrent loss of MLH1 and PMS2 was the most common pattern of abnormal expression (50/432, 12%) followed by concurrent loss of MSH2 and MSH6 (33/432, 8%). Of 55 cases with abnormal PMS2 expression, 5 (9%) demonstrated isolated loss of PMS2 expression. Of 47 cases with abnormal MSH6 expression, 14 (30%) demonstrated isolated loss of MSH6 expression. Isolated loss of MLH1 or MSH2 was not observed. Colorectal carcinomas more frequently demonstrated abnormal expression of PMS2 (39/59, 66%). Skin sebaceous neoplasms more frequently demonstrated abnormal expression of MSH6 (18/24, 75%, respectively). A total of 65 tumors with abnormal mismatch repair protein expression were tested for microsatellite instability (MSI): 47 (72%) MSI high, 9 (14%) MSI low, and 9 (14%) microsatellite stable (MSS). Abnormal MSH6 expression accounted for 14/18 (78%) cases that were MSS or MSI low. Our findings confirm the utility of a two-antibody approach using PMS2 and MSH6 in colorectal carcinoma and indicate that this approach is effective in extraintestinal neoplasms associated with Lynch syndrome.

▶ Hereditary deficits in mismatch repair (MMR) proteins are responsible for hereditary nonpolyposis colorectal cancer (Lynch) syndrome and the variant syndrome Muir-Torre, which may have cutaneous sebaceous tumors. Two now frequently used methods of identifying high-risk patients with these conditions include immunohistochemical (IHC) detection for loss of expression of commonly affected MMR proteins and microsatellite instability (MSI) testing. Both methods may miss some patients. IHC studies may miss lesser-known MMR proteins nonfunctional proteins that retain antigenicity, and MSI testing may miss cases where low levels of microsatellite instability are produced. Nevertheless, the increasing quality of IHC studies and their widespread availability have prompted many groups to screen for patients with this method. The study includes a relatively large series (49) of sebaceous neoplasms, a distinctive feature for Muir-Torre syndrome. The increased rate of MMR protein abnormality in men and a trunk/extremity location that has been reported previously is confirmed by this series. Many patients presenting with a sebaceous neoplasm included in the series were discovered to have MMR abnormalities, thus demonstrating the value of screening at least some (if not all) patients with a sebaceous neoplasm. In the preselected group of patients determined to be at higher risk for MMR abnormalities, 55% were found to have a deficit in at least 1 protein. The larger finding of the study, IHC for 2 of the proteins (PMS2, MSH6) is as adequate as IHC for all 4 (including MLH1, MSH2) of the MMR proteins in patients with extracolonic tumors, added significant support for this 2-marker approach. IHC studies are complex tests, and some have noted the occasional technical difficulty in performing this test. The authors discovered a difficulty with PMS2 in the retrospective portion of their study, and several observers have noted MSH6 to be particularly fickle. Thus, if this more efficient 2-maker panel is preferred, when loss of MMR expression is detected or equivocal, the authors' advice to perform IHC studies for the other markers is prudent to support the diagnosis; this is also worthwhile for identification of the specific protein involved. MSI testing could also be used as another means for supporting IHC results and should be considered for further screening of patients strongly suspected to harbor an MMR protein mutation, even in the face of negative IHC studies.

J. Wisell, MD

Mitotic Activity Within Dermal Melanocytes of Benign Melanocytic Nevi: A Study of 100 Cases With Clinical Follow-up
Ruhoy SM, Kolker SE, Murry TC (Virginia Mason Med Ctr, Seattle, WA; Providence Portland Med Ctr, OR; Laboratory Medicine Consultants, Las Vegas, NV)
Am J Dermatopathol 33:167-172, 2011

It is generally accepted that otherwise benign intradermal or compound melanocytic nevi may show mitotic activity within dermal melanocytes. However, it is not known whether there is any clinical significance to this finding. Our objective is to analyze and describe the clinicopathologic features of benign nevi with mitotic activity (NMA). To do this, we collected 100 consecutive NMA during the usual course of business in our private dermatopathology practice. These cases were seen between the years 2000 and 2008. We then collected clinical and pathologic data on these cases and compared the findings with 100 control nevi without mitotic activity (CN). We compared these nevi with regard to demographic features, clinical history provided by clinician, and clinical follow-up, as well as anatomic site and season of biopsy, type of nevus, and selected histologic features (ie, trauma). We also estimate the incidence of NMA and describe the amount and location of mitotic figures within the NMA. Our results indicate that the incidence of NMA is 0.91%. Most (80) NMA revealed only one mitotic figure, whereas some (20) NMA revealed more than one mitotic figure. Most NMA (89) showed mitotic activity in the upper portion of the nevus, whereas some (11) showed mitotic activity in the lower portion of the nevus. NMA patients were of younger age than the CN patients ($P = 0.0019$). Compared with CN, the NMA were more likely to be from the extremities ($P = 0.0113$) or head and neck ($P = 0.0237$) and less likely to be from the trunk ($P < 0.001$). The NMA were also more likely to show histologic features suggesting a congenital onset ($P < 0.001$) and were more likely to be Spitz nevi ($P = 0.0185$). Compared with the CN, the NMA were more often reexcised ($P = 0.0073$) and more often, there was residual nevus in the reexcision specimen ($P = 0.13$), although the latter finding was not statistically significant. Anecdotally, 2 of our NMA were identified adjacent to invasive melanomas; however, on clinical follow-up, we were unable to detect any increased incidence of melanoma.

▶ Mitotic figures have long been considered an important discriminator between benign and malignant melanocytic lesions. However, as is known by those of us involved in the daily histopathologic diagnosis of skin lesions, mitoses—like virtually all histopathologic features when taken in isolation—are far from being a solitary indicator for melanoma. Melanocytic mitotic figures have been examined in the literature, particularly in regard to their prognostic significance when discovered in melanoma. They have also been detailed in benign lesions, including their presence in Spitz nevi, blue nevi, and during pregnancy. This study, along with at least 3 other recent reports,[1-3] sought to clearly define the presence, features, and associations of mitoses in otherwise banal nevi. This most recent study has also added clinical follow-up information. Younger patients, head and neck or extremities, congenital histologic features, and Spitz nevi were all more likely to be associated with mitotic activity. This confirms some of the findings from the series published in 2010,[1] including the tendency toward younger patients and Spitz nevi to have mitoses. In contrast, the earlier study did not find evidence of congenital nevi to be more often mitotically active. The 2010 study also found signs of traumatization to correlate significantly with mitotically active lesions, providing evidence for what others had previously suggested.[3] The current study, however, did not corroborate this finding, instead finding equal numbers of traumatized and nontraumatized nevi with mitoses. Interestingly, patients with mitotically active nevi were much more likely to have the lesion reexcised than those in the control group, suggesting that the report of an occasional mitotic figure may have resulted in treatment differences. Although not generating as much interest as mitotic figures in malignant melanocytic lesions, this report adds to understanding of proliferative activity in otherwise benign nevi.

J. Wisell, MD

References

1. Glatz K, Hartmann C, Antic M, Kutzner H. Frequent mitotic activity in banal melanocytic nevi uncovered by immunohistochemical analysis. *Am J Dermatopathol.* 2010;32:643-649.

2. Jensen SL, Radfar A, Bhawan J. Mitoses in conventional melanocytic nevi. *J Cutan Pathol.* 2007;34:713-715.
3. Selim MA, Vollmer RT, Herman CM, Pham TT, Turner JW. Melanocytic nevi with nonsurgical trauma: a histopathologic study. *Am J Dermatopathol.* 2007;29: 134-136.

Proliferative Nodules Arising Within Congenital Melanocytic Nevi: A Histologic, Immunohistochemical, and Molecular Analyses of 43 Cases

Phadke PA, Rakheja D, Le LP, et al (Massachusetts General Hosp and Harvard Med School, Boston; Univ of Texas Southwestern Med Ctr, Dallas; et al)

Am J Surg Pathol 35:656-669, 2011

The histopathologic interpretation of proliferative nodules (PNs) in congenital melanocytic nevi can present significant challenges as some PNs may exhibit atypical features that make the distinction from melanoma difficult. We compared histologic features, Ki-67%, PHH3, and CD117% expression levels by immunohistochemistry in 18 benign and 25 atypical PNs (from 41 patients) with that of background congenital nevi (of these 43 cases), 10 congenital nevi, and 3 dermal melanomas arising in congenital melanocytic lesions. In addition, we evaluated the presence of *BRAF, GNAQ, HRAS, KRAS,* and *NRAS* mutations in all groups using the SNaP-shot Multiplex System. Follow-up was available on 19 patients (9 benign and 10 atypical PNs) (range, 2 to 20 y; median, 8 y) and all were alive with no evidence of disease. The specific histologic features of atypical PNs, such as sharp demarcation ($P < 0.001$), expansile growth ($P < 0.001$), epidermal effacement ($P < 0.001$), nuclear pleomorphism ($P < 0.001$), and increased mitoses ($P < 0.001$), differed significantly from those of benign PNs. Immunohistochemical results showed that Ki-67% and PHH3 scores, but not CD117% expression, were significantly higher ($P < 0.05$) in atypical PNs. Molecular analyses showed that the PNs and background congenital melanocytic nevi of the giant congenital nevi possess more frequent *NRAS* mutations and infrequent *BRAF* mutations when compared with those of the remaining cases. These findings suggest that histologic features and Ki-67 and PHH3 expression levels are the strongest parameters to distinguish between benign versus atypical PNs. The immunohistochemical results suggest that atypical PNs are distinct borderline lesions residing between benign PNs and dermal melanomas. Although numerous mutations are detected in the samples, the diagnostic use of molecular analysis in this regard is limited.

▶ Congenital melanocytic nevi (CMN) are a common lesion, present in more than 1% of the population in some series. Rarely a nodule is found developing within a CMN, and some have classified these nodular proliferations into presumably entirely benign nodules, characterized by only rare mitoses and poor demarcation from the background lesion, and a more worrisome nodule with increased proliferation and sharp surrounding delineation. Because CMN have an overall associated risk for the development of melanoma that correlates with increasing size, these more worrisome nodular proliferations pose a troublesome, although uncommon, diagnostic challenge for pathologists. Despite this difficulty, this area has only been lightly addressed, with a handful of previously published reports that include outcome information. This current series provides a relatively large number of cases and includes both contemporary methods and some clinical follow-up. Proliferative nodules are divided into atypical and nonatypical varieties. They found that use of immunohistochemical proliferative markers similarly stratifies these lesions into 2 groups, adding support for the histologic classification of proliferative nodules. They found no clear association with any of the currently popular melanoma-associated genetic mutations, but they did develop further this nascent body of knowledge for the genetic basis of proliferative nodules, atypical and otherwise. The true significance of atypical features in proliferative nodules remains unclear, but the proliferative rate more similar to 3 patients with dermal melanoma suggests that these features should not be overlooked, for both clinical reasons and the opportunity to further understand the pathogenesis of melanocytic neoplasia.

J. Wisell, MD

Poikilodermatous mycosis fungoides: A study of its clinicopathological, immunophenotypic, and prognostic features

Abbott RA, Sahni D, Robson A, et al (Guy's and St Thomas' Natl Health Service Foundation Trust, London, UK)
J Am Acad Dermatol 65:313-319, 2011

Background.—Poikilodermatous mycosis fungoides (MF) is a variant of MF, and its clinicopathological, immunophenotypic, molecular, and prognostic features have not previously been defined in the literature.

Objective.—The purpose of this study was to improve the data available for this variant of MF thus enabling clinicians to apply the appropriate treatment and follow-up.

Methods.—In a retrospective single center study we evaluated the clinical, histopathological, immunohistochemical, and molecular characteristics of patients with predominant (>50%) poikilodermatous lesions of MF.

Results.—In all, 49 patients were identified. The median age at diagnosis was 44 years (15-81 years). Of 49 patients, 43 (88%) had early stage disease (≤ IIA) at diagnosis. No patients had stage IV disease at presentation. A frequent association was coexistence of lymphomatoid papulosis (9/49; 18%). Histopathology review showed a high number of cases with CD8$^+$ CD4$^-$ atypical lymphocytes (38%). After diagnosis most patients were treated with expectant or skin-directed therapy. Psoralen plus ultraviolet A therapy was most frequently used and had high response rates (83%). Five (10%) of 49 received systemic therapy. The mean follow-up was 11 years, 10 months (1->40 years). In all, 47 (96%) of 49 patients had stable disease and two (4%) of 49 had progressive disease. No patients died during follow-up.

Limitations.—As a tertiary center our patient cohort may be expected to have more advanced and aggressive disease.

Conclusion.—Poikilodermatous MF represents a distinct clinicopathological entity from classic patch/plaque MF. It presents at a younger age and is more frequently associated with lymphomatoid papulosis. There is an increased number of cases with predominantly CD8$^+$ CD4$^-$ atypical lymphocytes. Overall there is a good response to phototherapy and the overall prognosis appears favorable.

▶ The 2005 World Health Organization/European Organization for Research and Treatment of Cancer (WHO/EORTC) classification of cutaneous lymphomas recognizes lists 2 subtypes of mycoses fungoides (MF), pagetoid reticulosis and folliculotropic MF, and 1 variant, granulomatous slack skin.[1] However, a much larger number (> 30) of clinicopathologic variants have been offered in the literature.[2] In a clarifying action, the WHO/EORTC only included those types they believed to have clinical behavior distinct from the classical (Alibert-Bazin) type of MF. Yet the myriad descriptions and characterizations of the various forms and presentations of MF related in the literature serves to convey the occasional difficulty in establishing the correct diagnosis, often imitating other clinical dermatologic entities. Because the clinical morphologic appearances of dermatologic conditions generally contain extensive overlap with histologic features, the mimicry follows the biopsy from the clinic to the microscope. One such orphaned "variant" is MF with poikilodermatous clinical features, which predominantly include distinct lesions characterized by dyspigmentation, atrophy, and telangiectasia. Although the series included a large (49) number of patients, only a minority (13) were histologically characterized in the review. Several of these cases were found to have keratinocytic apoptosis and other features imitating interface dermatitis, confirming previous reports from similar patients. This presents a potentially confounding histologic finding to the unwary. Interestingly, this collection of patients also had a conspicuously higher rate of CD8-expressing tumor cells (38%) than classical MF, which is usually characterized by CD4-expressing cells. To the credit of the WHO/EORTC classification, this series did not show a prognosis that differed with the expected outcome of classical MF. Yet cagey clinicians and histopathologists may still appreciate the continued description of these unique MF patients to aid in a rapid diagnosis and facilitate identification of optimal treatments.

J. Wisell, MD

References

1. Willemze R, Jaffe ES, Burg G, et al. WHO-EORTC classification for cutaneous lymphomas. *Blood.* 2005;105:3768-3775.
2. Cerroni L, Gatter K, Kerl H. *An Illustrated Guide to Skin Lymphoma.* Malden, MA: Blackwell Pub; 2004. 22, ISBN 1405113766.

Superficial Ewing's sarcoma family of tumors: a clinicopathological study with differential diagnoses

Machado I, Llombart B, Calabuig-Fariñas S, et al (Valencia Univ, Spain; Instituto Valenciano de Oncología, Valencia, Spain)
J Cutan Pathol 38:636-643, 2011

Background.—Superficial/cutaneous Ewing's sarcoma family of tumors (ESFT) are rare and have a relatively favorable prognosis compared with deep-seated tumors. The aim of the present study is to describe the clinicopathological characteristics of six genetically confirmed ESFT presenting a superficial location.

Methods.—Clinical data, radiology, histopathology, immunohistochemistry, molecular study [reverse transcriptase-polymerase chain reaction (RT-PCR)/fluorescence in situ hybridization], treatment and follow-up data were retrieved.

Results.—Locations included fingers (2), back (1), neck (1), thigh (1) and subcutaneous breast (1). Two tumors showed conventional morphology, one consisted of primitive neuroectodermal tumor and three tumors showed atypical vascular morphology with hemosiderin deposition and pigmentation. All cases showed CD99, FLI-1, HNK-1 and CAV-1 positivity. RT-PCR revealed the *EWS/Fli1* gene fusion in all cases. Treatment was by wide excision in all cases; one received chemotherapy (CT) and one CT and radiotherapy. Available follow-up revealed the following: two patients with metastasis and death at 5 months and 2 years and one local recurrence at 18 years.

Conclusions.—Superficial ESFT appears to have a relatively favorable prognosis but further studies with additional series, a larger number of cases and more extensive follow-up are necessary to confirm this statement.

▶ Lesions within the Ewing's sarcoma family of tumors (ESFT) pose difficulty for those who interpret skin biopsies, but only rarely or never evaluate deeper soft tissue and bone lesions. ESFT involving the superficial tissues are staggeringly rare and can be easily confused with uncommon variants of tumors frequently seen in the skin, such as melanoma and fibrous histiocytic tumors. The rise of widely available molecular testing has both aided the diagnosis, allowing for the direct testing of characteristic translocations, and complicated the differential diagnosis because these translocations are not entirely specific for ESFT. This series, although comprising only 6 cases, is among the larger series that have been published and includes clinical data, immunohistochemistry, and molecular studies. Some have suggested that a superficial location of these tumors may portend a better prognosis, possibly related to an earlier diagnosis inherent in superficially placed lesions. Of the patients in this series, 3 had sufficient clinical follow-up, 2 of whom have died of their disease. The authors make the important observation that deeply seated ESFT are aggressively treated with surgery, chemotherapy, and radiation therapy, whereas the patients included in this and past reports who have died from superficial ESFT were treated less aggressively, sometimes only with excision. Further data regarding treatment of these rare tumors with their associated outcomes is needed, and series like this report, although limited, are valuable. It is also important for the vigilant practicing pathologist to remain aware of these tumors, including those who may only see the more superficial variants.

J. Wisell, MD

Pseudomyogenic Hemangioendothelioma: A Distinctive, Often Multicentric Tumor With Indolent Behavior
Hornick JL, Fletcher CDM (Harvard Med School, Boston, MA)
Am J Surg Pathol 35:190-201, 2011

A 1992 report described 5 keratin-positive spindle cell neoplasms with multifocal presentation in a single limb, which were proposed at that time to be a variant of epithelioid sarcoma. This tumor type is not widely recognized and is incompletely characterized. We examined 50 cases of this distinctive tumor to evaluate histologic, immunophenotypic, and clinical features. There was a 4.6:1 male predominance (mean age, 31 y; 82% ≤40 y). Half of the patients presented with painful nodules and the other half with painless nodules. Mean tumor size was 1.9 cm (range, 0.3 to 5.5 cm). Tumors arose in the lower limb (54%), the upper limb (24%), trunk (18%), or head and neck (4%). Thirty-three (66%) were multifocal lesions (ranging from 2 to 15 lesions), including 32 cases with involvement of multiple tissue planes. Of 205 total lesions, 64 (31%) involved the dermis, 42 (20%) involved the subcutis, 70 (34%) lesions involved muscle, and 29 (14%) lesions involved bone; all the lesions had infiltrative margins. The tumors were composed of loose fascicles and sheets of plump spindle cells with vesicular nuclei, variably prominent nucleoli, and abundant brightly eosinophilic cytoplasm, some with a strikingly rhabdomyoblast-like appearance. In all cases, a minority of cells were epithelioid. Twenty-seven tumors contained a prominent neutrophilic inflammatory infiltrate. Most tumors showed only mild nuclear atypia; 6 tumors contained foci of notably pleomorphic cells. The median mitotic rate was 1 per 10 HPF (range, 1 to 10). Seven tumors showed vascular invasion; 7 tumors had areas of necrosis. By immunohistochemistry, all tumors were diffusely positive for AE1/AE3 and FLI1; 22 of 47 tumors were variably positive for CD31. Focal positivity was seen for CAM5.2 (21 of 35), smooth muscle actin (14 of 42), epithelial membrane antigen (7 of 49 weak), and PAN-K (MNF116) (1 of 47). All were negative for CD34, desmin, and S100 protein and showed intact INI1 expression. Follow-up was available for 31 patients and ranged from 9 months to 17 years (mean, 4 y). Most lesions were treated by local excision. Eighteen (58%) patients had local recurrence or developed additional nodules in the same region, all but one, within 1 year of first presentation. Eight patients had postoperative radiation therapy and 6 patients had chemotherapy. Four patients had amputations for multifocal disease. One patient had a regional lymph node metastasis, and, thus far, only 1 patient has developed distant metastases (disseminated), 16 years after primary tumor excision. At the time of the last follow-up, 27 patients were alive with no evidence of the disease, 1 patient was alive with unknown disease status, 2 patients were alive with recurrent disease, and 1 patient died of the disease. In summary, we describe a distinctive type of rarely metastasizing ("intermediate") tumor affecting mainly young men and usually characterized by multifocality in different tissue planes of a limb. Although sharing some features with epithelioid sarcoma (skin/soft tissue of distal extremities, young adults, keratin positive), it differs by having predominantly myoid-appearing spindle cell morphology, expression of FLI1, common reactivity for CD31, lack of epithelial membrane antigen, CD34, and PAN-K expression, and intact INI1. The overall immunophenotypic findings favor endothelial differentiation. Despite the ominous presentation, follow-up thus far suggests an indolent clinical course with a small risk of distant metastasis. Although the precise nosologic status of this tumor type is uncertain, we propose the interim designation "pseudomyogenic hemangioendothelioma."

▶ This report details a collection of tumors and attempts to refine their taxonomy. These and similar tumors were initially believed to be at least closely related to, if not outright, epithelioid sarcomas (ES). This initial obfuscation stems from similar clinical presentations of young to middle-age patients with often multifocal tumors involving extremities. The histology, nicely delineated by the authors, is quite different than ES. These tumors show fascicles and sheets of plump tumor cells as opposed to nodules of epithelioid cells. The immunohistochemical features, particularly FLI1, CD31, and INI expression, also militate against ES. Although not necessarily indicated by the histologic features, the immunohistochemical studies suggest endothelial differentiation, which contributes to the rational for the proposed classification as a type of hemangioendothelioma. Interestingly, these tumors were uniformly negative for CD34, which not only further distinguished them from true ES, but also likened them to a series of tumors titled "epithelioid sarcoma-like hemangioendothelioma."[1] Since the publication of this article, the likely possibility that these 2 entities are indeed the same has been discussed, as has optimal terminology. Regardless of the appellation, the argument for distinction of these lesions from ES is compelling, given the apparently much more aggressive behavior of the latter.

J. Wisell, MD

Reference

1. Billings SD, Folpe AL, Weiss SW. Epithelioid sarcoma-like hemangioendothelioma. *Am J Surg Pathol.* 2003;27:48-57.

Melanocytes in nonlesional sun-exposed skin: A multicenter comparative study

Hendi A, Wada DA, Jacobs MA, et al (Private Practice, Chevy Chase, MD; Mayo Clinic, Rochester, MN; et al)
J Am Acad Dermatol 65:1186-1193, 2011

Background.—There are limited data regarding melanocyte density and distribution on sun-exposed skin of the head and neck, in particular, comparing morphology (hematoxylin-eosin [H&E] staining) and immunohistochemistry (Melan-A staining) on formalin-fixed tissue. Furthermore, comparisons of melanocyte density between distinct geographic populations have not been made using these methods. This information would be useful for physicians who use histologic criteria to diagnose and treat lentigo maligna.

Objective.—We aimed to characterize the density and distribution of melanocytes using Melan-A and H&E stains on nonlesional sun-exposed skin of the face and neck, and compare the results between patients seen in Florida and Minnesota. We also aimed to quantify the presence and extent of features considered characteristic of melanoma in these noncancerous specimens of sun-damaged skin. The overall goal was to be able to provide this information to physicians who perform histopathologic interpretations of skin biopsy specimens to potentially prevent the overdiagnosis of melanoma.

Methods.—In all, 100 patients undergoing Mohs micrographic and reconstructive surgery for basal cell and squamous cell carcinoma were enrolled, 50 each at the two sites. Permanent tissue sections were prepared from sun-exposed skin without clinical lesions. Melanocyte density and distribution were quantified.

Results.—The overall median and 90th percentile, respectively, of melanocytes per high-power field was 9 and 14 on the H&E-stained sections and 11 and 19 on the Melan-A-stained sections. The means were 9.3 and 12.0, respectively ($P < .001$). There was evidence that melanocyte densities were higher in patients in Florida than in Minnesota, at least using H&E staining. There was evidence of lower melanocyte densities with increasing age, more so for Melan-A than H&E staining, and higher densities in men using Melan-A. Confluence was noted in 24% of cases using H&E and 45% using Melan-A. More than two thirds of these were classified as having mild confluence, whereas the others demonstrated higher amounts of confluence (3-8 melanocytes). Only 37 patients had a follicle present; of these, 7 patients had follicular extension although this did not extend beyond 1 mm in depth. Cytologic atypia was noted in 19 of the 100 patients; pagetoid spread was found in 3.

Limitations.—This was a selected population of patients; results may not be generalizable to the wider population. Variables such as contours of the epidermis (rete density), density of hair follicles, and epidermal thickness may affect the reproducibility of the results. Melanomas were not included for comparison.

Conclusion.—Relatively high melanocyte density, mild to moderate confluence of melanocytes, focal pagetosis, superficial follicular extension (<1.0 mm), and mild or moderate cytologic atypia may be observed in the absence of a melanocytic neoplasm. It is important for physicians to be aware of these findings so that such features are interpreted appropriately when making a histologic assessment that may ultimately influence therapy and outcome.

▶ This article follows a previous article by the same author,[1] this time using paraffin-embedded tissue instead of frozen section tissue from 2 distinctly separate geographic areas. This investigation combines with at least 3 additional articles published this year[2-4] addressing the same issue that poses a near-daily challenge for those interpreting biopsies from sun-damaged skin, a group that includes pathologists, dermatologists, dermatopathologists, and Mohs surgeons. Melanoma in situ occurring on sun-exposed sites (lentigo maligna) has features that overlap with the changes seen in sun-damaged skin, namely, increased densities of melanocytic cells and increased melanocytic atypia, along with other less commonly shared findings, such as nesting and pagetoid spread. This study provides a quantitative basis for evaluating skin from sun-exposed sites and finds on average 9.3 and 12 melanocytes per 0.5 mm by hematoxylin and eosin stains and Melan-A immunohistochemical studies, respectively. These numbers should not be translated into clinical practice too exactly, as differences in geography, immunohistochemical study performance, and staining characteristics may vary. The authors stress the importance of integrating all of the histopathologic— and possibly the immunohistochemical—characteristics to reach or refute a diagnosis of lentigo maligna. Such a diagnosis should not rely on a single feature, particularly increased melanocytes. The similar recent study by Madden et al[2] notes that melanocyte number alone is only somewhat useful; they found features such as nesting to be more reliable but acknowledge that this too may be seen in otherwise nonlesional sun-damaged skin, although in isolation. The authors of the study at hand (Hendi et al) did not identify keratinocytic cells labeling with Melan-A, a possible hazard that has been previously reported. Kim et al[3] more directly address this latter issue and assert that Melan-A significantly overestimates melanocytic density, preferring the MiTF marker in this setting. Madden and colleagues[2] did not address this latter issue.

J. Wisell, MD

References

1. Hendi A, Brodland DG, Zitelli JA. Melanocytes in long-standing sun-exposed skin: quantitative analysis using the MART-1 immunostain. *Arch Dermatol.* 2006;142:871-876.
2. Madden K, Forman SB, Elston D. Quantification of melanocytes in sun-damaged skin. *J Am Acad Dermatol.* 2011;64:548-552.
3. Kim J, Taube JM, McCalmont TH, Glusac EJ. Quantitative comparison of MiTF, Melan-A, HMB-45 and Mel-5 in solar lentigines and melanoma in situ. *J Cutan Pathol.* 2011;38:775-779.
4. Black WH, Thareja SK, Blake BP, Chen R, Cherpelis BS, Glass LF. Distinction of melanoma in situ from solar lentigo on sun-damaged skin using morphometrics and MITF immunohistochemistry. *Am J Dermatopathol.* 2011;33:573-578.

p16 Expression: A marker of differentiation between childhood malignant melanomas and Spitz nevi

Al Dhaybi R, Agoumi M, Gagné I, et al (Univ of Montreal, Quebec, Canada)
J Am Acad Dermatol 65:357-363, 2011

Background.—Childhood malignant melanomas frequently present as nodular melanomas with Spitzoid features. Spitz nevus and Spitzoid melanoma overlap clinically and histopathologically and there have been many attempts to differentiate between them. Spitz nevi differ from melanomas by their immunohistochemical pattern of expression of cell cycle and apoptosis regulators such as the p16 protein.

Objective.—The aim of this study was to evaluate in a childhood population the expression of p16 in nodular malignant melanoma of Spitzoid type, Spitz nevi, and a control group of benign compound melanocytic nevi.

Methods.—We performed immunohistochemical studies for expression of p16 in 6 Spitzoid malignant melanomas, 18 Spitz nevi, and 12 compound melanocytic nevi in children younger than 18 years. Statistical analysis was used to compare p16 expression, mitotic count/mm^2, and Ki-67 index of childhood nodular malignant melanomas and Spitz nevi.

Results.—All the childhood melanoma cases were associated with loss of p16 without any correlation with their Breslow thickness whereas all the Spitz nevi and benign melanocytic nevi had strong positive nuclear and cytoplasmic expression of p16 staining. We found a statistically significant difference in p16 expression, mitotic counts, and Ki-67 index when comparing the Spitzoid melanomas with the Spitz nevi.

Limitations.—This study is limited by the small number of malignant melanomas, which are known to be rare in childhood.

Conclusion.—p16 Expression in childhood nodular Spitzoid malignant melanomas and Spitz nevi, in conjunction with clinical and histopathological evaluation, may be a useful tool in differentiating between these two entities.

▶ This report adds to the growing knowledge of the important cell cycle regulatory protein p16 and its role in melanoma. Investigators have previously found loss of p16 expression by immunohistochemistry to be helpful in differentiating benign from malignant melanocytic lesions.[1] The current series supplies striking evidence to this argument by reporting their entire collection of childhood spitzoid melanomas to be negative for p16 expression but showing all of their Spitz and conventional nevi to demonstrate at least some p16 labeling. However, some important caveats should be noted. First, they collected 6 cases of Spitzoid melanoma; this does not indicate a poor effort by the authors; indeed, these are uncommon malignancies among the already uncommon pediatric solid malignancies. Second, these 6 tumors show striking proliferation rates, reported as an average of 6 mitoses per square millimeter and an average Ki-67 rate of close to 50%. This suggests a particularly aggressive collection of tumors. The previous studies of melanomas of different types, almost all in older patients, show generally lower proliferation and more variable p16 labeling. Even given these limitations, this study broadens the scope of diagnostic p16 use to include these often diagnostically difficult childhood Spitzoid lesions.

J. Wisell, MD

Reference

1. Karim RZ, Li W, Sanki A, et al. Reduced p16 and increased cyclin D1 and pRb expression are correlated with progression in cutaneous melanocytic tumors. *Int J Surg Pathol.* 2009;17:361-367.

Specificity of *IRF4* translocations for primary cutaneous anaplastic large cell lymphoma: a multicenter study of 204 skin biopsies
Wada DA, Law ME, Hsi ED, et al (Mayo Clinic, Rochester, MN; Cleveland Clinic Foundation, OH; et al)
Mod Pathol 24:596-605, 2011

Current pathologic criteria cannot reliably distinguish cutaneous anaplastic large cell lymphoma from other CD30-positive T-cell lymphoproliferative disorders (lymphomatoid papulosis, systemic anaplastic large cell lymphoma with skin involvement, and transformed mycosis fungoides). We previously reported *IRF4* (interferon regulatory factor-4) translocations in cutaneous anaplastic large cell lymphomas. Here, we investigated the clinical utility of detecting *IRF4* translocations in skin biopsies. We performed fluorescence *in situ* hybridization (FISH) for *IRF4* in 204 biopsies involved by T-cell lymphoproliferative disorders from 182 patients at three institutions. In all, 9 of 45 (20%) cutaneous anaplastic large cell lymphomas and 1 of 32 (3%) cases of lymphomatoid papulosis with informative results demonstrated an *IRF4* translocation. Remaining informative cases were negative for a translocation (7 systemic anaplastic large cell lymphomas; 44 cases of mycosis fungoides/Sézary syndrome (13 transformed); 24 peripheral T-cell lymphomas, not otherwise specified; 12 CD4-positive small/medium-sized pleomorphic T-cell lymphomas; 5 extranodal NK/T-cell lymphomas, nasal type; 4 gamma-delta T-cell lymphomas; and 5 other uncommon T-cell lymphoproliferative disorders). Among all cutaneous T-cell lymphoproliferative disorders, FISH for *IRF4* had a specificity and positive predictive value for cutaneous anaplastic large cell lymphoma of 99 and 90%, respectively ($P = 0.00002$, Fisher's exact test). Among anaplastic large cell lymphomas, lymphomatoid papulosis, and transformed mycosis fungoides, specificity and positive predictive value were 98 and 90%, respectively ($P = 0.005$). FISH abnormalities other than translocations and *IRF4* protein expression were seen in 13 and 65% of cases, respectively, but were nonspecific with regard to T-cell lymphoproliferative disorder subtype. Our findings support the clinical utility of FISH for *IRF4* in the differential diagnosis of T-cell lymphoproliferative disorders in skin biopsies, with detection of a translocation favoring cutaneous anaplastic large cell lymphoma. Like all FISH studies,

IRF4 testing must be interpreted in the context of morphology, phenotype, and clinical features.

▶ This study adds to the author's previous report[1] of translocations of the interferon regulatory factor-4 (IRF4) gene in primary cutaneous anaplastic large cell lymphoma (ALCL). Differentiating this latter condition from other CD30-positive proliferations in the skin can be challenging. The histologic differential diagnosis for these types of proliferations may include primary cutaneous ALCL, systemic ALCL with cutaneous involvement, transformation of mycosis fungoides (MF), lymphomatoid papulosis (LyP) and rarely cutaneous classic Hodgkin lymphoma. With significant histologic overlap, some of these disorders can only be reliably separated with prolonged clinical follow-up. This study suggests that fluorescence in situ hybridization (FISH) studies, but not immunohistochemistry, for IRF4 may be the most useful nonclinical feature yet discovered that could be used to help separate cutaneous and systemic ALCL, transformed MF, and LyP. Translocations were found predominantly in cases of primary cutaneous ALCL (9 of 45 cases). However, as the authors note, this alone does not separate these entities completely. The only other large study to evaluate IRF4 FISH in this setting[2] found 2 of 24 transformed MF cases to contain an IRF4 translocation. This current series included a solitary case of LyP out of 32 with a translocation. Interestingly, infrequently finding the translocation in these latter 2 disorders raises questions about how the 3 are related. For example, the identification of the case of LyP with this translocation could also be used for the argument that LyP (particularly type C) and primary cutaneous ALCL are closely related diseases that would be better considered as a continuum rather than 2 clearly separate entities. Although no case of systemic ALCL involving the skin has been found to harbor the translocation, the previous study[1] by this group included a solitary case of systemic ALCL without cutaneous involvement, but with the translocation suggesting that finding the IRF4 translocation should also not absolutely exclude systemic ALCL. This study and the prior 2 studies cited below indicate IRF4 FISH may be a welcome addition in these cases that are often difficult for the histopathologist to classify.

J. Wisell, MD

References

1. Feldman AL, Law M, Remstein ED, et al. Recurrent translocations involving the IRF4 oncogene locus in peripheral T-cell lymphomas. *Leukemia.* 2009;23:574-580.
2. Pham-Ledard A, Prochazkova-Carlotti M, Laharanne E, et al. IRF4 gene rearrangements define a subgroup of CD30-positive cutaneous T-cell lymphoma: a study of 54 cases. *J Invest Dermatol.* 2010;130:816-825.

6 Lung and Mediastinum

Thymic Carcinoma Associated With Multilocular Thymic Cyst: A Clinicopathologic Study of 7 Cases
Weissferdt A, Moran CA (MD Anderson Cancer Ctr, Houston, TX)
Am J Surg Pathol 35:1074-1079, 2011

We present 7 cases of thymic carcinoma associated with a multilocular thymic cyst (MTC). The patients were 5 men and 2 women aged 22 to 71 years (mean, 49.3 y). Clinically, 6 patients presented with chest, sternal, or upper extremity pain, and in 1 patient the tumor was an incidental finding. Grossly, 4 tumors were described as multilobulated solid-cystic masses, whereas 3 cases were described as solid tumors with a white-yellow cut surface and areas of hemorrhage and necrosis. The tumor size ranged from 7.0 to 10.0 cm (mean, 8.1 cm). Histologically, 4 cases were classified as squamous cell carcinoma, and 1 each as sarcomatoid (spindle) cell carcinoma, papillary carcinoma, and basaloid carcinoma. In addition to the tumor component, prominent MTC changes were observed in the adjacent remnant thymic tissue. Immunohistochemical studies were conducted in 2 cases of squamous cell carcinoma. The neoplastic cells were positive for cytokeratin (CK), CK5/6, and p63, and showed variable reactivity for CK7 and CD5. Clinical follow-up showed that 4 patients were alive and well, 2 to 63 months after diagnosis, and 3 patients were alive with disease, 13 to 33 months after diagnosis. This study expands the morphologic spectrum of thymic carcinoma associated with MTC, detects a higher incidence than previously believed, and highlights the importance of adequate sampling and proper evaluation of all cystic lesions of the anterior mediastinum so as not to mistake malignancy for a benign cystic process.

▶ Thymic cysts are rare and may be unilocular or multilocular. Multilocular thymic cysts often have a predominant inflammatory component and have a tendency to recur. Cystic changes also occur in a variety of neoplasms of the anterior mediastinum, and these neoplasms include germ cell tumors, thymomas, and lymphomas. Multilocular thymic cysts also occur with thymic carcinomas, and consequently thymic carcinomas must be included in the differential of rarer malignancies with multicystic components. Challenges in identifying the malignant component presumably would occur in fine-needle aspiration sampling (when only the cystic component is sampled) and during an intraoperative consultation frozen section. Extensive sampling also would be recommended of all multilocular thymic cystic lesions. For additional reading, please see the reference section.[1,2]

S. S. Raab, MD

References

1. Snover DC, Levine GD, Rosai J. Thymic carcinoma. Five distinctive histological variants. *Am J Surg Pathol.* 1982;6:451-470.
2. Suster S, Rosai J. Multilocular thymic cyst: an acquired reactive process. Study of 18 cases. *Am J Surg Pathol.* 1991;15:388-398.

High-grade neuroendocrine carcinomas of the lung highly express enhancer of zeste homolog 2, but carcinoids do not

Findeis-Hosey JJ, Huang J, Li F, et al (Univ of Rochester Med Ctr, NY; Univ of California, Los Angeles)
Hum Pathol 42:867-872, 2011

Enhancer of zeste homolog 2, the catalytic subunit of polycomb repressive complex 2, is a histone methyltransferase and plays an important role in cell proliferation and cell cycle regulation. It has been shown to be overexpressed in a number of malignant neoplasms. This study aimed to determine the expression pattern of enhancer of zeste homolog 2 in neuroendocrine tumors of the lung and the potential of enhancer of zeste homolog 2 to serve as a biomarker to segregate carcinoids from high-grade neuroendocrine carcinomas. Fifty-four cases, including 25 typical carcinoids, 7 atypical carcinoids, 9 large-cell neuroendocrine carcinomas, and 13 small-cell lung carcinomas, were immunohistochemically studied using a monoclonal antibody against enhancer of zeste homolog 2. All 13 small-cell lung carcinomas demonstrated moderate to strong nuclear staining with 12 exhibiting more than 90% of tumor cells staining. All 9 large-cell neuroendocrine carcinomas were moderately to strongly positive for enhancer of zeste homolog 2, with 6 cases having staining in more than 80% of tumor cells. In contrast, all 25 typical carcinoids and 6 atypical carcinoids showed only rare scattered enhancer of zeste homolog 2–positive tumor cells, with 1 case of atypical carcinoid exhibiting moderate staining in 40% of tumor cells. A subsequent validation study of the 14 specimens of lung or mediastinal lymph node biopsy and fine-needle aspiration, including 6 small-cell lung carcinomas, 2 large-cell neuroendocrine carcinomas, 5 typical carcinoids, and 1 atypical carcinoid, was performed. Enhancer of zeste homolog 2 was diffusely and strongly positive in all small-cell lung carcinomas and large-cell neuroendocrine carcinomas, even with severe crush artifact, whereas it was only positive in rare tumor cells in carcinoids. These findings support the formulation that enhancer of zeste homolog 2 may play an important role in the regulation of biologic behavior of high-grade neuroendocrine carcinomas and as a diagnostically useful marker in distinguishing high-grade neuroendocrine carcinomas from carcinoids.

▶ On large excisional pulmonary or mediastinal specimens, the classification of neuroendocrine tumors into high and low grade types generally is not difficult. However, on biopsy specimens and fine-needle aspiration specimens, this separation may be exceedingly challenging, especially in scenarios of tiny amounts of tissue or sampling artifacts, such as tissue crushing. Finding a neuroendocrine immunohistochemical study that facilitates in this assessment has been difficult. Interobserver variation studies of this separation have shown surprisingly low agreement. Although pathologists often agree on diagnoses such as small cell carcinoma and carcinoid, they may not agree on diagnoses such as small cell carcinoma and atypical carcinoid. The data presented by Findeis-Hosey and colleagues show that the zeste homolog 2 marker offers the potential to make the diagnostic distinction between high-grade neuroendocrine tumors (small cell carcinoma and large cell neuroendocrine carcinoma) and low-grade neuroendocrine tumors (carcinoids). The application of zeste homolog 2 to actual practice needs to be further evaluated before recommending its use. For additional reading, please see the reference section.[1,2]

S. S. Raab, MD

References

1. Travis WD. Lung tumours with neuroendocrine differentiation. *Eur J Cancer.* 2009;45:251-266.
2. den Bakker MA, Willemsen S, Grünberg K, et al. Small cell carcinoma of the lung and large cell neuroendocrine carcinoma interobserver variability. *Histopathology.* 2010;56:356-363.

Pax8 Expression in Thymic Epithelial Neoplasms: An Immunohistochemical Analysis
Weissferdt A, Moran CA (MD Anderson Cancer Ctr, Houston, TX)
Am J Surg Pathol 35:1305-1310, 2011

Pax8 is a transcription factor associated with the embryonic development of the thyroid gland, kidney, and the Müllerian system and plays a role in the tumorigenesis of these organs. Pax8 has been shown to be expressed immunohistochemically in a high percentage of tumors of thyroid, renal, and Müllerian origin in both primary and metastatic sites. The diagnostic utility of Pax8 protein expression in thymic epithelial neoplasms has not been comprehensively studied. This study examines the immunohistochemical expression of Pax8 in a series of thymic epithelial neoplasms, including 31 thymic carcinomas, 30 World Health Organization (WHO) type A thymomas, and 30 WHO type B thymomas (B1, B2, B3). Positive immunoreactivity for Pax8 was noted in 77% of thymic carcinomas, 100% of WHO type A thymomas, and 93% of WHO type B thymomas. Consistent but weaker staining for Pax8 was also identified in the epithelial cells of remnant thymic tissue located in the periphery of the tumors. This study expands the spectrum of tumors expressing Pax8 to include thymic epithelial neoplasms. The consistent expression of this marker in these tumors is a valuable diagnostic tool that can be of use in the differential diagnosis of anterior mediastinal neoplasms. As Pax8 expression has been demonstrated to be limited to organs the development of which depends on this transcription factor, the possibility that the organogenesis of the thymic gland also depends on this factor should be explored.

▶ Weissferdt and Moran present a straightforward study evaluating immunohistochemical Pax8 expression in thymic carcinomas and World Health Organization type A and type B thymomas. In this limited series, a high immunohistochemical expression frequency for Pax8 is seen in all these thymic tumors. As Pax8 also is expressed in other epithelial neoplasms (eg, thyroid and renal), the authors conclude that their findings have potential benefit in the evaluation of mediastinal lesions to confirm the tumor site of origin. Thus, theoretically, Pax8 could be added to a panel of immunohistochemical studies to exclude or confirm various metastases and other primary tumors. The jury is still out on the clinical utility until this theoretical study is performed. Many immunohistochemical markers appear sensitive and specific in single marker evaluations but fail when applied in panels applied prospectively in real clinical practice. Of important note is that this study was conducted on tissue blocks from thymectomy surgical specimens and not on biopsy tissues, which may be the predominant specimen type in which the differentiation will need to occur. For additional reading, please see the reference section.[1,2]

S. S. Raab, MD

References

1. Bowen NJ, Logani S, Dickerson EB, et al. Emerging roles for PAX8 in ovarian cancer and endosalpingeal development. *Gynecol Oncol.* 2007;104:331-337.
2. Ozcan A, Shen SS, Hamilton C, et al. PAX 8 expression in non-neoplastic tissues, primary tumors, and metastatic tumors: a comprehensive immunohistochemical study. *Mod Pathol.* 2011;24:751-764.

Small Neuroendocrine Lesions in Intrathoracic Lymph Nodes of Patients With Primary Lung Adenocarcinoma: Real Metastasis?
Li F, Wang X, Xu H, et al (Univ of Rochester Med Ctr, MN; et al)
Am J Surg Pathol 34:1701-1707, 2010

The presence of individual neuroendocrine cells in rare peripancreatic lymph nodes (LNs) suggests that neuroendocrine tumor or nested neuroendocrine cell proliferation can arise in situ from neuroendocrine cells native to any LN. However, it is very difficult to ascertain whether any neuroendocrine lesion in LNs is a primary tumor or a metastasis from adjacent organs. We encountered 4 cases of neuroendocrine proliferation in intrathoracic LNs (ILNs) of patients with primary lung adenocarcinoma. All patients had a single lung mass without mediastinal lymphadenopathy based on computed tomography and positron emission tomography imaging. Mediastinal staging was done by either mediastinoscopy or thoracotomy and none of them had metastasis from adenocarcinoma in any LN. One patient had three ILNs positive for neuroendocrine proliferation measuring 1.7, 1.8, and 4.0 mm, respectively and a minute tumorlet less than 1.0 mm in the lung. Three other patients had small areas of neuroendocrine proliferation no more than 1 mm in single ILN without any lung neuroendocrine lesion. Neuroendocrine cells in ILNs often formed nests of varying size with similar morphology to carcinoid tumorlet in the lung. Small clusters of neuroendocrine cells without any particular pattern were often seen together with these nests. These cells were positive for neuroendocrine markers: synaptophysin, chromogranin, and CD56. They were also positive for CK7 and TTF-1. It is interesting to note, single cells positive for neuroendocrine markers and TTF-1 were identified near or away from these neuroendocrine nests or clusters. These findings suggest that neuroendocrine lesion can be incidentally identified in ILNs. Close clinical follow-up is warranted as metastasis from or synchronous lesions in adjacent organs cannot be excluded.

▶ Li and coauthors report the finding of small foci of neuroendocrine cells in intrathoracic lymph nodes in patients who do not have a history or clinical findings of a primary neuroendocrine tumor. Do these represent metastases from an unknown tumor, differentiation of a metastasis from a nonneuroendocrine tumor, or a spectrum of normal? The impression that I get from the conclusions of this article is that these lesions represent a spectrum of normal findings similar to what has been seen in peripancreatic lymph nodes. In the lung, a problem arises in patients who have a low-grade neuroendocrine tumor, such as a carcinoid tumor, and a small lymph node focus of neuroendocrine cells. Traditionally, these foci have been considered as metastases, but in light of the authors' findings, this may be incorrect. The authors do not really provide a solution but want to make us aware of the dilemma. For additional reading, please see the reference section.[1,2]

S. S. Raab, MD

References

1. Francioni F, Rendina EA, Venuta F, Pescarmona E, De Giacomo T, Ricci C. Low grade neuroendocrine tumors of the lung (bronchial carcinoids)—25 years experience. *Eur J Cardiothorac Surg.* 1990;4:472-476.
2. Herrmann ME, Ciesla MC, Chejfec G, DeJong SA, Yong SL. Primary nodal gastrinomas. *Arch Pathol Lab Med.* 2000;124:832-835.

Lymphomatoid Granulomatosis: Insights Gained Over 4 Decades
Katzenstein A-LA, Doxtader E, Narendra S (SUNY Upstate Med Univ, Syracuse)
Am J Surg Pathol 34:e35-e48, 2010

Lymphomatoid granulomatosis is a rare lymphoproliferative disease involving predominantly the lung, and there is uncertainty about its relationship to lymphoma. It affects mainly middle-aged adults, although there is a wide age range, and men are affected almost twice as often as women. Multiple nodular, usually bilateral, infiltrates are seen radiographically, and extrapulmonary involvement, especially of skin and nervous system, occurs in more than one third of the patients. Mortality rates are high, and treatment modes are not well established. Morphologically, there is a nodular polymorphous mononuclear cell infiltrate with prominent vascular infiltration and often necrosis. Varying numbers of large, often atypical, CD20-positive B-lymphocytes are present within a background containing numerous CD3-positive small T lymphocytes and scattered admixed plasma cells and histiocytes. Evidence of Epstein-Barr virus infection can be shown in most cases by in-situ hybridization for Epstein-Barr virus RNA. The infiltrate is graded as 1 to 3 based on the proportion of large B cells. Morphologically, there is overlap in grades 2 and 3 with variants of large B-cell lymphoma, and many such cases show evidence of monoclonality by polymerase chain reaction. It is suggested that lymphoma (T-cell rich large B-cell or diffuse large B-cell) be diagnosed in addition to lymphomatoid granulomatosis in grades 2 and 3 to appropriately communicate the nature of the disease to clinicians (Table 3).

▶ Katzenstein and colleagues provide a thorough review of lymphomatoid granulomatosis, including the challenges in establishing the diagnosis. Table 3 shows the algorithm for reaching the diagnosis that relies heavily on

TABLE 3.—Algorithm LYGfor Diagnosing[†]

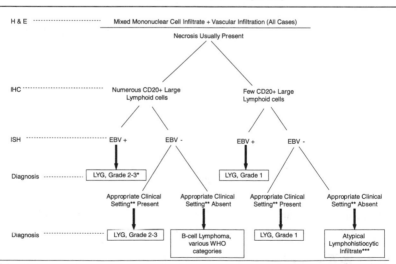

*Patients with prior organ transplant or methotrexate treatment should be diagnosed as posttransplant lymphoproliferative disorder or iatrogenic immunodeficiency-associated lymphoproliferative disorder, respectively, rather than LYG.
**Appropriate clinical setting includes any one or combination of multiple nodules radiographically, skin involvement, or nervous system (usually central) involvement.
***Special stains and cultures should be performed in all cases to exclude infection.
†See text for explanation.
EBV indicates Epstein-Barr virus; H&E, hematoxylin and eosin; IHC, immunohistochemistry; ISH, in-situ hybridization; LYG, lymphomatoid granulomatosis; WHO, World Health Organization.

the knowledge of the clinical setting. For additional reading, please see reference list.[1,2]

S. S. Raab, MD

References

1. Liebow AA, Carrington CR, Friedman PJ. Lymphomatoid granulomatosis. *Hum Pathol.* 1972;3:457-558.
2. Nicholson AG, Wotherspoon AC, Diss TC, et al. Lymphomatoid granulomatosis: evidence that some cases represent Epstein-Barr virus-associated B-cell lymphoma. *Histopathology.* 1996;29:317-324.

Optimal Immunohistochemical Markers for Distinguishing Lung Adenocarcinomas From Squamous Cell Carcinomas in Small Tumor Samples
Terry J, Leung S, Laskin J, et al (BC Cancer Agency, Vancouver, Canada; et al)
Am J Surg Pathol 34:1805-1811, 2010

The histologic subtype of non-small cell lung carcinoma is important in selecting appropriate chemotherapy for patients with advanced disease. As many of these patients are not operative candidates, they are treated medically after biopsy for diagnosis. Inherent limitations of small biopsy samples can make distinguishing poorly differentiated lung adenocarcinoma (ADC) from squamous cell carcinoma (SCC) difficult. The value of histochemical and immunohistochemical markers to help separate poorly differentiated ADC from SCC in resection specimens is well established; however, the optimal use of markers in small tissue samples has only recently been examined and the correlation of marker expression in small tissue samples with histologic subtype determined on resection specimens has not been well documented. We address this issue by examining the expression of 9 markers (p63, TTF1, CK5/6, CK7, 34βE12, Napsin A, mucicarmine, NTRK1, and NTRK2) on 200 cases of ADC and 225 cases of SCC in tissue microarray format to mimic small tissue specimens. The single best marker to separate ADC from SCC is p63 (for SCC: sensitivity 84%, specificity 85%). Logistic regression analysis identifies p63, TTF1, CK5/6, CK7, Napsin A, and mucicarmine as the optimal panel to separate ADC from SCC. Reduction of the panel to p63, TTF1, CK5/6, and CK7 is marginally less effective but may be the best compromise when tissue is limited. We present an algorithm for the stepwise application of p63, TTF1, CK5/6, CK7, Napsin A, and mucicarmine in situations in which separation of ADC from SCC in small specimens cannot be accomplished by morphology alone (Fig 3).

▶ The field of pathology has not formally determined the best practices of immunohistochemical study use. These best practices include the clinical scenarios in which immunohistochemical studies should be examined and the immunohistochemical panels applied. Terry et al examined immunohistochemical studies in lung core biopsy specimens, although these may vary greatly in reflecting the

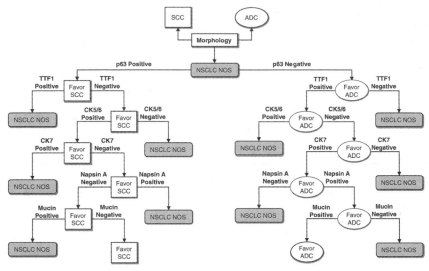

FIGURE 3.—A simplified binary scheme to classify and report NSCLC in small samples (biopsies and cell blocks) based on sequential addition of markers from the optimal 6-marker panel identified by logistic regression analysis. ADC indicates adenocarcinoma; NSCLC NOS, non-small cell lung carcinoma not otherwise specified; SCC, squamous cell carcinoma. (Reprinted from Terry J, Leung S, Laskin J, et al. Optimal immunohistochemical markers for distinguishing lung adenocarcinomas from squamous cell carcinomas in small tumor samples. *Am J Surg Pathol.* 2010;34:1805-1811, with permission from Lippincott Williams & Wilkins.)

concept of "small" tumor samples. Thus, an underlying question (not answered) is when do we apply immunohistochemical studies to separate lung adenocarcinomas from squamous cell carcinomas? Some pathologists apply immunohistochemical studies to all cases, others apply them to only limited subsets, and others forgo definitive classification. Terry and colleagues investigated immunohistochemical panels (with mucicarmine) and recommended an algorithm involving a stepwise application of specific stains (Fig 3). Terry et al reported that their recommended panel should be applied when the separation of adenocarcinoma and squamous cell carcinoma cannot be accomplished by morphology alone, but their study did not involve these types of cases (they investigated all core biopsy tissues). From their data, it appears that the panel of TTF1, cytokeratin 5/6, and cytokeratin 7 achieve a high sensitivity alone and the other stains only add a very small incremental value. For additional reading, please see reference list.[1,2]

S. S. Raab, MD

References

1. Hirsch FR, Spreafico A, Novello S, Wood MD, Simms L, Papotti M. The prognostic and predictive role of histology in advanced non-small cell lung cancer: a literature review. *J Thorac Oncol.* 2008;3:1468-1481.
2. Loo PS, Thomas SC, Nicolson MC, Fyfe MN, Kerr KM. Subtyping of undifferentiated non-small cell carcinomas in bronchial biopsy specimens. *J Thorac Oncol.* 2010;5:442-447.

7 Cardiovascular

Importance of specimen length during temporal artery biopsy

Ypsilantis E, Courtney ED, Chopra N, et al (Queen Elizabeth Hosp, King's Lynn, UK; Conquest Hosp, Hastings, UK; et al)
Br J Surg 98:1556-1560, 2011

Background.—Variations in surgical technique of temporal artery biopsy (TAB) performed for diagnosis of giant cell arteritis (GCA) may contribute to high false-negative rates. This was a retrospective analysis of a large database that explored potential associations between specimen length and diagnostic sensitivity of TAB.

Methods.—Histopathological reports and medical records of patients who underwent TAB in six hospitals between 2004 and 2009 were reviewed.

Results.—A total of 966 biopsies were analysed. The median postfixation specimen length was 1 (range $0 \cdot 1 - 8 \cdot 5$) cm and 207 biopsies ($21 \cdot 4$ per cent) were positive for GCA. Significant variation in prebiopsy erythrocyte sedimentation rate (ESR), arterial specimen length and positive results was noted amongst hospitals. Multivariable analysis revealed that patient age, ESR value and specimen length were independent predictors of GCA. Positive biopsies had significantly longer median specimen length compared with negative biopsies: $1 \cdot 2$ (range $0 \cdot 3 - 8 \cdot 5$) *versus* $1 \cdot 0$ ($0 \cdot 2 - 8 \cdot 0$) cm respectively ($P = 0 \cdot 001$). Receiver operating characteristic (ROC) analysis identified postfixation specimen length of at least $0 \cdot 7$ cm as the cut-off length with highest positive predictive value for a positive biopsy (area under ROC curve $0 \cdot 574$). Biopsies with specimen length of $0 \cdot 7$ cm or more had a significantly higher rate of positive results than smaller specimens ($24 \cdot 8$ *versus* $12 \cdot 9$ per cent respectively; odds ratio $2 \cdot 17$, $P = 0 \cdot 001$).

Conclusion.—Specimen length and ESR were independent prognostic factors of a positive TAB result. A uniform referral practice and standard specimen length of approximately 1 cm could help eliminate discrepancies in the results of TAB.

▶ The take-home message for surgical pathologists of this article by Ypsilantis et al is that the length of the temporal artery biopsy tissue (in toto, if fragmented) should be reported in the pathology report. According to Ypsilantis and colleagues, the optimal biopsy specimen should be greater than 0.7 cm. A limitation in the manuscript is the failure to report or analyze important tissue preparation metrics, such as the number of levels (the authors only report that the minimum number of levels was 3), tissue sections on the levels, the depth of cutting into the block (eg, exhausting the block), and the number of cross sections grossly prepared. The authors have not examined the relationship of the false-negative frequency to the amount of tissue histologically examined (dependent on different analytic protocols). Once again, specimen quality is a major factor that affects diagnostic accuracy, and specimen quality is affected by clinical and laboratory factors. For additional reading, please see the reference section.[1,2]

S. S. Raab, MD

References

1. Mahr A, Saba M, Kambouchner M, et al. Temporal artery biopsy for diagnosing giant cell arteritis: the longer, the better? *Ann Rheum Dis.* 2006;65:826-828.
2. Zhou L, Luneau K, Weyand CM, Biousse V, Newman NJ, Grossniklaus HE. Clinicopathologic correlations in giant cell arteritis: a retrospective study of 107 cases. *Ophthalmology.* 2009;116:1574-1580.

Endomyocardial biopsy—when and how?
Veinot JP (Univ of Ottawa Heart Inst, Ontario, Canada)
Cardiovasc Pathol 20:291-296, 2011

Endomyocardial biopsy is a commonly performed useful procedure utilized for the evaluation of cardiac tissue. Biopsy may be used to monitor transplant rejection, but it has many other applications including the evaluation of myocarditis, cardiomyopathy, chest pain, arrhythmia, and secondary involvement by systemic diseases. Drug toxicity may be evaluated and neoplasms may be biopsied. Recent developments include advances in myocardial and viral molecular biology and advances in image or electrophysiology guided biopsy. The utility of endomyocardial biopsy is reviewed with consideration of these advances.

▶ Veinot has provided a superb summary of the value and description of the endomyocardial biopsy. In some academic centers, endomyocardial biopsy is performed in transplant patients and in a few other cases, although in other institutions, endomyocardial biopsy is performed infrequently. Veinot reports that the infrequency of the performance of the endomyocardial biopsy procedure has resulted in decreased pathologist expertise, which, in turn, may result in fewer procedures, as the nondefinitive diagnosis frequency increases. The field of endomyocardial tissue biopsy interpretation could implement a system of expert telepathology centers on which less experienced pathologists could rely. The article by Veinot describes a variety of lesions that may be diagnosed definitively and lesions that are more challenging. It is worth keeping a copy of this article if you do not see endomyocardial biopsies frequently and do not have a more detailed textbook. The photomicrographs are relatively few but are good examples of common and rare disease. For additional reading, please see the reference section.[1,2]

S. S. Raab, MD

References

1. Veinot JP. Diagnostic endomyocardial biopsy pathology—general biopsy considerations, and its use for myocarditis and cardiomyopathy: a review. *Can J Cardiol.* 2002;18:55-65.
2. Nippoldt TB, Edwards WD, Holmes DR Jr, Reeder GS, Hartzler GO, Smith HC. Right Ventricular endomyocardial biopsy: clinicopathologic correlates in 100 consecutive patients. *Mayo Clin Proc.* 1982;57:407-418.

8 Soft Tissue and Bone

Low-Grade Fibromyxoid Sarcoma: A Clinicopathologic Study of 33 Cases With Long-Term Follow-Up

Evans HL (Univ of Texas M.D. Anderson Cancer Ctr, Houston)
Am J Surg Pathol 35:1450-1462, 2011

Cases listed in the U.T.M.D Anderson Cancer Center files as low-grade fibromyxoid sarcoma and originally diagnosed before 2004 were reviewed. They were included in the study if the diagnosis was confirmed and if there was adequate histologic material and clinical information with at least 5 years of follow-up. Thirty-three cases met the study criteria. The patients were 6 to 52 years old at the time of diagnosis (median, 29 y); 19 were male and 14 were female. The most common tumor locations were the shoulder area (5), thigh (5), and inguinal area (4). Tumor size varied from 1.5 to 16 cm (median, 9.4 cm) in those cases in which it was known. The typical histologic findings were contrasting fibrous and myxoid areas, moderate to low cellularity, bland-appearing spindle cells with no or slight nuclear pleomorphism and rare mitotic figures, and a swirling, whorled growth pattern. Prominent vascularity in myxoid areas and perivascular hypercellularity were fairly common, whereas larger hypercellular zones were sometimes seen in primary tumors but were more frequent in recurrences (local) and metastases. Hypercellular regions sometimes had round rather than spindle cells, a diffuse sheet-like cell arrangement, and/or a somewhat increased mitotic rate. Very hypocellular fibrotic areas were also observed and sometimes had thick collagen bundles. Pericollagenous rosettes were present in 6 cases but not in all specimens from these. Other growth pattern variations included storiform, fascicular-herringbone, and patternless areas; uncommonly noted were cell clusters, strands, palisades, and a retiform network. Additional unusual features were moderate nuclear pleomorphism (seen mostly in recurrent and metastatic tumors), cysts, osseous metaplasia, and a tigroid pattern with alternating fibrous and myxoid strips. One patient had a recurrence with features of sclerosing epithelioid fibrosarcoma, whereas 2 had dedifferentiated recurrences with anaplastic predominantly round cells and numerous mitotic figures. Fourteen patients died of tumor after 3 (this patient's tumor became dedifferentiated) to 42 years (median, 15 y). Nineteen patients were alive at last follow-up of 5½ to 70 years (median, 13 y), 6 with tumor and 13 without. Twenty-one patients had recurrence after intervals of up to 15 years (median, 3½ y), and 15 had metastases (mostly in the lungs and pleura) after periods of up to 45 years (median, 5 y). Except for dedifferentiation, which led to short survival after it occurred, histologic differences were not related to tumor behavior or patient survival. The 4 patients whose neoplasms measured <3.5 cm were all tumor free at last follow-up.

▶ This article by Evans is a beautifully illustrated series of 33 cases of low-grade fibromyxoid sarcomas with long-term (> 5 years) follow-up. Most of the photomicrographs depict various histologic presentations of the primary tumor or recurrences. As low-grade fibromyxoid sarcomas have variable growth patterns, degrees of cellularity, and unusual features (eg, osseous metaplasia), the ability to make a definitive diagnosis on an initial core biopsy may be quite challenging. The typical appearance is that of a neoplasm of moderate to low cellularity of spindle cells with no or little nuclear pleomorphism and fibrous and myxoid appearing zones. The mitotic rate is low (0 to 1 mitotic figures per 10 high-power fields). Although the findings generally appear benign, the tumor is capable of malignant behavior, and several of the patients in this series died of their disease. Evans believes that low-grade fibromyxoid sarcoma may be related to epithelioid fibrosarcoma. This series focuses on the follow-up and the variety of appearances and not on providing a differential diagnoses. For additional reading, please see the reference section.[1,2]

S. S. Raab, MD

References

1. Evans HL. Low-grade fibromyxoid sarcoma. A report of 12 cases. *Am J Surg Pathol.* 1993;17:595-600.
2. Goodlad JR, Mentzel T, Fletcher CD. Low grade fibromyxoid sarcoma: clinico-pathological analysis of eleven new cases in support of a distinct entity. *Histopathology.* 1995;26:229-237.

Percutaneous CT-guided biopsy of the musculoskeletal system: Results of 2027 cases
Rimondi E, Rossi G, Bartalena T, et al (Istituto Ortopedico Rizzoli, Bologna, Italy; Univ of Bologna, Italy; et al)
Eur J Radiol 77:34-42, 2011

Introduction.—Biopsy of the musculoskeletal system is useful in the management of bone lesions particularly in oncology but they are often challenging procedures with a significant risk of complications. Computed tomography (CT)-guided needle biopsies may decrease these risks but doubts still exist about their diagnostic accuracy. This retrospective analysis of the experience of a single institution with percutaneous CT-guided biopsy of musculoskeletal lesions evaluates the results of these biopsies for bone lesions either in the appendicular skeleton or in the spine, and defines indications.

Materials and Methods.—We reviewed the results of 2027 core needle biopsies performed over the past 18 years at the authors' institution. The results obtained are subject of this paper.

TABLE 6.—Accuracy Rates Versus Histotype Regardless Site, Lesion Size and Needle Gauge

Histotype	I CT-Guided Biopsy 1567 (77.3%)	II CT-Guided Biopsy 340 (16.8%)	Open Biopsy 120 (5.9%)
Primary benign	360	63	39
Pseudotumoral	66	39	27
Primary malignant	334	39	1
Systemic malignant	111	11	33
Secondary malignant	320	33	1
Inflammatory disease	202	53	9
Other[a,b]	174	102[b]	10
	Overall accuracy 1097 (94.1%)		*Percutaneous biopsy failure 120 (5.9%)*

[a]Paget's disease, gout, metabolic disease (e.g. hyperparathyroidism).
[b]41 Cases further defined by the second percutaneous biopsy included in this group (see text): aspecific non-pathologic diagnoses as stress fractures, osteoporotic fragments with bone resorption, edema in irradiated bone, bone sclerosis or necrosis, and subchondral cystic lesion in osteoarthritis.

Results.—In 1567 cases the correct diagnosis was made with the first CT-guided needle biopsy (77.3% accuracy rate), in 408 cases the sample was not diagnostic and in 52 inadequate. Within 30 days these 408 patients underwent another biopsy, which was diagnostic in 340 cases with a final diagnostic accuracy of 94%. Highest accuracy rates were obtained in primary and secondary malignant lesions. Most false negative results were found in cervical lesions and in benign, pseudotumoral, flogistic, and systemic pathologies. There were 22 complications (18 transient paresis, 3 haematomas, 1 retroperitoneal haematoma) which had no influence on the treatment strategy, nor on patient outcome.

Conclusion.—This technique is reliable and safe and should be considered nowadays the gold standard for biopsies of the musculoskeletal system (Table 6).

▶ Pathology groups are seeing an increase in the number of tissues from core needle biopsies of the musculoskeletal system, as the needle biopsy technique is safer and more efficient to perform than the open biopsy. Table 6 shows the diagnostic accuracy and classification by general disease process. Sclerotic bone lesions (prevalently intracompartmental) had a higher inadequate frequency compared with lytic and mixed lytic-sclerotic lesions. In addition, a higher percentage of spinal lesions (11%) required open biopsy compared with lesions from other sites. Of the 52 cases that were initially inadequate, an open biopsy found 15 aneurysmal bone cysts and 26 systemic disease (eg, lymphoma or plasma cell dyscrasia). Sufficient details are not provided to determine if initial failures in the computed tomography—guided methods were secondary to sampling, processing, interpretation, or a combination of problems. It would be interesting to determine if changes in sampling technique would further affect adequacy or if the utilization of touch preparations or combined fine-needle aspiration/core biopsy would affect the quality of sampling. For additional reading, please see the reference section.[1,2]

S. S. Raab, MD

References

1. Skrzynski MC, Biermann JS, Montag A, Simon MA. Diagnostic accuracy and charge-savings of outpatient core needle biopsy compared with open biopsy of musculoskeletal tumors. *J Bone Joint Surg Am.* 1996;78:644-649.
2. Yang YJ, Damron TA. Comparison of needle core biopsy and fine-needle aspiration for diagnostic accuracy in musculoskeletal lesions. *Arch Pathol Lab Med.* 2004;128:759-764.

BCL-6 expression in mesenchymal tumours: an immunohistochemical and fluorescence in situ hybridisation study

Walters MP, McPhail ED, Law ME, et al (Mayo Clinic, Rochester, MN)
J Clin Pathol 64:866-869, 2011

The BCL-6 proto-oncogene encodes a transcriptional repressor protein. Among normal tissues, BCL-6 expression is confined to germinal center B-cells and a subpopulation of T-helper cells. Little is known about BCL-6 expression in mesenchymal tissues. We examined a series of solitary fibrous tumor (SFT) and other mesenchymal tumors for BCL-6 expression. Immunohistochemistry for BCL-6 was performed on 64 mesenchymal tumors [26 SFT (19 benign/uncertain, 7 malignant), 6 synovial sarcomas (SS), 5 gastrointestinal stromal tumors (GIST), 5 malignant peripheral nerve sheath tumors (MPNST), 5 leiomyosarcomas (LMS), 9 leiomyomas (LM) 4 desmoid tumors (DT), 4 perineuriomas (PN)]. Nuclear immunoreactivity was considered positive. Six BCL-6 positive SFT were also tested for BCL-6 gene rearrangement/amplification by FISH. Nuclear expression of BCL-6 was seen in 13/26 SFT, 5/5 LMS, 1/9 LM, 5/6 SS, 1/5 GIST, 1/5 MPNST, 1/4 PN, and 0/5 DT. BCL-6 expression was significantly more frequent in malignant (6/7) as compared with benign/uncertain SFT (6/19) (p=0.02) and in LMS (5/5) as compared with LM (1/9) (p=0.003). FISH for BCL-6 rearrangement/amplification was negative in all tested cases. We have observed BCL-6 expression in 50% or more of SFT, SS, and LMS, and in a lesser percentage of LM, GIST, MPNST and PN. Significantly more frequent expression of BCL-6 in malignant compared with benign/uncertain SFT and in LMS compared with LM suggests abnormalities in the BCL-6 signaling pathway may contribute to malignant transformation in at least some mesenchymal tumors. It is unlikely that BCL-6 expression in mesenchymal tumors is due to BCL-6 gene amplification or rearrangement. amplification or rearrangement (Table 1).

▶ The article by Walters et al is a classic example of a weakly designed immunohistochemical investigation in which a newer antibody is applied to a group of tumors to evaluate the reactivity pattern. Presumably, if this pattern is unique, we could use the marker to differentiate tumor types. The findings indicate that BCL-6 should not be used for the immunohistochemical classification of smooth muscle neoplasms (Table 1). This is not a surprise, as not a lot of immunohistochemical markers are useful for this neoplasm group. The authors also reported

TABLE 1.—Immunohistochemical Results

Tumour Type	BCL-6 Positive (%)	Staining Intensity
SFT, benign or uncertain malignant potential (n=19)	7 (37)	1+: 4
		2+: 3
SFT, malignant (n=7)	6 (86)	1+: 3
		2+: 3
Perineurioma (n=4)	1 (25)	1+
Synovial sarcoma (n=6)	5 (83)	1+: 4
		3+: 1
GIST (n=5)	1 (20)	2+
Desmoid fibromatosis (n=4)	0 (0)	
MPNST (n=5)	1 (20)	2+
Leiomyoma (n=9)	1 (11)	1+
Leiomyosarcoma (n=5)	5 (100)	1+: 2
		2+: 3

BCL-6, B-cell lymphoma-6; SFT, solitary fibrous tumour; GIST, gastrointestinal stromal tumour; MPNST, malignant peripheral nerve sheath tumour.

greater expression in histologically malignant than benign cases, although the data do not indicate that this finding should be used in the diagnostic subclassification. For additional reading, please see the reference section.[1,2]

S. S. Raab, MD

References

1. Dent AL, Vasanwala FH, Toney LM. Regulation of gene expression by the proto-oncogene BCL-6. *Crit Rev Oncol Hematol.* 2002;41:1-9.
2. Dent AL, Shaffer AL, Yu X, Allman D, Staudt LM. Control of inflammation, cytokine expression, and germinal center formation by BCL-6. *Science.* 1997;276:589-592.

9 Female Genital Tract

Correlation between invasive pattern and immunophenotypic alterations in endocervical adenocarcinoma
Stewart CJR, Crook ML, Little L, et al (King Edward Memorial Hosp, Perth, Western Australia, Australia)
Histopathology 58:720-728, 2011

Aims.—To assess the immunophenotypic changes associated with epithelial-mesenchymal transition (EMT) in endocervical adenocarcinoma, and correlate the findings with tumour morphology including growth pattern.

Methods and Results.—Twenty-seven endocervical adenocarcinomas were studied using a panel of immunohistochemical markers to vimentin, cyclin D1, E-cadherin, beta-catenin, p16 protein and cytokeratin 7. There were 24 moderately differentiated and three poorly differentiated tumours. Fourteen of the moderately differentiated carcinomas showed a focal infiltrative component, typically towards the deep tumour margin (invasive front), comprising attenuated glands, small cell clusters and single cells. These foci typically showed cytological alteration including loss of cellular polarity and cytoplasmic eosinophilia, while immunohistochemistry demonstrated reduced cell membrane E-cadherin and beta catenin labelling, and expression of cyclin D1 and, in some cases, vimentin. Similar immunophenotypic changes were focally observed at the deep aspect of some larger 'conventional' tumour glands. No consistent changes were observed in the poorly differentiated carcinomas.

Conclusions.—Endocervical adenocarcinomas that demonstrate an infiltrative growth pattern show immunophenotypic changes consistent with EMT. Frequently, these are accompanied by a morphological alteration in the tumour cells and the changes exhibit a specific micro-anatomical distribution. Epithelial-mesenchymal transition may represent an important mechanism in the progression of some endocervical neoplasms (Fig 3).

▶ In this article, the authors build on their previous work studying the distribution of cyclin D1 in endocervical lesions and specifically apply the distribution of multiple immunohistochemical stains to the concept of epithelial-mesenchymal transition (EMT). EMT is thought to play a role in the growth of invasive carcinomas; the histologic correlate of this process is increased expression of mesenchymal markers at the invading front of carcinomas. Of note, the authors describe various histomorphologic changes in invasive foci of endocervical adenocarcinomas such as nuclear enlargement, cytoplasmic

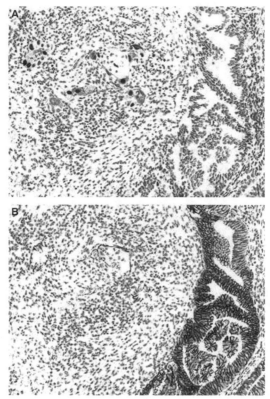

FIGURE 3.—Infiltrative tumour elements (left field) show cyclin D1 expression (A) and fragmentation of E-cadherin expression (B), whereas an adjacent conventional tumour gland (right field) shows retained membranous E-cadherin staining and minimal cyclin D1 reactivity. (Reprinted from Stewart CJR, Crook ML, Little L, et al. Correlation between invasive pattern and immunophenotypic alterations in endocervical adenocarcinoma. *Histopathology.* 2011;58:720-728, with permission from Blackwell Publishing Limited.)

eosinophilia, and loss of polarization, which are more readily detected on hematoxylin and eosin (H&E)-stained sections than by immunohistochemistry, highlighting the importance of an initial detailed and thorough examination of a tumor by conventional light microscopy. Whether an endocervical adenocarcinoma is in situ or invasive is a frequently encountered problem, however, and the addition of immunohistochemical stains to aid in recognition of invasive foci would be most welcome. Cyclin D1 seems to offer some utility in this matter; the authors found that it consistently labeled the infiltrative neoplastic elements of the tumors included in the study, including some subtle areas that were overlooked on initial H&E diagnosis (Fig 3). Of the other markers tested, E-cadherin also proved useful, showing an inverse staining pattern—namely, there was some degree of loss of membranous staining in infiltrative foci or at the deep edges of conventional tumor glands. The authors raise the possibility that various histomorphologies of endocervical adenocarcinoma may in fact be due to distinct mechanisms of tumor growth, of which EMT is only one. This is an intriguing theory, although not further explored in the current study. It does lend evidence to the idea that EMT occurs in at least some endocervical adenocarcinomas and that Cyclin D1 and E-cadherin may have practical utility in the evaluation of infiltrative growth in these cancers. For further reading, see the reference section.[1,2]

M. D. Post, MD

References

1. Al-Nafussi A. Histopathological challenges in assessing invasion in squamous, glandular neoplasia of the cervix. *Curr Diagn Pathol.* 2006;12:364-393.
2. Iwatsuki M, Mimori K, Yokobori T, et al. Epithelial—mesenchymal transition in cancer development and its clinical significance. *Cancer Sci.* 2010;101:293-299.

Significant Variation in the Assessment of Cervical Involvement in Endometrial Carcinoma: An Interobserver Variation Study
McCluggage WG, Hirschowitz L, Wilson GE, et al (Belfast Health and Social Care Trust, Northern Ireland; Birmingham Women's Hosp, UK; Manchester Univ Hosps NHS Foundation Trust, Manchester, England; et al)
Am J Surg Pathol 35:289-294, 2011

The histologic assessment of cervical involvement in endometrial carcinoma may be problematic for a number of reasons, but an accurate evaluation of this is important for correct staging, dictating the need for adjuvant therapy, and prognostication. In this study, we assessed interobserver variation in the evaluation of cervical involvement in hysterectomy specimens of endometrial carcinoma among 6 specialist gynecologic pathologists. Seventy-six cases of endometrial carcinoma enriched for cases exhibiting some perceived issue in the assessment of cervical involvement were used. In all the cases, a single slide of the primary tumor in the uterine corpus and a single slide of the cervix were circulated among the 6 participants who filled in a proforma. On the basis of the responses, the tumors were staged according to the 1988 International Federation of Gynecology and Obstetrics (FIGO) staging system (I, IIA, IIB) and the 2009 FIGO staging system (I, II). Using the 1988 FIGO staging system, the unweighted and weighted κ values between individual observers ranged from 0.3115 to 0.6139 (average 0.4675) and from 0.3492 to 0.6533 (average 0.5065), respectively. The κ values between observers for the 2009 FIGO staging system ranged from 0.3481 to 0.6862 (average 0.4908). Although enriched for problematic cases, our study shows that there is at most a fair-to-good agreement among specialist gynecologic pathologists in the assessment of cervical involvement in endometrial carcinoma. Problematic factors include determination of the junction between the lower uterine segment and upper endocervix, the distinction between "floaters" and true cervical glandular involvement, the distinction between cervical glandular involvement and stromal involvement, and the distinction between cervical glandular involvement and reactive non-neoplastic lesions of the endocervical

TABLE 2.—Kappa Values Between Individual Observers

	Unweighted 1988	Weighted 1988	2009
1 vs 2	0.6031	0.6533	0.6862
1 vs 3	0.5219	0.5444	0.5111
1 vs 4	0.4325	0.4753	0.3712
1 vs 5	0.6139	0.6425	0.5709
1 vs 6	0.4505	0.4854	0.4704
2 vs 3	0.4534	0.4724	0.4896
2 vs 4	0.3115	0.3853	0.3658
2 vs 5	0.4948	0.5629	0.5350
2 vs 6	0.3709	0.4907	0.4246
3 vs 4	0.4775	0.5369	0.4497
3 vs 5	0.4566	0.4501	0.4775
3 vs 6	0.3564	0.3492	0.3481
4 vs 5	0.4889	0.5102	0.5554
4 vs 6	0.4198	0.4773	0.5353
5 vs 6	0.5601	0.5576	0.5709

glands. There is a need for specialist pathology groups dealing with gynecologic cancers to develop and disseminate recommendations regarding the assessment of cervical involvement in endometrial carcinoma (Table 2).

▶ In evaluation of hysterectomy specimens for endometrial carcinoma, one variable that must always be reported is the presence or absence of cervical involvement. Based on the previous (1988) Fédération Internationale de Gynécologie Obstétrique (FIGO) staging system, a distinction was made between endocervical glandular versus endocervical stromal involvement (Stage IIA vs IIB), whereas the updated (2009) FIGO staging system only considers stromal involvement (Stage II). Although typically straightforward, there are instances in which it is difficult to determine whether the cervix is involved by carcinoma and whether it involves exclusively the glandular component. The authors (all experts in gynecologic pathology) here undertook a study of interobserver variability in 76 cases of endometrial carcinoma with respect to cervical involvement (Table 2). This was deliberately enriched for difficult or problematic cases, and therefore the finding that there was only fair-to-good agreement (kappa value 0.4–0.75) in the majority of cases may be artificially lowered. However, it does highlight the need for some standardization and/or publication of guidelines for use in general practice. What also became clear as a result of evaluating these cases was that various pathologists had different opinions as to what constitutes cervical (vs lower uterine segment) involvement and how to define stromal (vs deep glandular) involvement. Given the potential for markedly different therapies based on whether an endometrial carcinoma is staged as FIGO I or FIGO II (often observation vs adjuvant radiotherapy), improving the reproducibility of this variable is essential. Not surprisingly, there was a greater degree of agreement using the 2009 staging system, because exclusively glandular involvement by endometrial carcinoma remains within the definition of Stage I disease. However, the authors point out that some oncologists will administer vaginal brachytherapy in this situation, necessitating the need for a standardized approach and reporting schema. A final area of contention that arose was whether the presence of carcinoma exclusively in vascular spaces was sufficient to "upstage"; however, per reported communication, it is not. This conundrum, as well as the presence of exclusively vascular space invasion in the parametrium or adnexa, arises frequently enough to warrant wider dissemination of standardized guidelines. One suggested avenue for the development and dissemination of this information is via the International Society of Gynecologic Pathologists. For further reading, see the reference section.[1,2]

M. D. Post, MD

References

1. Pecorelli S. Revised FIGO staging for carcinoma of the vulva, cervix, and endometrium. *Int J Gynaecol Obstet.* 2009;105:103-104.
2. Jordan LB, Al-Nafussi A. Clinicopathological study of the pattern and significance of cervical involvement in cases of endometrial adenocarcinoma. *Int J Gynecol Cancer.* 2002;12:42-48.

Mutation and Loss of Expression of *ARID1A* in Uterine Low-grade Endometrioid Carcinoma
Guan B, Mao T-L, Panuganti PK, et al (Johns Hopkins Univ School of Medicine, Baltimore, MD; Natl Taiwan Univ College of Medicine, Taipei; et al)
Am J Surg Pathol 35:625-632, 2011

ARID1A is a recently identified tumor suppressor gene that is mutated in approximately 50% of ovarian clear cell and 30% of ovarian endometrioid carcinomas. The mutation is associated with loss of protein expression as assessed by immunohistochemistry. In this study, we evaluated *ARID1A* immunoreactivity in a wide variety of carcinomas to determine the prevalence of *ARID1A* inactivation in carcinomas. Mutational analysis of *ARID1A* was carried out in selected cases. Immunoreactivity was not detected (corresponding to inactivation or mutation of *ARID1A*) in 36 (3.6%) of 995 tumors. Uterine low-grade endometrioid carcinomas showed a relatively high-frequency loss of *ARID1A* expression, as 15 (26%) of 58 cases were negative. The other tumor that had a relatively high-frequency loss of *ARID1A* expression was gastric carcinoma (11%). Mutational analysis showed 10 (40%) of 25 uterine endometrioid carcinomas; none of 12 uterine serous carcinomas and none of 56 ovarian serous and mucinous carcinomas harbored somatic *ARID1A* mutations. All mutations in endometrioid carcinomas were nonsense or insertion/deletion mutations, and tumors with *ARID1A* mutations showed complete loss or clonal loss of *ARID1A* expression. In conclusion, this study is the first large-scale analysis of a wide variety of carcinomas showing that uterine low-grade endometrioid carcinoma is the predominant tumor type harboring *ARID1A* mutations and frequent loss of *ARID1A* expression. These findings suggest that the molecular pathogenesis of low-grade uterine endometrioid carcinoma is similar to that of ovarian low-grade endometrioid and clear cell carcinoma, tumors that have previously been shown

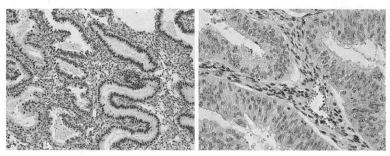

FIGURE 2.—*ARID1A* immunoreactivity in representative carcinoma types (right panel) and their normal tissue counterparts (left panel). Negative staining (undetectable level) of *ARID1A* in an International Federation of Gynecology and Obstetrics grade I endometrioid carcinoma (A). (Reprinted from Guan B, Mao T-L, Panuganti PK, et al. Mutation and loss of expression of *ARID1A* in uterine low-grade endometrioid carcinoma. *Am J Surg Pathol.* 2011;35:625-632, with permission from Lippincott Williams & Wilkins.)

to have a high-frequency loss of expression and mutation of *ARID1A* (Fig 2A).

▶ *ARID1A* has been shown to be mutated in endometriosis-related clear cell carcinoma and endometrioid ovarian carcinoma; however, a systematic study of its mutation in other tumor types had not previously been undertaken. The authors tested 995 tumors and normal tissues via tissue microarray using immunohistochemistry looking for loss of expression. They found 26% of uterine low-grade endometrioid carcinomas had lost *ARID1A* expression (confirmed via whole-tissue sections; Fig 2A). While it is generally tricky to evaluate loss of expression, the authors sidestep that issue by considering any level of *ARID1A* immunoreactivity as a positive case. They then took a subset of uterine low-grade endometrioid carcinomas and performed mutational analysis, finding that complete loss of expression by immunohistochemistry significantly correlated with mutational status. Their results suggest that *ARID1A* mutation may contribute to the development of carcinomas from endometrial-derived tissue. This is an intriguing concept, as the molecular link between intrauterine cancers and extrauterine endometriosis has not yet been studied in detail.

Some limitations of the study include the number and distribution of tumor types included (eg, 221 high-grade serous carcinomas were studied in comparison with only 58 grade 1 endometrioid adenocarcinomas and 17 type II endometrial cancers). Further, loss of *ARID1A* expression by immunohistochemistry was also observed at some frequency in other tumor types (11% of gastric carcinomas and 10% of pulmonary squamous cell carcinomas), potentially limiting its utility. While *ARID1A* shows promise in further elucidating the molecular pathways leading to the development of type I endometrial cancers and endometriosis-associated ovarian cancers, its utility in routine pathology practice remains to be seen. For further reading, see the reference section.[1,2]

M. D. Post, MD

References

1. Wiegand KC, Shah SP, Al-Agha OM, et al. ARID1A mutations in endometriosis-associated ovarian carcinomas. *N Engl J Med*. 2010;363:1532-1543.
2. Jones S, Wang TL, Shih IM, et al. Frequent mutations of chromatin remodeling gene ARID1A in ovarian clear cell carcinoma. *Science*. 2010;330:228-231.

Immunoexpression of PAX 8 in Endometrial Cancer: Relation to High-Grade Carcinoma and *p53*

Brunner AH, Riss P, Heinze G, et al (Med Univ of Vienna, Austria)
Int J Gynecol Pathol 30:569-575, 2011

PAX 8 is a crucial transcription factor for organogenesis of the thyroid gland, kidney, and the Müllerian system and plays an essential role in cell proliferation. The purpose of this study was to evaluate the association between *p53* and PAX 8 expression and the clinical value of PAX 8 in endometrial carcinoma. We detected 106 consecutive patients with primary endometrial carcinoma (type I/ endometrioid, n=84; type II/ nonendometrioid, n=20; rare subtypes, n=2) who were treated at our institution between 1999 and 2009. Of the 106 patients, 97 cases were eligible for further investigations. PAX 8 and *p53* expression were assessed using immunohistochemistry from paraffin-embedded tissue blocks. Results were correlated with clinical data. PAX 8 immunoreaction was found in 70 of 97 (72.1%) patients, including 56 of 77 (72.7%) endometrioid carcinomas and 13 of 18 (72.2%) type II carcinomas. A positive correlation was observed between PAX 8 and *p53* expression ($P=0.0005$), histologic type ($P=0.04$), and histologic grade ($P=0.02$). No association was found between PAX 8 expression and tumor stage, vascular space involvement, lymph node involvement, and age of the patients. Furthermore, using univariate and multivariate analyses, no statistically significant relationship could be evaluated between patient survival data and PAX 8 expression. PAX 8 is expressed in the vast majority of endometrial carcinomas both of endometrioid and nonendometrioid type. PAX 8 overexpression correlates with *p53* expression and high-grade endometrial carcinomas but seems not to be useful as a prognostic parameter (Fig 1).

▶ Paired-box (PAX) transcription factors play a role in normal and neoplastic development. Recent studies have found that 1 of the 9 genes, *PAX 8*, is frequently expressed in renal, thyroid, and Mullerian neoplasms. In fact, reactivity was seen in 87% of ovarian neoplasms. The expression of *PAX 8* in endometrial cancer and its potential use as a prognostic marker has not been studied previously. This article details the results of immunostaining of 97 cases of endometrial carcinoma (both type I and type II histologic subtypes) with *PAX 8* and *p53* (Fig 1). The authors then examine the significance of the staining pattern with respect to different clinicopathologic and prognostic parameters. They found that, although *PAX 8* staining was significantly associated with nonendometrioid and high-grade carcinomas, it was not significantly

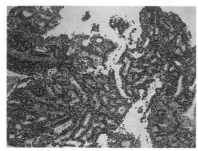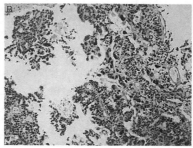

FIGURE 1.—(A) Positive immunohistochemical staining for PAX 8 in an endometrioid endometrial (type I) carcinoma (magnification: 100×). (B) Immunohistochemical staining for PAX 8 in a serous endometrial (type II) carcinoma. Strong nuclear reactivity is shown in many of the neoplastic nuclei (magnification: 100×). (Reprinted from Brunner AH, Riss P, Heinze G, et al. Immunoexpression of PAX 8 in endometrial cancer: relation to high-grade carcinoma and *p53*. *Int J Gynecol Pathol.* 2011;30:569-575, with permission from International Society of Gynecological Pathologists.)

associated with other studied variables. This is in contrast with PAX 8 expression in ovarian cancer, where survival analyses showed that overexpression was an unfavorable prognostic indicator. The study does provide the first solid evidence of the relationship between *PAX 8* and the functional restricted *p53* mechanism (protein overexpression as determined by immunohistochemical staining); however, lack of prognostic significance limits its adoption in routine clinical use. The role of PAX 8 in precursor lesions in the endometrium is unclear and warrants further study, as its possible influence on *p53* expression or function may contribute to antiapoptotic pathways in endometrial tumorigenesis. For further reading, see the reference section.[1,2]

M. D. Post, MD

References

1. Alkushi A, Köbel M, Kalloger SE, Gilks CB. High-grade endometrial carcinoma: serous and grade 3 endometrioid carcinomas have different immunophenotypes and outcomes. *Int J Gynecol Pathol.* 2010;29:343-350.
2. Chi N, Epstein JA. Getting your PAX straight: PAX proteins in development and disease. *Trends Genet.* 2002;18:41-47.

IMP2 Expression Distinguishes Endometrioid From Serous Endometrial Adenocarcinomas

Zhang L, Liu Y, Hao S, et al (Univ of Massachusetts Med Ctr, Worcester)
Am J Surg Pathol 35:868-872, 2011

Among various endometrial adenocarcinomas, endometrioid carcinoma can be very difficult to separate from serous carcinomas. Various biomarkers have been studied with proven value, including p53, Ki-67, and p16. In this study, we present data on another biomarker, IMP2, which we believe is sensitive and specific. Using 320 endometrial biopsy cases, we demonstrate that IMP2 is normally expressed in all proliferative and inactive endometrial

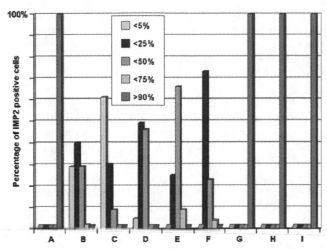

FIGURE 2.—Illustration of the percentages of tumor cells that lost IMP2 expression in lesions of benign (A), endometrioid carcinoma regardless grade (B), FIGO-I endometrioid carcinoma (C), FIGO-II endometrioid carcinoma (D), FIGO-III endometrioid carcinoma (E), endometrioid component of mixed carcinoma (F), serous carcinoma regardless mixed or pure (G), pure serous carcinoma (H), serous component of mixed carcinoma (I). (Reprinted from Zhang L, Liu Y, Hao S, et al. IMP2 expression distinguishes endometrioid from serous endometrial adenocarcinomas. *Am J Surg Pathol.* 2011;35:868-872, with permission from Lippincott Williams & Wilkins.)

glandular cells. The pattern of such expression is unchanged in serous carcinomas. IMP2 expression is, however, lost in all cases of endometrioid carcinomas by at least 25% to >95% of tumor cell populations. Therefore, loss of IMP2 expression can differentiate endometrioid from serous carcinomas. Such finding of IMP2 expression remained the same in mixed endometrioid and serous carcinomas; IMP2 expression is lost in all endometrioid components by at least 25% of tumor cell population, whereas it remained diffuse and strong in all serous components of carcinomas (Fig 2).

▶ A not infrequently encountered problem in gynecologic pathology is the discrimination between endometrioid and serous carcinomas of the endometrium, particularly in sometimes scanty biopsy specimens. Currently, the combination of Ki-67, p53, and p16 are felt to provide useful information; however, no single marker (or even a complete panel) has proven entirely satisfactory. The authors here introduce the use of a member of a family of mRNA binding proteins, which is normally expressed in many adult human tissues as an extremely sensitive and specific marker to distinguish between endometrioid and serous endometrial adenocarcinoma. Based on 320 biopsy specimens, they found that loss of IMP2 cytoplasmic staining in > 25% of malignant cells had a 100% sensitivity and specificity in separating the 2 morphologies (Fig 2). Interestingly, low-grade endometrioid adenocarcinomas (FIGO grade I) had preferential loss of IMP2 expression beyond that seen in higher-grade tumors (FIGO grades II and III). This suggests that IMP2 is involved in the early pathogenesis of type I endometrial carcinomas, although no sufficient explanation currently exists as to how expression is regained in the higher-grade tumors. On the surface, this appears to provide an excellent new tool for use in a situation with profound clinical implications. It does, however, also raise some as-yet unanswered questions. The diagnoses of the test cases used here were confirmed by 2 pathologists, but no mention is made of whether these were classic examples of the entities or more difficult cases. It would be interesting to take cases that had discordant diagnoses and evaluate performance of the antibody on such cases. It would also be of interest to test other type II carcinomas of the endometrium, such as clear cell carcinoma or carcinosarcoma to further elucidate the putative role of IMP2 in development solely of type I cancers. While there are still questions remaining to be answered, including the actual mechanism by which IMP2 participates in endometrial carcinogenesis, this commercially available marker offers a powerful addition to the arsenal of immunohistochemistry we often rely on to distinguish between these entities. For further reading, see the reference section.[1,2]

M. D. Post, MD

References

1. Ioffe OB. Recent developments and selected diagnostic problems in carcinomas of the endometrium. *Am J Clin Pathol.* 2005;124:S42-S51.
2. Nielsen FC, Nielsen J, Christiansen J. A family of IGF-II mRNA binding proteins (IMP) involved in RNA trafficking. *Scand J Clin Lab Invest Suppl.* 2001;234: 93-99.

Should grade 3 endometrioid endometrial carcinoma be considered a type 2 cancer—A clinical and pathological evaluation
Voss MA, Ganesan R, Ludeman L, et al (Cheltenham General Hosp, Gloucestershire, UK; Birmingham Women's Hosp NHS trust, UK; et al)
Gynecol Oncol 2011 [Epub ahead of print]

Objective.—Endometrial cancer is classified into: Type I estrogen-dependent endometrioid adenocarcinoma, with good prognosis and type 2 non-estrogen-dependent cancer with serous or clear cell histology and poor prognosis. Grade 3 endometrioid cancers (G3 EEC), share features of type 1 and type 2 cancer and have not been classified as either. This study compares immunohistochemistry and survival in G3 EEC and type 2 cancers.

Methods.—Clinicopathological data compared with immunohistochemistry and survival in 156 consecutive patients with poor prognosis cancer—G3 EEC, uterine papillary serous (UPSC) and clear cell carcinoma (CC), sarcoma, carcinosarcoma and endometrial tumors of mixed histology. 131 (84%) datasets were complete, 25 tumors comprising sarcoma, carcinosarcoma or mixed histologies were excluded. Tissue microarray constructed and tested for estrogen receptor (ER), progesterone receptor (PR), p53 and human epidermal growth factor receptor-2 (Her-2).

Results.—There was no significant difference in the mean age for G3 EEC (n = 68) and USPC+CC (n = 38), (68.01 and 67.08 respectively, p = 0.697) or stage at diagnosis (p = 0.384). For ER, PR, p53 and Her-2, there was no significant difference in marker positivity between G3 EEC and UPSC+CC (p = 0.612, 0.132, 0.16 and 0.132 respectively). With a mean follow-up time 148 months Disease specific and recurrence-free survival between G3 EEC and USPC+CC was similar (p = 0.842 and 0.863).

Conclusion.—G3 EEC and UPSC+CC share similar clinical, immuno-histochemistry and poor survival. G3 EEC is better characterised as type 2 cancer and should be treated with similar adjuvant therapy to UPSC/CC.

▶ This article examines the clinical and immunohistochemical differences between grade 3 endometrioid carcinomas and more classic morphologies of type II endometrial cancers, such as serous and clear cell carcinomas. It is stated that in their practice, type II cancers receive adjuvant radiotherapy and chemo-therapy, whereas type I (endometrioid) cancers receive radiotherapy alone. Therefore, determining how best to classify grade 3 endometrioid carcinomas has major implications for patient care. In this evaluation of 78 cases of grade 3 endometrioid carcinomas and 42 cases of serous or clear cell endometrial carci-nomas, the authors found no significant difference in age, stage at time of presentation, overall or recurrence-free survival, or hormone receptor status between the 2 groups. Particularly in light of the similarly abysmal survival rate, this suggests that grade 3 endometrioid carcinomas should be classified and treated in the same category as serous and clear cell endometrial cancers. One noted limitation of the study is that some cases underwent what would currently be considered incomplete staging; however, standard of care at the time of those operations was different. Additionally, the authors note variability in immunohistochemical scoring schema, potentially limiting the ability to compare this with other studies. At the time of publication, there are ongoing studies in both Great Britain and the United States to evaluate optimal manage-ment for patients with these tumors. Although more work remains to be done to further understand the molecular underpinnings of high-grade endometrial tumors, based on the currently available genetic and clinical parameters, it seems as though the majority of grade 3 endometrioid carcinomas fit best into the type II category of endometrial cancers. For further reading, see the reference section.[1,2]

M. D. Post, MD

References

1. Llobet D, Pallares J, Yeramian A, et al. Molecular pathology of endometrial carci-noma: practical aspects from the diagnostic and therapeutic viewpoints. *J Clin Pathol.* 2009;62:777-785.
2. Doll A, Abal M, Rigau M, et al. Novel molecular profiles of endometrial cancer-new light through old windows. *J Steroid Biochem Mol Biol.* 2008;108:221-229.

Liposarcoma Arising in Uterine Lipoleiomyoma: A Report of 3 Cases and Review of the Literature

McDonald AG, Dal Cin P, Ganguly A, et al (Massachusetts General Hosp, Boston; Brigham and Women's Hosp, Boston, MA; et al)
Am J Surg Pathol 35:221-227, 2011

Background.—Primary sarcomas of the uterus are uncommon, leiomyosarcoma being the most frequent. Most uterine sarcomas arise de novo, with malignant transformation of a benign mesenchymal tumor being a very rare event, and is reported only in leiomyomata.

Design.—The clinicopathologic features of 3 uterine liposarcomas arising in association with a lipoleiomyoma were studied. Immunohistochemistry for desmin, h-caldesmon, S100, and MDM2, and fluorescence in situ hybridization for the t(12;16) (q13;p11) were performed in all cases.

Result.—Patients ranged in age from 49 to 70 (mean, 59) years. The tumors were centered in the myometrium, ranged in size from 10 to 18.5 cm, and showed a gelatinous cut surface with foci of necrosis. On microscopic examination, the tumors had well-circumscribed pushing margins. One neoplasm was uniformly hypocellular with a prominent myxoid background, and a striking delicate vascular network. Another neoplasm showed alternating hypocellular (myxoid) and hypercellular areas, whereas the third tumor was uniformly hypercellular with a hyalinized background. In the myxoid areas, the cells were small and spindle with oval nuclei and inconspicuous nucleoli. In the hypercellular areas, the cells were pleomorphic with large, hyperchromatic nuclei. Mitotic activity ranged from <3 to 7/10 high-power fields. Lipoblasts were present in all tumors but were more common in the hypercellular areas. Two tumors merged imperceptibly with a lipoleiomyoma (1 typical and 1 with bizarre nuclei), whereas the third tumor showed an infarcted area composed of ghost mature adipocytes admixed with hyalinized smooth muscle most consistent with an infarcted lipoleiomyoma. Tumors were classified as myxoid, mixed myxoid and pleomorphic, and pleomorphic liposarcoma, respectively. The benign and malignant adipose components were positive for S100, whereas the benign smooth muscle component stained for desmin and h-caldesmon. MDM2 immunostain was positive in the 2 cases with a pleomorphic liposarcoma component. Fluorescence in situ hybridization analysis was successfully completed in only 1 of 3 tumors (pure pleomorphic liposarcoma), which failed to show the t(12;16) and HMAG2 amplification. The patients are alive and well 1, 2, and 20 years after initial surgery with no adjuvant therapy.

Conclusions.—Primary liposarcomas of the uterus are extremely rare and are most likely to arise from malignant transformation of a lipoleiomyoma. These tumors should be added to the differential diagnosis of benign lipomatous tumors, myxoid mesenchymal tumors, and malignant mixed Müllerian tumors (if pleomorphic) of the uterus.

▶ This article describes the clinicopathologic and immunohistochemical features of 3 cases of primary uterine liposarcoma arising in lipoleiomyoma. Uterine sarcomas are exceedingly rare, and the majority of these are leiomyosarcomas, followed by endometrial stromal sarcomas. To date, only 10 cases of uterine liposarcoma have been reported. Uterine sarcoma is thought to typically arise de novo rather than from a precursor lesion, although the combination of this case series and recent studies showing leiomyosarcomas originating in leiomyomas raises the possibility that pathologists should afford more time and extensive sampling to "fibroid uterus" specimens than is often granted.

Interestingly, liposarcoma of the soft tissues is uncommonly of the myxoid variant, while 2 of the 3 cases presented here and an additional 7 of 10 previously reported cases had a myxoid liposarcoma component or were pure myxoid liposarcomas. This suggests that there may be a different pathogenetic mechanism at play when liposarcomas arise in the uterus. Similarly, soft tissue, well-differentiated, and dedifferentiated liposarcomas are characterized by MDM2 overexpression and myxoid/round-cell liposarcomas contain a DDIT3 rearrangement either by t(12;16) or t(12;22). In the current series, 2 of the 3 cases showed MDM2 overexpression (positive immunohistochemical staining), despite different phenotypes. The 1 case in which fluorescence in situ hybridization analysis was successfully completed (pure pleomorphic liposarcoma) did not show DDIT3 rearrangement or HMGA2 overexpression.

While uterine liposarcoma is likely to remain a rare and esoteric diagnosis, the addition of another 3 cases to the available literature and the mounting evidence that some sarcomas do arise via progression from benign mesenchymal lesions should alert pathologists to the possibility of this diagnosis when confronted by a strikingly myxoid, adipocytic, or hypercellular region within a uterine mass. For further reading, see the reference section.[1,2]

M. D. Post, MD

References

1. Fletcher CDM, Unni KK, Mertens F, et al. *Pathology and Genetics of Tumours of Soft Tissue and Bone*. Lyon, France: IARC Press; 2002.
2. Sieiński W. Lipomatous neometaplasia of the uterus: report of 11 cases with discussion of histogenesis and pathogenesis. *Int J Gynecol Pathol*. 1989;8:357-363.

Correlation of macroscopic and microscopic pathology in risk reducing salpingo-oophorectomy: Implications for intraoperative specimen evaluation

Rabban JT, Mackey A, Powell CB, et al (Univ of California San Francisco; et al)
Gynecol Oncol 121:466-471, 2011

Objective.—A minority of risk-reducing salpingo-oophorectomy (RRSO) specimens from BRCA mutation carriers will contain clinically occult carcinoma that is detectable only using a specialized pathologic evaluation protocol. Although intraoperative detection of cancer may alter immediate surgical management, technical complications impairing pathologic diagnosis may result if fresh tissue dissection and frozen sections are performed on unselected RRSO specimens. We hypothesize that macroscopic specimen findings may predict which RRSO specimens contain cancer and therefore may guide selection of specimens for intraoperative pathologic evaluation. The aim of this study was to correlate the macroscopic and microscopic pathologic findings in RRSO.

Methods.—RRSO specimens from 134 women with a BRCA mutation were retrospectively classified by their grossly visible findings (cysts and/or nodules versus grossly unremarkable). Correlation of the gross findings with the microscopic finding of occult tubal and/or ovarian carcinoma was performed by re-examination of all pathology slides.

Results.—While 46% of RRSO had visible ovarian cysts and 34% had visible tubal/paratubal cysts, no cyst contained cancer on microscopic examination. Carcinoma was detected in 2/22 (9%) visible ovarian nodules and in 2/8 (25%) visible tubal nodules. Conversely, among all 11 RRSO specimens containing cancer, 7 (64%) had no corresponding visible abnormality.

Conclusion.—Frozen section evaluation of a solid nodule may be valuable in patients consented for immediate surgical staging. Otherwise it is best to avoid intraoperative dissection or frozen section of RRSO that are macroscopically normal or contain only cysts; such specimens should remain undissected for immediate formalin-fixation as the first step of the specialized pathology evaluation protocol.

▶ Increasingly frequent specimens in a surgical pathology practice include risk-reducing salpingo-oophorectomy (RRSO) specimens from women with demonstrated germline *BRCA1* or *BRCA2* mutations, as up to 10% of these patients will have carcinoma. Evaluation of these specimens for minute occult cancers or precancerous lesions requires special handling to include extensive sectioning and microscopic evaluation of the entirety of the ovary, fallopian tube (with an emphasis on the fimbriated end), and soft tissues.[1] Some surgeons will ask for intraoperative consultation on these specimens, presumably with the intent of carrying out a staging procedure in the event of detection of an occult carcinoma.[2] In this article, the authors attempt to establish guidelines for the appropriate situations in which to acquiesce to the surgeon's request. They found, via retrospective review of 134 cases, that 46% and 36% (n = 62 and 46) had macroscopically visible ovarian or tubal/paratubal cysts, respectively, but that none of these contained malignancy. In contrast, of the 16% and 6% (n = 22 and 8) that had grossly visible ovarian or tubal/paratubal solid nodules, a total of 4 contained carcinoma. All of the grossly visible nodules that were malignant were greater than 5 mm. In contrast, of the 11 patients found to have carcinoma, 7 (63%) had no associated grossly visible abnormality. The authors point out the potential detriments of evaluating these specimens intraoperatively, including perturbation of the delicate ovarian surface/fimbrial epithelium where these high-grade serous carcinomas often arise, "warped" fixation of freshly cut tissue limiting the surface area later observable, and frozen section artifact that may confound immediate interpretation or reduce antigenicity for future immunohistochemical studies. Based on their findings, the authors propose practical guidelines for the intraoperative gross or microscopic examination of these specimens. Essentially, they recommend that the only situation in which a frozen specimen be undertaken is in the event of a nodule greater than 5 mm. This corresponds to experience at my institution, in which the surgeons routinely request gross evaluation, which can typically be performed with a minimal amount of specimen handling.

M. D. Post, MD

References

1. Medeiros F, Muto MG, Lee Y, et al. The tubal fimbria is a preferred site for early adenocarcinoma in women with familial ovarian cancer syndrome. *Am J Surg Pathol.* 2006;30:230-236.
2. Mehrad M, Ning G, Chen EY, Mehra KK, Crum CP. A pathologist's road map to benign, precancerous, and malignant intraepithelial proliferations in the fallopian tube. *Adv Anat Pathol.* 2010;17:293-302.

FOXL2 Is a Sensitive and Specific Marker for Sex Cord-Stromal Tumors of the Ovary

Al-Agha OM, Huwait HF, Chow C, et al (Vancouver General Hosp, British Columbia, Canada; et al)
Am J Surg Pathol 35:484-494, 2011

Sex cord-stromal tumors (SCSTs) of the ovary are relatively uncommon tumors. Diagnosis of SCST rests primarily on the histomorphology of these tumors, and tumors with an atypical or unconventional appearance can pose diagnostic challenges. Previously, we had identified FOXL2 (402C→G) mutation as being characteristic of adult granulosa cell tumors (aGCTs). However, molecular screening for this mutation is not always possible and adds time and cost to the diagnostic process. In this study, we investigated the potential diagnostic use of immunostaining for FOXL2 on formalin-fixed paraffin-embedded tissue sections. Using a commercially available polyclonal antiserum against FOXL2 protein, immunoexpression of FOXL2 was tested in 501 ovarian tumor samples, including 119 SCSTs, using whole tissue sections and tissue microarrays. Staining was correlated with FOXL2 mutation status. In addition, we compared FOXL2 immunoexpression with that of α-inhibin and calretinin, the 2 traditional immunomarkers of SCST, in a subset of 89 SCSTs. FOXL2 immunostaining was present in 95 of 119 (80%) SCSTs, including >95% of aGCTs, juvenile granulosa cell tumors, fibromas, and sclerosing stromal tumors. Only 50% of Sertoli-Leydig cell tumors (N = 40) expressed FOXL2. One of 11 steroid cell tumors and 3 of 3 female adnexal tumors of probable Wolffian origin showed FOXL2 immunoreactivity, whereas all other non-SCSTs tested (N = 368) were negative for FOXL2 expression. Thus, the sensitivity and specificity of FOXL2 immunoreactivity for SCST are 80% and 99%, respectively. The FOXL2 (402C→G) mutation was confirmed to be both a sensitive and relatively specific indicator of aGCT. Forty-five of 119 SCSTs were mutation positive. These cases were 39 of 42 (93%) aGCTs, 3 of 40 Sertoli-Leydig cell tumors, 2 of 5 thecomas, and 1 of 4 (25%) SCSTs of unclassified type. SCSTs harboring a FOXL2 mutation consistently immunoexpressed

TABLE 2.—Correlation of FOXL2 (402C→G) Mutation With FOXL2 Immunoexpression

Tumors With Mutant FOXL2	No. Cases (n)	FOXL2 Immunoexpression
aGCT	39	39/39 (100%)
SLCT	3	2/3 (66.7%)
Thecoma	2	2/2 (100%)
SCST, unclassified	1	1/1 (100%)
Total	45	44/45 (98%)

FOXL2 (44 of 45, 98%), but FOXL2 immunostaining was also seen in many SCSTs that lacked a mutation (49 of 73, 67%). FOXL2 immunostaining showed higher sensitivity for the diagnosis of SCST, compared with α-inhibin and calretinin, and FOXL2 staining was typically more intense in positive cases compared with either α-inhibin or calretinin. In the SCSTs that were negative for FOXL2 expression, α-inhibin and/or calretinin immunostaining yielded positive results. In conclusion, FOXL2 is a relatively sensitive and highly specific marker for SCST. FOXL2 staining is present in almost all SCSTs with a FOXL2 mutation, and also in a majority of SCSTs without a mutation. FOXL2, together with α-inhibin and calretinin, forms an immunomarker panel that will result in positive staining with 1 or more markers in essentially all cases of SCST (Table 2).

▶ The authors previously showed that a C to G mutation in FOXL2, a transcription factor expressed as a nuclear protein, is strongly associated with adult granulosa cell tumor but recognize that molecular testing is impractical in most surgical cases in which a sex-cord stromal tumor (SCST) enters the differential diagnosis. Here they investigate the utility of FOXL2 immunohistochemistry to diagnose SCST in problematic cases, stressing that the majority of cases can be accurately diagnosed solely on the basis of hematoxylin and eosin staining. Via tissue microarray (339 cases) and whole tissue sections (161 cases), they looked at FOXL2 expression in 501 ovarian tumors, which included 119 SCST. They found that 80% of these were positive for nuclear FOXL2 staining, whereas mutational analysis of all SCST showed only 38% of SCST to harbor the classic mutation (Table 2). Additionally, FOXL2 was shown to be a better marker of sex-cord stromal differentiation than either calretinin or alpha-inhibin, although using a panel of all 3 markers, 100% of SCST showed some positivity. Interestingly, all 3 female adnexal tumors of probably Wolffian origin (FATWO) studied showed immunoreactivity with FOXL2, suggesting additional work is needed to definitively establish the origin of this tumor. The authors hypothesize that based on current evidence, FOXL2 mutation should be considered a diagnostic criterion for a diagnosis of adult granulosa cell tumor regardless of growth pattern. This is a distinct and likely controversial shift away from the paradigm in gynecologic pathology in which expert consultation is considered the gold standard. The article does provide compelling evidence for incorporation of this commercially available antibody into the workup of challenging ovarian tumors when SCST is in the differential, but additional experience will need to be acquired before incorporation of the test can be used in lieu of standard histomorphologic analysis. For further reading, see the reference section.[1,2]

M. D. Post, MD

References

1. Shah SP, Köbel M, Senz J, et al. Mutation of FOXL2 in granulosa-cell tumors of the ovary. *N Engl J Med.* 2009;360:2719-2729.
2. Cocquet J, Pailhoux E, Jaubert F, et al. Evolution and expression of FOXL2. *J Med Genet.* 2002;39:916-921.

Patterns of Low-grade Serous Carcinoma With Emphasis on the Nonepithelial-lined Spaces Pattern of Invasion and the Disorganized Orphan Papillae
Silva EG, Deavers MT, Malpica A (The Univ of Texas MD Anderson Cancer Ctr, Houston)
Int J Gynecol Pathol 29:507-512, 2010

Low-grade serous carcinoma is a relatively recent recognized entity. The cytologic features of this type of carcinoma have been described in detail; however, the different histologic patterns of this carcinoma have not been discussed yet. We reviewed the hematoxylin and eosin-stained slides and studied the different patterns of invasion and the histologic features of areas that were not obviously invasive of 40 cases of ovarian pure low-grade serous carcinoma. Destructive areas of invasion were present in all cases; however, in 25 of the 40 cases obvious invasive areas were mixed with foci that were difficult to recognize as invasive. The obvious areas of invasion were characterized by the presence of tumor cells within nonepithelial-lined spaces, which are clefts in the stroma surrounding the tumor cells. The different patterns of the tumor cells within the nonepithelial-lined spaces and the frequency that they are found were: groups or nests (nidi pattern) in 100% of the cases, micropapillae in 70%, these 2 patterns frequently were mixed, macropapillae in 25%, large solid groups in 5%, and single cells in 3%. The 2 patterns difficult to recognize as invasive because of the absence of nonepithelial-lined spaces were disorganized orphan papillae within epithelial-lined spaces present in 40% of the cases, and small irregular glands with a haphazard distribution infiltrating the tissue eliciting desmoplastic stromal reaction present in 22% of the cases. Calcifications were present in all cases, and mucin in 70% of the cases. Areas of stromal invasion characterized by tumor cells within nonepithelial-lined spaces or clefts are seen in all low-grade carcinomas. Within these spaces, small groups of tumor cells are found frequently mixed with micropapillae. In 62% of the cases, in addition to obvious areas of invasion, there were 2 patterns difficult to recognize as invasive, disorganized orphan papillae, and irregular well-developed glands (Fig 7).

▶ This article presents the largest descriptive study to date of low-grade serous carcinoma, a relatively recently described entity with distinct clinical, morphologic,

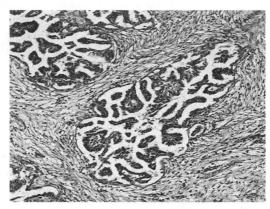

FIGURE 7.—Disorganized orphan papillae within a space lined by epithelial cells. (Reprinted from Silva EG, Deavers MT, Malpica A. Patterns of low-grade serous carcinoma with emphasis on the nonepithelial-lined spaces pattern of invasion and the disorganized orphan papillae. *Int J Gynecol Pathol.* 2010;29:507-512, with permission from International Society of Gynecological Pathologists.)

and genetic characteristics that differ from the more common and readily recognized high-grade serous carcinoma. Namely, low-grade serous carcinoma is distinguished by the presence of minimal nuclear atypia (less than a 3-fold difference in size) and fewer than 12 mitotic figures per 10 high-power fields.[1] Through observation of 40 cases, the authors describe 6 common patterns of invasion, including the universally observed nested pattern as well as micropapillary, macropapillary, solid scanty cells around calcifications, and single cell infiltration. They additionally detail 2 more difficult patterns to recognize, that of "orphan" papillae (Fig 7) and well-formed glands. Recognition of invasion is quite important in clinical practice to differentiate the neoplasm in question from the closely related serous borderline tumor.[2] Interestingly, the authors also note the frequent presence of mucin in these neoplasms (70% of cases), suggesting a closer relationship to serous borderline tumors than high-grade serous carcinomas. This finding also serves as a potential diagnostic pitfall in routine evaluation of small specimens. The main contribution of the article is to make practicing pathologists aware of the varying morphologic appearances that may be encountered in low-grade serous carcinomas. Accurate diagnosis has major consequences, including treatment decisions and appropriate counseling of patients regarding disease course and outcomes.

M. D. Post, MD

References

1. Malpica A, Deavers MT, Lu K, et al. Grading ovarian serous carcinoma using a two-tier system. *Am J Surg Pathol.* 2004;28:496-504.
2. Singer G, Stöhr R, Cope L, et al. Patterns of p53 mutations separate ovarian serous borderline tumors and low- and high- grade carcinomas and provide support for a new model of ovarian carcinogenesis: a mutational analysis with immunohistochemical correlation. *Am J Surg Pathol.* 2005;29:218-224.

Emergence of CA125 Immunoreactivity in Recurrent or Metastatic Primary Ovarian Mucinous Neoplasms of the Intestinal Type

Miller K, Millar J, McCluggage WG (Belfast Health and Social Care Trust, Northern Ireland)
Am J Surg Pathol 35:1331-1336, 2011

Primary ovarian mucinous carcinomas are uncommon and usually present as unilateral stage 1 neoplasms. The vast majority are of the so-called intestinal or enteric type and arise from a preexisting intestinal-type mucinous borderline neoplasm. The overall prognosis is good. However, a minor proportion recurs or metastasizes, and this is associated with a poor prognosis. The vast majority of primary ovarian intestinal-type mucinous carcinomas and borderline tumors exhibit a variable degree of positivity with enteric markers and are CA125 negative. The primary purpose of this study was to describe the unusual phenomenon of CA125 immunoreactivity in 8 of 10 metastatic mucinous carcinomas arising after a diagnosis of primary ovarian mucinous carcinoma (n = 3) or mucinous borderline tumor of the intestinal type (n = 7) in which the primary neoplasms were mostly negative. The reasons underlying this emergent CA125 positivity are not clear, but we speculate it may be because while intestinal type mucinous borderline neoplasms and mucinous carcinomas exhibiting so-called expansile invasion are usually CA125 negative, focal positivity may be seen in areas of infiltrative stromal invasion, which may preferentially metastasize. CA125 positivity in the metastatic neoplasm may result in the pathologist considering an alternative primary site; however, this should not be the case. In our study, we found a 4.2% risk of malignant progression after a diagnosis of primary ovarian mucinous borderline tumor of the intestinal type. In light of this, we favor retaining the term "mucinous borderline tumor," because of this small, but not insignificant, risk of malignant transformation, which in most cases is likely secondary to a focus of invasion being unsampled at the time of reporting the primary neoplasms (Fig 3).

▶ This article explores the unusual phenomenon of CA125 immunoreactivity in recurrent or metastatic ovarian mucinous carcinomas, which are typically negative for that marker. The authors observed that, among the 5.7% (n = 10) of primary ovarian mucinous borderline tumors or carcinomas that recurred or metastasized, 8 showed more than 50% of tumor cells staining with CA125. In contrast, only 3 of the 9 primary neoplasms were CA125-positive, and these in less than 10% of tumor cells. The reason for this discordance between primary tumor and metastasis is uncertain. One possibility is that the neoplasms develop aberrant CA125 expression as they progress, and another is that the metastasis may be derived from an unsampled CA125-positive focus of the primary tumor. The latter is favored, because the authors note that areas of expansile invasion in mucinous carcinomas are typically CA125-negative, whereas the infiltrative invasion pattern is more likely to show expression (Fig 3). It is known that this latter pattern is associated with a worse prognosis,

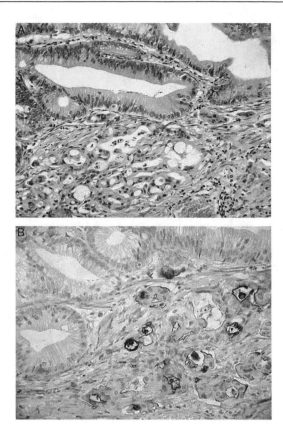

FIGURE 3.—Primary ovarian mucinous carcinoma, which exhibits both expansile (top) and infiltrative (bottom) stromal invasions (A). The area of expansile invasion is CA125 negative, whereas the infiltrative invasion is positive (B). (Reprinted from Miller K, Millar J, McCluggage WG. Emergence of CA125 immunoreactivity in recurrent or metastatic primary ovarian mucinous neoplasms of the intestinal type. *Am J Surg Pathol.* 2011;35:1331-1336, with permission from Lippincott Williams & Wilkins.)

and the finding of CA125-positive areas within a mucinous carcinoma could potentially be regarded as an adverse prognostic indicator. Typical workup of a mucinous ovarian lesion does not include CA125, because it is expected to be negative; however, based on the current study, it is worth considering whether this marker should be added to a panel, particularly when considering the presence of invasive foci. For further reading, see the reference section.[1,2]

M. D. Post, MD

References

1. Hart WR. Mucinous tumors of the ovary: a review. *Int J Gynecol Pathol.* 2005;24: 4-25.
2. Tabrizi AD, Kalloger SE, Köbel M, et al. Primary ovarian mucinous carcinoma of intestinal type: significance of pattern of invasion and immunohistochemical expression profile in a series of 31 cases. *Int J Gynecol Pathol.* 2010;29:99-107.

Placenta weight percentile curves for singleton and twins deliveries

Almog B, Shehata F, Aljabri S, et al (McGill Univ, Montreal, Quebec, Canada; et al)
Placenta 32:58-62, 2011

Objective.—To establish updated placental percentile nomograms in a large North American population for singleton and twin gestations for the use of researchers and clinicians.

Study Design.—Data was extracted from our computerized registry; McGill Obstetrics and Neonatal Database (MOND). The registry includes all the obstetrical data on all deliveries at the McGill University, including placental weight, placental pathologies, maternal and perinatal complications. 20,635 singleton deliveries and 527 twin deliveries were included. Placental weight, gestational age at delivery, birth weight and gender were retrieved. Tables and figures for the 3rd, 10th, 25th, 50th, 75th 90th, and 97th percentile of placental weight by gestational age, placental weight by birth weight and placental to birth weight ratio by gestational age were produced.

Results.—Tables and figures are presented for placental percentiles curves according to gestational age, gestational weight and gender for singleton and twin deliveries. In addition, tables and figures are presented for the ratio of placental weight to birth weight.

Conclusions.—Population percentile curves have been produced for placental weight and for the ratio of placental weight to birth weight to for singleton and twin deliveries.

▶ Placental pathology is an often neglected area, with many surgical pathology reports containing a minimal amount of information. There is increasing evidence that placental weight and birth/placental weight ratio may have important implications for maternal and neonatal health as well as predicting susceptibility to certain adulthood diseases such as hypertension.[1] This article establishes detailed curves for normal placental weights and birth/placental weight ratios by gestational age based on a large cohort of deliveries (n = 21 162). They include both singleton (n = 20 635) and twin (n = 527) deliveries, although only dichorionic-diamnionic twins were evaluated, and no distinction is made between fused and separate discs. The authors state the need to update this type of information every 5 to 10 years to account for shifting patient demographics; however, what is "normal" within a particular population at a single time provides limited data for longitudinal studies and fails to account for absolute effects of high or low weights on development of disease. Although placental weight charts have been published previously (in our practice, Pinar et al[2] is used), this study adds the birth/placental weight ratio, which is an increasingly recognized indicator of placental efficiency. When deranged, it can be associated with a multitude of adulthood diseases. The main limitation of using this ratio is the lack of readily available information regarding infant birth weight at the time of placental examination. While virtually every placental pathology report makes mention of the placental weight, it is equally important to use growth curves, such as those developed here, to give an indication of the percentile for gestational age and, if possible, the birth/placental weight ratio. Incorporation of these elements into pathology reports will offer increased clinical utility and may direct preventive health care efforts in the future.

M. D. Post, MD

References

1. Risnes KR, Romundstad PR, Nilsen TI, Eskild A, Vatten LJ. Placental weight relative to birth weight and long-term cardiovascular mortality: findings from a cohort of 31,307 men and women. *Am J Epidemiol.* 2009;170:622-631.
2. Pinar H, Sung CJ, Oyer CE, Singer DB. Reference values for singleton and twin placental weights. *Pediatr Pathol Lab Med.* 1996;16:901-907.

Placental Mesenchymal Dysplasia Presenting as a Twin Gestation With Complete Molar Pregnancy
Starikov R, Goldman R, Dizon DS, et al (Women & Infants Hosp, Providence, RI; The Warren Alpert Med School of Brown Univ, Providence, RI; Albany Med College, NY)
Obstet Gynecol 118:445-449, 2011

Background.—Placental mesenchymal dysplasia is a rare abnormality characterized by placentomegaly, grapelike cystic vesicles, and villous hyperplasia. The clinical and ultrasonographic presentation may mimic molar pregnancy, provoking incorrect diagnoses and unnecessary therapeutic interventions.

Case.—A 36-year-old nulliparous woman presented for prenatal ultrasonography that indicated the presence of one gestational sac containing both fetus and cystic mass, concerning for partial molar pregnancy. Amniocentesis returned a 46,XX karyotype, suggesting a twin gestation with complete mole. The patient was monitored closely and, because of fetal growth restriction, was induced successfully at term and delivered a healthy newborn. Histopathologic findings of the placenta were consistent with placental mesenchymal dysplasia.

Conclusion.—Although placental mesenchymal dysplasia is often confused with molar pregnancy, it is important to consider both in a differential to avoid inappropriate treatments (Table 2).

▶ Management of pregnancies complicated by abnormal ultrasound findings is at best a complicated topic, with the potential for over- or undertreatment of the mother. This article, although a case report, highlights the importance of placental examination, particularly in instances in which there has been a radiographic anomaly. Although the ultimate diagnosis in this case, placental mesenchymal dysplasia,[1] is entirely benign without any risk of persistence or malignancy, the

TABLE 2.—Differential Diagnoses

Diagnosis	bhCG	Karyotype	DNA Index	p57 Expression	Vascular Flow	Dilated Villi	Cystic Spaces	Trophoblastic Proliferation	Invasive Potential
Placental Mesenchymal Dysplasia	Normal/high	Usually 46,XX	1.00	+	−	+	Diffuse	−	−
Partial mole	Varies	triploid	1.50	+	−	+	Diffuse	+	+
Twin with complete mole	High	46,XX	1.00	−	−	+	Diffuse	+	+
Partial mosaic	Varies	Diploid/triploid	1.00>1.50	+	−	Varies	Varies	Varies	−
Chorioangioma	Normal	Diploid	1.00	+	+	−	Confined	Varies	−
Spontaneous abortion with hydropic change	Varies	Varies	Varies	+	−	+	Confined	Varies	−

bhCG, beta human chorionic gonadotropin.

pregnancy described herein was initially thought to contain a complete mole. Because up to 20% of complete hydatidiform moles will recur or progress, future management of the patient varies dramatically. There are a variety of entities that may enter the differential diagnosis of a cystic or otherwise abnormal-appearing placenta. Fortunately, simple gross and microscopic examination via hematoxylin and eosin—stained slides is usually sufficient to obtain the diagnosis (Table 2). When needed, ancillary techniques, such as immunohistochemistry for p57 (to rule out the presence of a complete mole) or fluorescence in situ hybridization analysis (to rule out the presence of a triploid partial mole) can be used.[2]

M. D. Post, MD

References

1. Parveen Z, Tongson-Ignacio JE, Fraser CR, Killeen JL, Thompson KS. Placental mesenchymal dysplasia. *Arch Pathol Lab Med.* 2007;131:131-137.
2. Chilosi M, Piazzola E, Lestani M, et al. Differential expression of p57Kip2, a maternally imprinted cdk inhibitor, in normal human placenta and gestational trophoblastic disease. *Lab Invest.* 1998;78:269-276.

Eosinophilic/T-cell Chorionic Vasculitis: A Clinicopathologic and Immunohistochemical Study of 51 Cases
Jacques SM, Qureshi F, Kim CJ, et al (Hutzel Women's Hosp, Detroit, MI; et al)
Pediatr Dev Pathol 14:198-205, 2011

We report 51 placentas diagnosed with eosinophilic/Tcell chorionic vasculitis (E/TCV), an unusual form of chorionic vasculitis characterized by an infiltrate composed predominantly of CD3+ T cells and eosinophils. The placentas were all 3rd trimester, with 48 (94.1%) being term. Forty-seven (92.2%) were singleton placentas, and the remaining 4 were twins. The E/TCV was limited to 1 chorionic surface vessel in 40 (78.4%) and involved 50% or less of the vessel circumference in 30 (58.8%) placentas. The inflammation faced the intervillous space in 12 (23.5%) and the amniotic cavity in 8 (15.7%) and had no distinct predominant direction in the remaining 31 (60.8%) placentas. Twelve (25.5%) placentas showed mural thrombi or intramural fibrin in association with the E/TCV. One hundred six term singleton placentas were selected as the control group, and the 47 singleton placentas with E/TCV made up the study group for comparison of demographic and histopathologic features. Villitis of unknown etiology was identified more frequently in study group placentas (20 [42.6%]) compared with control group placentas (14 [13.2%]) ($P < 0.001$). Vascular changes of fetal vascular thrombo-occlusive disease were identified away from the E/TCV more frequently in study group placentas (8 [17.0%]) compared with control group placentas (4 [3.8%]) ($P = 0.008$). There were no significant differences in the frequencies of other placental lesions studied, including acute inflammatory lesions and lesions related to maternal underperfusion. There were no significant differences in maternal age, race, parity, birth weight, allergy history, blood type, or medication use.

▶ Eosinophilic/T-cell chorionic vasculitis (E/TCV) is an uncommon and focal placental entity, the pathogenesis and associations of which are unclear. This is the largest study to date of this finding; it places particular emphasis on clinicopathologic and demographic features in an attempt to determine clinical relevance. Unfortunately, there is only minimal such evidence to be found. The authors found a statistically significant increase in co-incidence of villitis of unknown etiology (VUE) in cases of E/TCV, although none of the cases in the study (n = 47) or control (n = 106) groups were classified as diffuse high-grade VUE, the subtype most associated with adverse fetal outcomes. Thus, the significance of this association remains unclear. Interestingly, E/TCV was not observed before 34 weeks gestational age, similar to the finding that VUE is a disease of late third trimester. There was a statistically significant higher incidence of vascular changes of fetal vascular thrombo-occlusive disease seen in cases of E/TCV, however, the significance of this remains unknown, and the total number of placentas with these findings was small (8 or 17% of the study group and 4 or 3.8% of the control group). Other inflammatory conditions, including maternal and fetal responses to amniotic fluid infection (acute chorioamnionitis and umbilical cord/chorionic plate vasculitis, respectively), were not significantly different between study and control populations.

The authors posit that this entity is likely more common than even they detected (0.6%) with extensive sampling because of its focality. Although a histologically interesting diagnosis with potential implications for understanding the way fetal chronic inflammatory responses occur, this study did not show practical utility of the diagnosis as a marker for adverse fetal outcome. Whether it has as yet undetermined clinical associations remains to be seen. For further reading, see the reference section.[1,2]

M. D. Post, MD

References

1. Fraser RB, Wright JR Jr. Eosinophilic/T-cell chorionic vasculitis. *Pediatr Dev Pathol.* 2002;5:350-355.
2. Redline RW. Clinically and biologically relevant patterns of placental inflammation. *Pediatr Dev Pathol.* 2002;5:326-328.

10 Urinary Bladder and Male Genital Tract

Epithelial Proliferations in Prostatic Stromal Tumors of Uncertain Malignant Potential (STUMP)
Nagar M, Epstein JI (The Johns Hopkins Hosp, Baltimore, MD)
Am J Surg Pathol 35:898-903, 2011

Stromal tumors of uncertain malignant potential (STUMPs) are rare tumors characterized by an atypical, unique stromal proliferation of the prostate. Various stromal proliferations of STUMPs have been described; however, epithelial proliferations occurring within the STUMP have not been systematically described to date. We reviewed 89 cases of STUMP from our consultation service from 1990 to 2010. Nineteen cases without a glandular component were excluded. We next evaluated the glandular component of the remaining 70 cases of STUMP for glandular crowding and complexity, prostatic intraepithelial neoplasia (PIN), squamous metaplasia, urothelial metaplasia, basal cell hyperplasia, adenosis, and clear cell cribriform hyperplasia. In 58 cases (83%), the glandular component differed from glands on the same biopsy specimen uninvolved by STUMP. The most common abnormalities were glandular crowding in 35 of 70 (50%) and a very prominent basal cell layer in some glands in 32 of 70 (46%) cases. The next most frequent glandular variation from normal was prominent papillary infolding in 13 of 70 (19%) cases. Less-frequent epithelial changes within the STUMP were as follows: 10 of 70 (14%) showed cystically dilated glands; 7 of 10 (10%) had basal cell hyperplasia; 6 of 70 (9%) had urothelial metaplasia; 6 of 70 (9%) showed squamous metaplasia; 3 of 70 (4%) had cribriform hyperplasia; 3 of 70 (4%) had adenosis; and 1 case each showed high-grade PIN, low-grade PIN, and partial atrophy. The glandular component of STUMP was histologically normal in 12 (17%) cases. There was a tendency toward urothelial and squamous metaplasia in STUMPs with a phyllodes pattern, and a prominent basal cell layer in STUMPs with degenerative and cellular stroma. This is the first study to systematically describe the epithelial proliferations occurring in STUMP. This study suggests that, within STUMPs, there is epithelial-mesenchymal crosstalk, as has been described in benign prostate and in prostatic carcinogenesis. In unusual cases of STUMP, the epithelial proliferation may

TABLE 2.—Glandular Proliferations According to STUMP Subtype

	Degenerative	Cellular	Phyllodes
Crowded	25/43 (58%)	8/16 (50%)	1/10 (10%)
Prominent basal cells	22/43 (51%)	7/16 (44%)	3/10 (30%)
Papillary infolding	9/43 (21%)	4/16 (25%)	0/10 (0%)
Cystic glands	5/43 (12%)	1/16 (6%)	4/10 (40%)
Adenosis	2/43 (5%)	1/16 (6%)	0/10 (0%)
Cribriform hyperplasia	4/43 (9%)	2/16 (13%)	1/10 (10%)
Squamous metaplasia	2/43 (5%)	2/16 (13%)	2/10 (20%)
Urothelial metaplasia	1/43 (2%)	2/16 (13%)	3/10 (30%)
HGPIN	1/43 (2%)	0/16 (0%)	0/10 (0%)
LGPIN	0/43 (0%)	1/16 (6%)	0/10 (0%)
Basal cell hyperplasia	5/43 (12%)	2/16 (13%)	0/10 (0%)
Partial atrophy	0/43 (0%)	0/16 (0%)	0/10 (0%)

HGPIN indicates high-grade PIN; LGPIN, low-grade PIN.

predominate to the extent that it can mask the diagnosis of STUMP (Table 2).

▶ Prostatic stromal tumors of uncertain potential are rare, have been classified into 4 subtypes, and need to be distinguished from sarcomas (which show hypercellularity, atypia, mitotic activity, and necrosis). In this article, Nagar and Epstein describe the epithelial components; the glandular proliferations, classified by subtype, are shown in Table 2. For additional reading, please see reference list.[1,2]

S. S. Raab, MD

References

1. Gaudin PB, Rosai J, Epstein JI. Sarcomas and related proliferative lesions of specialized prostatic stroma: a clinicopathologic study of 22 cases. *Am J Surg Pathol.* 1998;22:148-162.
2. Bostwick DG, Hossain D, Qian J, et al. Phyllodes tumor of the prostate: long-term followup study of 23 cases. *J Urol.* 2004;172:894-899.

Epithelial Proliferations in Prostatic Stromal Tumors of Uncertain Malignant Potential (STUMP)

Nagar M, Epstein JI (The Johns Hopkins Hosp, Baltimore, MD)
Am J Surg Pathol 35:898-903, 2011

Stromal tumors of uncertain malignant potential (STUMPs) are rare tumors characterized by an atypical, unique stromal proliferation of the prostate. Various stromal proliferations of STUMPs have been described; however, epithelial proliferations occurring within the STUMP have not been systematically described to date. We reviewed 89 cases of STUMP from our consultation service from 1990 to 2010. Nineteen cases without a glandular component were excluded. We next evaluated the glandular

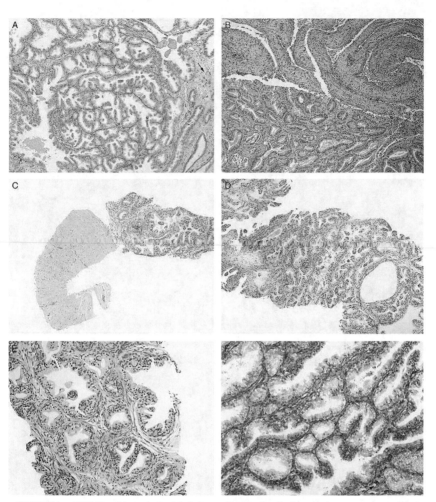

FIGURE 1.—STUMPs with marked epithelial crowding. A, A radical prostatectomy specimen showing marked crowding of glands, with only focal STUMP stroma with degenerative atypia (arrow) visible. B, A radical prostatectomy section with phyllodes pattern (upper half) and smaller, crowded glands (adenosis) (lower half). C, Prostate needle biopsy showing a discrete nodule of STUMP with a sharp interface between tumor and nontumor. D, Another core of the case shown in C showing marked crowding of benign glands almost obscuring the stromal component of a cellular STUMP. E, High magnification of D shows hypercellular stroma of a cellular STUMP. F, Marked crowding of benign glands with a prominent basal cell layer obscuring the stromal component of this STUMP with degenerative atypia (arrow). (Reprinted from Nagar M, Epstein JI. Epithelial proliferations in prostatic stromal tumors of uncertain malignant potential (STUMP). *Am J Surg Pathol.* 2011;35:898-903, with permission from Lippincott Williams & Wilkins.)

component of the remaining 70 cases of STUMP for glandular crowding and complexity, prostatic intraepithelial neoplasia (PIN), squamous metaplasia, urothelial metaplasia, basal cell hyperplasia, adenosis, and clear cell cribriform hyperplasia. In 58 cases (83%), the glandular component differed from glands on the same biopsy specimen uninvolved by STUMP. The most

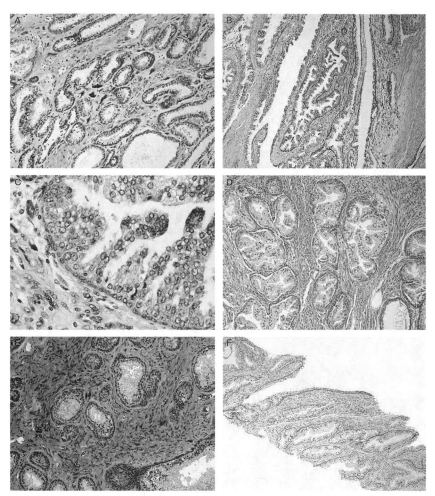

FIGURE 2.—STUMPs with prominent basal cell layer. A, STUMP with degenerative atypia with crowded small-to-medium-sized glands with a visible basal cell layer even at low magnification. B, STUMP with degenerative atypia with a high-grade PIN gland (center). C, Higher magnification of high-grade PIN seen in B with a prominent basal cell layer. D, STUMP with cellular stroma with moderately crowded benign glands and prominent basal cells. E, STUMP with degenerative atypia, cellular stroma, and focal basal cell hyperplasia. F, STUMP with cellular stroma on needle biopsy with cystically dilated glands having a prominent basal cell layer. (Reprinted from Nagar M, Epstein JI. Epithelial proliferations in prostatic stromal tumors of uncertain malignant potential (STUMP). *Am J Surg Pathol.* 2011;35:898-903, with permission from Lippincott Williams & Wilkins.)

common abnormalities were glandular crowding in 35 of 70 (50%) and a very prominent basal cell layer in some glands in 32 of 70 (46%) cases. The next most frequent glandular variation from normal was prominent papillary infolding in 13 of 70 (19%) cases. Less-frequent epithelial changes within the STUMP were as follows: 10 of 70 (14%) showed cystically dilated glands; 7 of 10 (10%) had basal cell hyperplasia; 6 of 70 (9%)

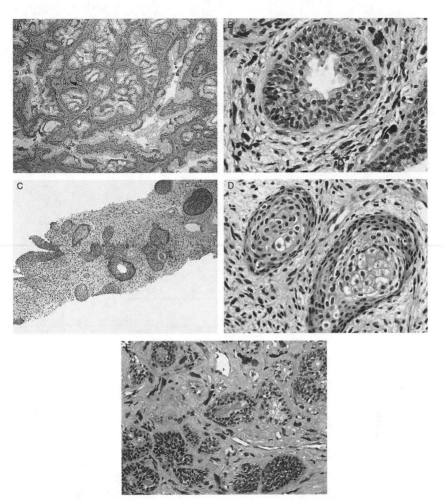

FIGURE 3.—Miscellaneous glandular findings in STUMPS. A, Cribriform hyperplasia in STUMP with degenerative atypia (arrow). B, Basal cell hyperplasia in a degenerative-type STUMP. C, Extensive urothelial and squamous metaplasia in STUMP with cellular stroma. D, Higher magnification of C showing urothelial and squamous metaplasia. E, Marked basal cell hyperplasia in STUMP with degenerative atypia. (Reprinted from Nagar M, Epstein JI. Epithelial proliferations in prostatic stromal tumors of uncertain malignant potential (STUMP). *Am J Surg Pathol.* 2011;35:898-903, with permission from Lippincott Williams & Wilkins.)

had urothelial metaplasia; 6 of 70 (9%) showed squamous metaplasia; 3 of 70 (4%) had cribriform hyperplasia; 3 of 70 (4%) had adenosis; and 1 case each showed high-grade PIN, low-grade PIN, and partial atrophy. The glandular component of STUMP was histologically normal in 12 (17%) cases. There was a tendency toward urothelial and squamous metaplasia in STUMPs with a phyllodes pattern, and a prominent basal cell layer in STUMPs with degenerative and cellular stroma. This is the first study to systematically describe the epithelial proliferations occurring in STUMP.

TABLE 1.—Glandular Proliferations in STUMP

Crowded glands	35/70 (50%)
Prominent basal cells	32/70 (46%)
Prominent papillary infolding	13/70 (19%)
Cystic glands	10/70 (14%)
Basal cell hyperplasia	7/70 (10%)
Cribriform hyperplasia	7/70 (10%)
Urothelial metaplasia	6/70 (9%)
Squamous metaplasia	6/70 (9%)
Adenosis	3/70 (4%)
HGPIN	1/70 (1%)
LGPIN	1/70 (1%)
Partial atrophy	1/70 (1%)
Normal	12/70 (17%)

HGPIN indicates high-grade PIN; LGPIN, low-grade PIN.

TABLE 2.—Glandular Proliferations According to STUMP Subtype

	Degenerative	Cellular	Phyllodes
Crowded	25/43 (58%)	8/16 (50%)	1/10 (10%)
Prominent basal cells	22/43 (51%)	7/16 (44%)	3/10 (30%)
Papillary infolding	9/43 (21%)	4/16 (25%)	0/10 (0%)
Cystic glands	5/43 (12%)	1/16 (6%)	4/10 (40%)
Adenosis	2/43 (5%)	1/16 (6%)	0/10 (0%)
Cribriform hyperplasia	4/43 (9%)	2/16 (13%)	1/10 (10%)
Squamous metaplasia	2/43 (5%)	2/16 (13%)	2/10 (20%)
Urothelial metaplasia	1/43 (2%)	2/16 (13%)	3/10 (30%)
HGPIN	1/43 (2%)	0/16 (0%)	0/10 (0%)
LGPIN	0/43 (0%)	1/16 (6%)	0/10 (0%)
Basal cell hyperplasia	5/43 (12%)	2/16 (13%)	0/10 (0%)
Partial atrophy	0/43 (0%)	0/16 (0%)	0/10 (0%)

HGPIN indicates high-grade PIN; LGPIN, low-grade PIN.

This study suggests that, within STUMPs, there is epithelial-mesenchymal crosstalk, as has been described in benign prostate and in prostatic carcinogenesis. In unusual cases of STUMP, the epithelial proliferation may predominate to the extent that it can mask the diagnosis of STUMP (Figs 1-3, Tables 1 and 2).

▶ This article focuses on a lesser-known entity in prostate pathology, stromal tumors of uncertain malignant potential (STUMPs). These are rare tumors characterized by an atypical stromal proliferation unique to the prostate (Figs 1 and 2). The authors describe 4 patterns of this in the prostate. The earlier literature[1] focused on the stromal component, whereas this study is focused on the epithelial component. A good differential diagnosis of epithelial stromal proliferations is depicted in Table 1. The STUMPs have also been subclassified into different categories (Table 2).

This is first of its kind, which throws light on benign epithelial proliferation occurring in STUMPs. Different associated epithelial proliferations within different patterns of STUMPs also reflect associated epithelial mesenchymal interactions. The study comprises quite a large number of cases, which is statistically significant.

S. A. Chandrakanth, MD, FRCPC

Reference

1. Epstein JI, Armas OA. Atypical basal cell hyperplasia of the prostate. *Am J Surg Pathol.* 1992;16:1205-1214.

Immunohistochemical Analysis in a Morphologic Spectrum of Urachal Epithelial Neoplasms: Diagnostic Implications and Pitfalls

Paner GP, McKenney JK, Barkan GA, et al (Univ of Chicago, IL; Stanford Univ Med Ctr, CA; Loyola Univ Med Ctr, Maywood, IL; et al)
Am J Surg Pathol 35:787-798, 2011

The vast majority of urachal epithelial neoplasms are adenocarcinomas with several described morphologic subtypes that include both enteric and nonenteric histologies. Adenocarcinoma from several other primaries may mimic any of these urachal adenocarcinoma subtypes in the bladder or at distant sites. However, data regarding the immunohistochemical profile of urachal carcinoma are limited, let alone its correlation with the different histologic subtypes that may have implications in the differential diagnostic workup with their morphologic mimics. Herein, we performed an immunohistochemical analysis in a broad spectrum of 39 urachal epithelial neoplasms (34 adenocarcinomas, 1 urothelial carcinoma, and 4 noninvasive mucinous cystic tumors), 13 urachal remnants, and 6 secondary colonic adenocarcinomas of the bladder, using an antibody panel that included novel and traditional gastrointestinal tract-associated markers. Expression levels of p63, CK7, CK20, CDX2, nuclear β-catenin, claudin-18, and Reg IV in urachal adenocarcinoma were as follows: 3%, 50%, 100%, 85%, 6%, 53%, and 85%. In urachal adenocarcinoma subtypes, expression levels of CDX2, nuclear β-catenin, claudin-18, and

TABLE 3.—Comparison of Urachal, Gastric, and Colonic Signet Ring Cell Carcinomas Immunoprofile Based on the Current and Other Published Studies

Tumor Type	CK7 (%)	CK20 (%)	CDX2 (%)	Claudin-18 (%)	Reg IV (%)
Urachal signet ring cell carcinoma, current study and[16]	3/8 (37)	8/8 (100)	6/8 (75)	4/6 (67)	6/6 (100)
Gastric signet ring cell carcinoma[11,38,55]	41/56 (73)	31/56 (55)	41/51 (80)	18/21 (86)	21/21 (100)
Colonic signet ring cell carcinoma[11,38,55]	6/30 (20)	28/30 (93)	22/25 (88)	6/16 (37)	16/16 (100)

Reg IV indicates regenerating islet-derived member 4.
Editor's Note: Please refer to original journal article for full references.

TABLE 4.—Comparison of Enteric Urachal Adenocarcinoma, Urachal Carcinoma Overall, Nonurachal Primary Bladder Adenocarcinoma, and Colonic Adenocarcinoma Immunoprofile Based on the Current and Other Published Studies

Tumor Type	CK7 (%)	CK20 (%)	CDX2 (%)	Nuclear β-catenin (%)	Claudin-18 (%)	Reg IV (%)
Urachal adenocarcinoma, enteric subtype, current study	4/11 (36)	11/11 (100)	10/11 (91)	1/11(9)	3/11 (27)	8/11 (73)
Urachal carcinoma, overall, current study and[19,64]	27/44 (61)	53/54 (98)	44/49 (90)	3/49 (6)	18/34 (53)	29/34 (85)
Nonurachal primary bladder adenocarcinoma[26,49,58,61,64,67]	39/56 (70)	39/56 (70)	9/25 (36)	0/17 (0)	—	—
Secondary colonic denocarcinoma to bladder, current study and[49,58,61,67]	1/52 (2)	50/52 (96)	46/46 (100)	17/22 (77)	0/6 (0)	2/6 (33)
Colonic adenocarcinoma, overall, current study and[3,6,12,13,14,19,29,32,34,41,44,45,49,58,61,64,65,67,69]	76/987 (8)	521/578 (90)	373/404 (92)	110/222 (50)	21/575 (4)	38/122 (31)

Reg IV indicates regenerating islet-derived member 4.
Editor's Note: Please refer to original journal article for full references.

Reg IV were as follows: mucinous (8/8, 0/8, 6/8, 8/8), enteric (10/11, 1/11, 3/11, 8/11), not otherwise specified (5/7, 0/7, 3/7, 5/7), and signet ring cell (4/6, 0/6, 4/6, 6/6) type. All urachal adenocarcinomas had membrano-cytoplasmic β-catenin staining and only 2 tumors had nuclear localization that were focal to moderate, in contrast to secondary colonic adenocarcinoma of the bladder, which mostly had both membrano-cytoplasmic and nuclear positivity. Claudin-18 positivity was observed only in frankly malignant tumors and not in noninvasive urachal tumors and urachal remnants. Reg IV expression seemed to be related to mucin production, which was often diffuse in mucinous and signet ring cell subtypes and focal in enteric subtype, with goblet cell-like reactivity similar to secondary colonic adenocarcinoma. p63 expression was present in urothelial urachal remnants (3/3) and contrasted with CDX2 expression seen in glandular (5/6) and mixed urothelial/glandular remnants (2/4). Thus, this study showed that CDX2 is expressed by urachal remnants of glandular type, noninvasive urachal mucinous cystic tumors and urachal adenocarcinomas, and can be diffuse in urachal adenocarcinomas, even without the classic enteric morphology. Nuclear localization of β-catenin can rarely occur in urachal adenocarcinoma; however, diffuse nuclear reactivity argues against its diagnosis. The novel gastrointestinal tract markers claudin-18 and Reg IV are both expressed in urachal adenocarcinoma, including in signet ring cell carcinoma, and thus refutes the suggested specificity for gastrointestinal tract signet ring cell carcinomas. An immunohistochemical panel that includes β-catenin and CK7 may have value in differentiating urachal adenocarcinoma of enteric morphology from colonic adenocarcinoma. Overall, this study suggests that the different morphologic presentations of urachal adenocarcinomas have a relatively similar or overlapping immunophenotype. Knowledge of the similarity in immunostaining to its different morphologic mimics may help avoid misdiagnosis in urachal adenocarcinoma (Tables 3 and 4).

▶ By light microscopy alone, primary urachal adenocarcinomas may be difficult to distinguish from adenocarcinomas from other sites. Paner and colleagues examined immunohistochemical expression for a number of markers to determine if an immunohistochemical panel could be developed for more definitive separation. The authors found that urachal carcinomas have a relatively similar or overlapping immunoprofile, although some stains may be used to favor or exclude a urachal adenocarcinoma. A summary of these data are shown in Tables 3 and 4. For additional reading, please see reference list.[1,2]

S. S. Raab, MD

References

1. Gopalan A, Sharp DS, Fine SW, et al. Urachal carcinoma: a clinicopathologic analysis of 24 cases with outcome correlation. *Am J Surg Pathol.* 2009;33:659-668.
2. Torenbeek R, Lagendijk JH, Van Diest PJ, Bril H, van de Molengraft FJ, Meijer CJ. Value of a panel of antibodies to identify the primary origin of adenocarcinomas presenting as bladder carcinoma. *Histopathology.* 1998;32:20-27.

Identification of Gleason Pattern 5 on Prostatic Needle Core Biopsy: Frequency of Underdiagnosis and Relation to Morphology

Fajardo DA, Miyamoto H, Miller JS, et al (The Johns Hopkins Med Insts, Baltimore, MD)
Am J Surg Pathol 35:1706-1711, 2011

The presence of a Gleason pattern 5 prostatic adenocarcinoma is associated with a worse outcome. This study assesses the accuracy of grading a tumor as having Gleason pattern 5 and the potential factors contributing to its undergrading. From the consultation service of one of the authors, we identified 59 consecutive needle biopsy cases comprising 138 parts that, upon review, were graded as having Gleason pattern 5. All cases were reported as the final diagnosis by the outside pathologist. They were sent for a second opinion at the behest of clinicians or patients and not because the pathologist was seeking a second opinion. Considering the highest Gleason score in a given multicore specimen as the overall Gleason score, Gleason pattern 5 was missed in 34 of 59 (57.6%) cases by the outside pathologist. Compared with the outside pathologist's diagnosis, the Gleason score rendered at the second opinion was increased in 101 of 138 (73.2%) parts, was decreased in 5 of 138 (3.6%) parts, and remained unchanged in 32 of 138 (23.2%) parts. Gleason pattern 5 was not identified by the initiating pathologist in 67 of 138 (48.6%) of the evaluated parts. The architectural patterns of pattern 5 were as follows: single cells (n = 104, 75.3%); solid sheets (n = 69, 50%); cords (n = 62, 44.9%); and comedonecrosis (n = 3, 2.2%). Pattern 5 was missed more frequently when it was not the primary pattern. The most common Gleason pattern 5 architectural type was single cells and the least common was comedonecrosis. None of the architectural patterns appeared to be more correctly identified than the others; however, the most accurate grading was when the primary pattern was 5 and was composed mostly of solid sheets. Owing to the important prognostic and therapeutic implications of Gleason pattern 5, pathologists must be attuned to its varied patterns and to the fact that it may often represent a secondary or tertiary component of the carcinoma (Table 5).

▶ Fajardo et al present data on the diagnostic precision (interobserver variability) for prostate core biopsies regarding the presence of Gleason pattern 5 prostatic adenocarcinoma, which is associated with worse outcome. An outside diagnosis

TABLE 5.—Identification of Gleason Pattern 5 When Gleason Pattern 5 is the Primary Pattern

Architectural Pattern	Pattern 5 Not Identified by Outside Pathologist (n = 15)	Pattern 5 Diagnosed by Outside Pathologist (n = 57)	Total
Single cells	9 (30.0%)	21 (70%)	30 (100%)
Solid sheets	2 (7.4%)	25 (92.6%)	27 (100%)
Cords	4 (26.7%)	11 (73.3%)	15 (100%)
Comedonecrosis	—	—	

is compared with an expert diagnosis. Fejardao et al present the data in terms of diagnostic accuracy, assuming that Johns Hopkins pathology is the gold standard. Undercalling and overcalling Gleason pattern 5 has important ramifications for patient management. Gleason pattern 5 has several architectural patterns that the authors indicate may be misinterpreted by outside pathologists (Table 5). For additional reading, please see reference list.[1,2]

S. S. Raab, MD

References

1. Allsbrook WC Jr, Mangold KA, Johnson MH, Lane RB, Lane CG, Epstein JI. Interobserver reproducibility of Gleason grading of prostatic carcinoma: general pathologist. *Hum Pathol.* 2001;32:81-88.
2. Glaessgen A, Hamberg H, Pihl CG, Sundelin B, Nilsson B, Egevad L. Interobserver reproducibility of percent Gleason grade 4/5 in prostate biopsies. *J Urol.* 2004; 171:664-667.

Routine dual-color immunostaining with a 3-antibody cocktail improves the detection of small cancers in prostate needle biopsies

Tolonen TT, Kujala PM, Laurila M, et al (Univ of Tampere and Tampere Univ Hosp, Finland)
Hum Pathol 42:1635-1642, 2011

We performed dual-color immunostaining with a 3-antibody cocktail (α-methylacyl coenzyme-A racemase, CK34betaE12, and p63) on prostate biopsies from 200 patients. Current practice (hematoxylin and eosin staining followed by dual-color immunostaining on selected cases) was compared with a protocol in which routine dual-color immunostaining was provided in all cases. In the original pathology reports, adenocarcinoma was diagnosed in 87/200 (43%) patients. Small foci interpreted as putative cancers were detected with dual-color immunostaining in 14/113 patients who were originally diagnosed with a nonmalignant lesion. All of the suggested cancerous foci were independently reevaluated by 5 pathologists. A diagnosis of adenocarcinoma was assessed by consensus in 8 cases, and atypical small acinar proliferation was diagnosed in 1 case. Consensus was not reached in 5 cases. Six of the foci reclassified as cancer were of Gleason score $3 + 3 = 6$, while 2 were graded as Gleason score $4 + 4 = 8$. The feasibility of routine dual-color immunostaining was also tested by analyzing the time spent on microscopic assessment. Because small, atypical lesions expressing α-methylacyl coenzyme-A racemase (blue chromogen) were easy to detect using dual-color immunostaining, the microscopic analysis of dual-color immunostaining and hematoxylin-eosin staining was faster than that of hematoxylin-eosin staining alone that was later followed by dual-color immunostaining in selected cases (median 251 seconds versus 299 seconds, $P < .0001$). We concluded that routine dual-color immunostaining of all prostate biopsies would produce better diagnostic sensitivity with a smaller microscopy workload for the pathologist. However, minute foci interpreted as cancer with dual-color immunostaining need to be

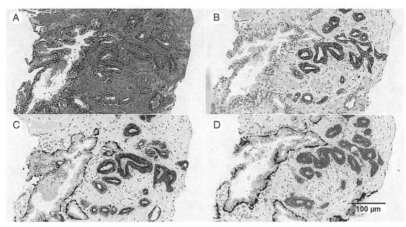

FIGURE 1.—A well-differentiated (Gleason score of 3+3 = 6) adenocarcinoma demonstrated by H&E staining (A), single-chromogen immunostaining of AMACR (B), blue-brown dual-chromogen immunos-taining of AMACR (blue) and basal cells (brown) (C), and (D) red-brown dual-chromogen immunostaining of AMACR (red) and basal cells (brown). A scale bar is included in the lower right corner. For interpretation of the references to color in this figure legend, the reader is referred to web version of this article. (Reprinted from Tolonen TT, Kujala PM, Laurila M, et al. Routine dual-color immunostaining with a 3-antibody cock-tail improves the detection of small cancers in prostate needle biopsies. *Hum Pathol*. 2011;42:1635-1642, Copyright 2011, with permission from Elsevier.)

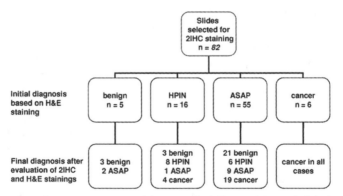

FIGURE 2.—A schematic representation of diagnostically challenging slides in which dual-color immu-nostaining (2IHC) was requested (*n* = 82). The initial diagnosis before 2IHC and the final diagnosis after evaluation of the slides stained by 2IHC. (Reprinted from Tolonen TT, Kujala PM, Laurila M, et al. Routine dual-color immunostaining with a 3-antibody cocktail improves the detection of small cancers in prostate needle biopsies. *Hum Pathol*. 2011;42:1635-1642, Copyright 2011, with permission from Elsevier.)

confirmed with hematoxylin-eosin staining, and minimal criteria for a defin-itive diagnosis of cancer are still lacking (Figs 1-3).

▶ This article emphasizes the value of triple cocktail in the routine diagnosis of prostatic adenocarcinoma as is used in suspicious cases of carcinoma. The stain is particularly helpful in the small number of cancers in which a dilemma appears between atypical acinar proliferation and small amount of cancers

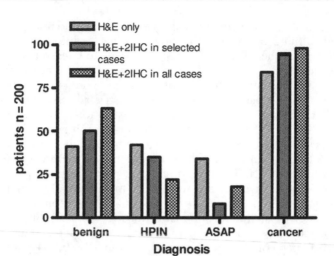

FIGURE 3.—The impact of routine dual-color immunostaining on the diagnostic distribution. Approximately half of the patients given HGPIN or ASAP as their worst diagnosis were resolved to a diagnosis of either benign or cancer with the aid of 2IHC. (Reprinted from Tolonen TT, Kujala PM, Laurila M, et al. Routine dual-color immunostaining with a 3-antibody cocktail improves the detection of small cancers in prostate needle biopsies. *Hum Pathol.* 2011;42:1635-1642, Copyright 2011, with permission from Elsevier.)

(Figs 1-3). The authors have noted this reduces the workload on pathologists and increases the diagnostic accuracy. Routine ordering also overcomes the delay in reporting, increases the cancer detection sensitivity, and offers improved diagnostic accuracy.

S. A. Chandrakanth, MD, FRCPC

Should Intervening Benign Tissue Be Included in the Measurement of Discontinuous Foci of Cancer on Prostate Needle Biopsy? Correlation With Radical Prostatectomy Findings
Karram S, Trock BJ, Netto GJ, et al (The Johns Hopkins Hosp, Baltimore, MD)
Am J Surg Pathol 35:1351-1355, 2011

Currently, there is no consensus as to the optimal method for measuring tumor length or percentage of cancer on a core when there are 2 or more foci of prostate cancer in a single core separated by benign intervening stroma. One option is to measure discontinuous foci of cancer as if they were 1 single continuous focus. The other option is to add the measurements of the individual separate foci of cancer, ignoring the extent of the intervening benign prostate tissue. The surgical pathology database at The Johns Hopkins Hospital was searched for outside consult cases of prostate needle biopsies reviewed between 2005 and 2010 when the patient came to our institution for radical prostatectomy (RP). Cases were restricted to those with biopsy Gleason score 6 in which there was at least 15% discordance between the outside and our institution in terms of the reported highest percentage of cancer per core per case. One hundred and nine patients were identified fulfiling our inclusion criteria. Seventy-nine showed the same Gleason score in the RP, and 30 had an upgrade to Gleason ≥ 7. Including all cases (scores 6, 7, and 8 at RP), there was no significant association between the maximum percentage of cancer per core with organ-confined disease or risk of positive surgical margins, regardless if the cores were measured at Hopkins or at the outside institutions. For cases with no upgrade at RP, the differences between the maximum percentage of cancer per core per case recorded at Hopkins and the outside institutions ranged from 15% to 80%, in which the mean and median differences were 35% and 30%, respectively. The maximum percentages of tumor involvement on a core per case given at our institution more strongly correlated with the presence of organ-confined disease ($P = 0.004$) compared with the percentages given at the outside institutions ($P = 0.027$). Surgical margin positivity was also associated with the maximum percentages of tumor involvement per core given at our institution ($P = 0.004$), whereas the outside percentages were not significant predictors of margin status ($P = 0.2$). In a multivariable analysis, maximum percentage of cancer per core per case measured at Hopkins which includes intervening benign prostate tissue in the measurement was also more predictive of stage and margins than ignoring intervening benign tissue. In summary, our study demonstrated that for prostate cancer in which the needle biopsy grade is representative of the entire tumor, quantifying cancer extent on biopsy by measuring discontinuous cancer on biopsy from one end to the other as opposed to "collapsing" the cancer by subtracting out the intervening benign prostate tissue correlates better with organ-confined disease and risk of positive margins.

▶ Karram and colleagues correlated 2 ways to measure extent of prostatic adenocarcinoma on core biopsy with radical prostatectomy outcomes (of organ-defined disease and margin status). The first way is to measure extent of prostatic adenocarcinoma by measuring the discontinuous extent of 2 or more foci of cancer (method 1), and the second way is to subtract out the discontinuous nontumor area from the final measure (method 2). It is important to note that this study involved only cases in which the initial cancer diagnosis on the core was Gleason score 6. I think the findings are not definitive. First, if the cancer on the radical prostatectomy specimen was upgraded to Gleason score > 6, there was no significant association between the maximum percentage of cancer per core with organ-confined disease or risk of positive surgical margins, regardless of measuring method. For those cases that did not get Gleason score upgraded, surgical margin positivity was statistically significantly associated with the maximum percentages of tumor involvement per core using the discontinuous measuring method (method 1) but not the subtracting method. For additional reading, please see reference list.[1,2]

S. S. Raab, MD

References

1. Brimo F, Vollmer RT, Corcos J, et al. Prognostic value of various morphometric measurements of tumour extent in prostate needle core tissue. *Histopathology.* 2008;53:177-183.
2. Epstein JI, Potter SR. The pathological interpretation and significance of prostate needle biopsy findings: implications and current controversies. *J Urol.* 2001;166: 402-410.

Plasmacytoid urothelial carcinoma of the urinary bladder: clinicopathologic, immunohistochemical, ultrastructural, and molecular analysis of a case series

Raspollini MR, Sardi I, Giunti L, et al (Univ Hosp Careggi, Viale G.B. Morgagni, Florence, Italy; "A. Meyer" Children Hosp, Florence, Italy; Division of Pathology-Dept of Critical Care Medicine and Surgery, Florence, Italy; et al)
Hum Pathol 42:1149-1158, 2011

A plasmacytoid variant of urothelial carcinoma has been recently recognized in the World Health Organization classification system. This is characterized by a discohesive growth of plasmacytoid cells with eccentric nuclei, extending in the bladder wall and often in the perivesical adipose tissue. Herein, we report the clinicopathologic, immunohistochemical, ultrastructural, and molecular features of a series of plasmacytoid urothelial carcinoma of the urinary bladder. Four bladder carcinomas characterized by epithelial cells with morphologic appearance resembling plasma cells were evaluated at the immunohistochemical, electron microscopic, and molecular genetic levels. Tumor cells stained with cytokeratins, epithelial membrane antigen, GATA-3 (endothelial transcription factor 3), CD15, p53, and p16. In addition, malignant cells strongly stained with CD138 in all the cases, whereas leukocyte common antigen and multiple myeloma 1/interferon regulatory factor 4 were completely negative, nor immunoreactivity was seen for either κ or λ light chains. The electron microscopic examination showed the presence of divergent squamous and glandular differentiation. At variance with conventional urothelial carcinoma, the analysis of exons 4-9 of *TP53* gene revealed no alteration in all the 4 tumors tested, and this can be of value in choosing additional chemotherapy after surgery. Plasmacytoid carcinoma of the bladder is a tumor entity, which can be characterized by specific immunohistochemical markers, including positivity for GATA-3, and presents phenotypic and genotypic peculiarities (Figs 1-5, Table 3).

▶ This is a very interesting article regarding plasma cytoid variant of urothelial carcinoma (Fig 1), an entity that was recently recognized in the World Health Organization classification. The authors have carried out various immunohistochemical stains and histochemical stains, analyzed the TP53 gene, and conducted electron microscopy examination (Figs 2-5, Table 3). Plasma cytoid carcinoma of the bladder is a less known entity.[1] It is important to recognize

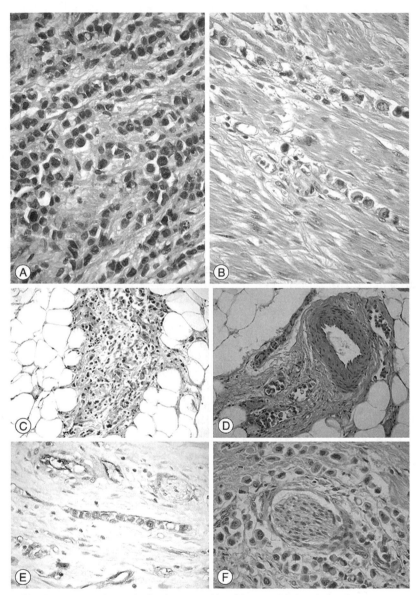

FIGURE 1.—A, Round to oval cells, characterized by a large peripheral nucleus and numerous mitoses with clear or eosinophilic cytoplasm and eccentrically placed enlarged hyperchromatic nuclei with small nucleoli, hematoxylin and eosin staining. B, The malignant cells were either isolated or in single-file pattern infiltrating the muscle, hematoxylin and eosin staining. C, Little clusters of tumor cells in the perivesical fat. Malignant cells in lymphatic vessels, hematoxylin and eosin staining (D) and D2-40 staining (E). F, Presence of tumor cells around nerves in a "coat-sleeve" pattern, hematoxylin and eosin staining (original magnification × 400). (Reprinted from Raspollini MR, Sardi I, Giunti L, et al. Plasmacytoid urothelial carcinoma of the urinary bladder: clinicopathologic, immunohistochemical, ultrastructural, and molecular analysis of a case series. *Hum Pathol.* 2011;42:1149-1158, Copyright 2011, with permission from Elsevier.)

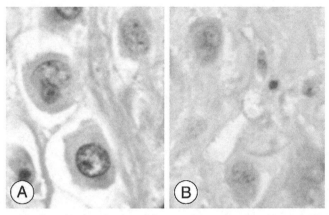

FIGURE 2.—Presence of both acid and neutral mucins that were turquoise blue with Alcian blue staining (A) or magenta with PAS D staining (B). For interpretation of the references to color in this figure legend, the reader is referred to web version of this article. (Reprinted from Raspollini MR, Sardi I, Giunti L, et al. Plasmacytoid urothelial carcinoma of the urinary bladder: clinicopathologic, immunohistochemical, ultrastructural, and molecular analysis of a case series. *Hum Pathol.* 2011;42:1149-1158, Copyright 2011, with permission from Elsevier.)

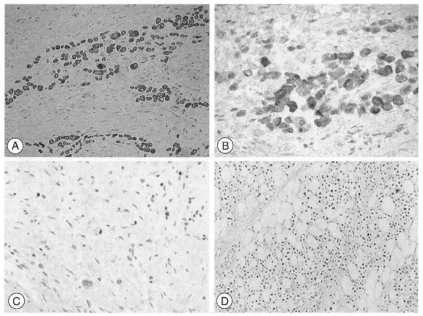

FIGURE 3.—A, Tumor cells strongly stained CK cocktail. B, Cytoplasm and membranes of malignant cells strongly stained with CD138. C, MUM1/IRF4 staining was completely negative in tumor cells, whereas the plasma cells in the bladder wall were positive internal control with MUM1/IRF4 positive staining. D, Tumor cells in the perivesical fat showed a positive staining for GATA-3. (Reprinted from Raspollini MR, Sardi I, Giunti L, et al. Plasmacytoid urothelial carcinoma of the urinary bladder: clinicopathologic, immunohistochemical, ultrastructural, and molecular analysis of a case series. *Hum Pathol.* 2011;42:1149-1158, Copyright 2011, with permission from Elsevier.)

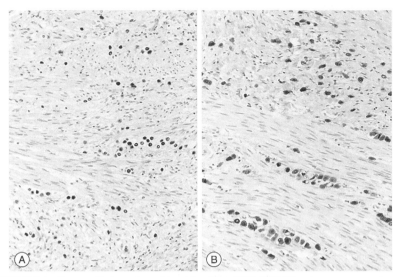

FIGURE 4.—Tumor cells showed a positive p53 staining (50%-60%) (A) and a strong expression with p16 staining (B). Reprinted from Raspollini MR, Sardi I, Giunti L, et al. Plasmacytoid urothelial carcinoma of the urinary bladder: clinicopathologic, immunohistochemical, ultrastructural, and molecular analysis of a case series. *Hum Pathol.* 2011;42:1149-1158, Copyright 2011, with permission from Elsevier.)

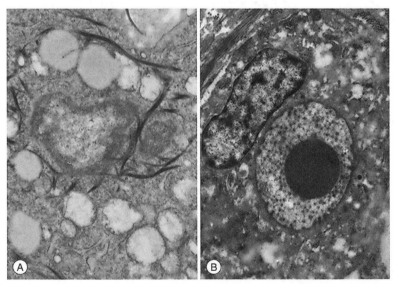

FIGURE 5.—A, Neoplastic cells frequently presented intracytoplasmic bundles of tonofilaments (original magnification × 10 400). B, Intracytoplasmic lumina with projecting microvilli, containing secretory material, was observed in all cases (original magnification × 10 400). These correspond to the paranuclear positivity for PAS and Alcian. (Reprinted from Raspollini MR, Sardi I, Giunti L, et al. Plasmacytoid urothelial carcinoma of the urinary bladder: clinicopathologic, immunohistochemical, ultrastructural, and molecular analysis of a case series. *Hum Pathol.* 2011;42:1149-1158, Copyright 2011, with permission from Elsevier.)

TABLE 3.—Immunohistochemical Staining Results

Antibody	Case 1	Case 2	Case 3	Case 4
AE1/AE3	+++ Cytoplasmic staining	+++ Cytoplasmic staining	+++ Cytoplasmic staining	+++ Cytoplasmic staining
CK7	+++ Cytoplasmic staining	+++ Cytoplasmic staining	+++ Cytoplasmic staining	+++ Cytoplasmic staining
CK20	+++ Cytoplasmic staining	+++ Cytoplasmic staining	+++ Cytoplasmic staining	+++ Cytoplasmic staining
High–molecular weight CK	+++ Cytoplasmic staining	+++ Cytoplasmic staining	+++ Cytoplasmic staining	+++ Cytoplasmic staining
CK8	+++ Cytoplasmic staining	+++ Cytoplasmic staining	+++ Cytoplasmic staining	+++ Cytoplasmic staining
EMA	+++ Cytoplasmic staining	+++ Cytoplasmic staining	+++ Cytoplasmic staining	+++ Cytoplasmic staining
GATA-3	++ Nuclear staining	++ Nuclear staining	++ Nuclear staining	++ Nuclear staining
CD15	++ Cytoplasmic staining	++ Cytoplasmic staining	++ Cytoplasmic staining	++ Cytoplasmic staining
THR	Negative	Negative	Negative	Negative
LCA	Negative	Negative	Negative	Negative
CD138	+++ Cytoplasmic and membrane staining	+++ Cytoplasmic and membrane staining	+++ Cytoplasmic and membrane staining	+++ Cytoplasmic and membrane staining
MUM1	Negative	Negative	Negative	Negative
κ Chain	Negative	Negative	Negative	Negative
λ Chain	Negative	Negative	Negative	Negative
Synaptophysin	Negative	Negative	Negative	Negative
Chromogranin	Negative	Negative	Negative	Negative
S-100	Negative	Negative	Negative	Negative
CD34	Negative	Negative	Negative	Negative
Podoplanin	Negative	Negative	Negative	Negative
Ki-67	Nuclear staining: 70%	Nuclear staining: 80%	Nuclear staining: 70%	Nuclear staining: 60%
p53	Nuclear staining: 50%	Nuclear staining: 60%	Nuclear staining: 50%	Nuclear staining: 60%
CD44	Negative	Negative	Negative	Negative
E-CAD	Negative	Negative	Negative	Negative
p16	+++ Nuclear staining	+++ Nuclear staining	+++ Nuclear staining	+++ Nuclear staining

this entity because it aids in the addition of chemotherapy after surgery. The authors have used various immunohistochemical stains consisting of urothelial lineage markers as well as urothelial-associated markers. These tumors appeared as large polypoid masses with large foundations. The data also confirmed that plasma cytoid carcinoma of the bladder has an urothelial phenotype, and it has been included in subtypes of urothelial carcinoma. The authors highlight the features associated with poor prognosis in these cases.

S. A. Chandrakanth, MD, FRCPC

Reference

1. Ro JY, Shen SS, Lee HI, et al. Plasmacytoid transitional cell carcinoma of urinary bladder: a clinicopathologic study of 9 cases. *Am J Surg Pathol.* 2008;32:752-757.

Initial High-grade Prostatic Intraepithelial Neoplasia With Carcinoma on Subsequent Prostate Needle Biopsy: Findings at Radical Prostatectomy
Al-Hussain TO, Epstein JI (The Johns Hopkins Hosp, Baltimore, MD)
Am J Surg Pathol 35:1165-1167, 2011

There are only a few small studies on men with an initial biopsy showing high-grade prostatic intraepithelial neoplasia (HGPIN) who later have cancer on repeat biopsy and then undergo radical prostatectomy. It is unknown whether this scenario impacts the prognosis of subsequent radical prostatectomy. We compared radical prostatectomy findings in 45 men with an initial diagnosis of HGPIN who subsequently were diagnosed with cancer with 18,494 men diagnosed with cancer who lacked an earlier diagnosis of HGPIN. All cases were retrieved from our institution between 1993 and 2008. The mean patient age was 60.2 years, and the mean serum prostate-specific antigen value was 9.0 ng/mL. For the 45 men with an initial HGPIN diagnosis, 21 of 45 (46.7%) men were found to have cancer within 6 months and 29 of 45 (64.4%) within 1 year after the diagnosis of HGPIN. Cancer involved a single core in 32 of 45 (71.1%) cases, and the maximum tumor volume was ≤5% in 57.8% of the 45 cases. Men with initial HGPIN had 84.4% organ-confined cancer, whereas cases without HGPIN had 65.4% organ-confined cancer ($P = 0.007$) at radical prostatectomy. For the RPs performed in men with an earlier diagnosis of HGPIN followed by cancer on biopsy, the mean and median tumor volumes were 0.3 cm^3 and 0.12 cm^3 (0.003 cm^3 to 1.46 cm^3). Favorable pathologic stage was maintained even when we restricted the analysis to men with only Gleason score 6 cancer on biopsy. In men with Gleason score 6 cancer on biopsy, men with an initial diagnosis of HGPIN had 88.9% organ confined versus 73.2% for men with no earlier biopsy diagnosis of HGPIN, ($P = 0.03$). At radical prostatectomy, although men with an earlier HGPIN diagnosis had less adverse findings in terms of Gleason score, surgical margin involvement, seminal vesicle involvement, and lymph node metastasis, the differences did not reach statistical significance. This was possibly due to the relatively small number of positive events in the men with no earlier HGPIN and due to the relatively small number of cases with earlier HGPIN. Prostatic adenocarcinomas discovered after an initial HGPIN diagnosis on biopsy are more likely to be organ confined, yet of similar grade, compared with cases diagnosed as cancer on the first biopsy. These findings likely reflect cancers associated with HGPIN, in which the cancers were missed on the initial biopsy as a result of smaller size.

▶ Like the diagnosis of atypical small acinar proliferation diagnosis, the diagnosis of high-grade prostatic intraepithelial neoplasia (HGPIN) is a risk diagnosis for invasive cancer on subsequent follow-up. In this article, Al-Hussain and Epstein provide additional data that men who have HPGIN on needle core biopsy have a higher risk of having adenocarcinoma; when HGPIN is observed on more than 2 core fragments, the risk increases to 30% to 40%. The authors argue that those men who have cancers associated with HGPIN have cancers that were most likely missed on core biopsy as a result of the cancer being of small size. Current prostate biopsy sampling techniques have expanded beyond the sextant biopsy procedures, and these more expansive techniques may detect smaller cancers. Thus, the import for pathologists is that the risk of cancer associated with HGPIN does not change as a result of this manuscript, although Al-Hussain and Epstein point out that cancers discovered after an initial HGPIN diagnosis are more likely to be organ confined. For additional reading, please see reference list.[1,2]

S. S. Raab, MD

References

1. Lee MC, Moussa AS, Yu C, Kattan MW, Magi-Galluzzi C, Jones JS. Multifocal high grade prostatic intraepithelial neoplasia is a risk factor for subsequent prostate cancer. *J Urol.* 2010;184:1958-1962.
2. Torenbeek R, Lagendijk JH, Van Diest PJ, et al. Value of a panel of antibodies to identify the primary origin of adenocarcinomas presenting as bladder carcinoma. *Histopathology.* 1998;32:20-27.

Initial High-grade Prostatic Intraepithelial Neoplasia With Carcinoma on Subsequent Prostate Needle Biopsy: Findings at Radical Prostatectomy
Al-Hussain TO, Epstein JI (The Johns Hopkins Hosp, Baltimore, MD)
Am J Surg Pathol 35:1165-1167, 2011

There are only a few small studies on men with an initial biopsy showing high-grade prostatic intraepithelial neoplasia (HGPIN) who later have cancer on repeat biopsy and then undergo radical prostatectomy. It is unknown whether this scenario impacts the prognosis of subsequent radical prostatectomy. We compared radical prostatectomy findings in 45 men with an initial diagnosis of HGPIN who subsequently were diagnosed with cancer with 18,494 men diagnosed with cancer who lacked an earlier diagnosis of HGPIN. All cases were retrieved from our institution between 1993 and 2008. The mean patient age was 60.2 years, and the mean serum prostate-specific antigen value was 9.0 ng/mL. For the 45 men with an initial

HGPIN diagnosis, 21 of 45 (46.7%) men were found to have cancer within 6 months and 29 of 45 (64.4%) within 1 year after the diagnosis of HGPIN. Cancer involved a single core in 32 of 45 (71.1%) cases, and the maximum tumor volume was ≤5% in 57.8% of the 45 cases. Men with initial HGPIN had 84.4% organ-confined cancer, whereas cases without HGPIN had 65.4% organ-confined cancer ($P = 0.007$) at radical prostatectomy. For the RPs performed in men with an earlier diagnosis of HGPIN followed by cancer on biopsy, the mean and median tumor volumes were 0.3 cm^3 and 0.12 cm^3 (0.003 cm^3 to 1.46 cm^3). Favorable pathologic stage was maintained even when we restricted the analysis to men with only Gleason score 6 cancer on biopsy. In men with Gleason score 6 cancer on biopsy, men with an initial diagnosis of HGPIN had 88.9% organ confined versus 73.2% for men with no earlier biopsy diagnosis of HGPIN, ($P = 0.03$). At radical prostatectomy, although men with an earlier HGPIN diagnosis had less adverse findings in terms of Gleason score, surgical margin involvement, seminal vesicle involvement, and lymph node metastasis, the differences did not reach statistical significance. This was possibly due to the relatively small number of positive events in the men with no earlier HGPIN and due to the relatively small number of cases with earlier HGPIN. Prostatic adenocarcinomas discovered after an initial HGPIN diagnosis on biopsy are more likely to be organ confined, yet of similar grade, compared with cases diagnosed as cancer on the first biopsy. These findings likely reflect cancers associated with HGPIN, in which the cancers were missed on the initial biopsy as a result of smaller size (Tables 1 and 2).

▶ This is one of the few studies showing the relation between high-grade prostatic intraepithelial neoplasia (HGPIN) and subsequent development of carcinoma.[1] The study comprises a large number of cases and correlates with other clinical parameters, including prostate-specific antigen levels (Table 1). At radical prostatectomy, more men with earlier diagnosis of HGPIN had organ-confined disease compared with men without HGPIN (Table 2), which is a significant finding. There is no difference in T stage between cancer with prior diagnosis of HGPIN and first-time diagnosis of cancer on a needle-core biopsy; in both groups the cancers were organ confined.

The major weakness of this study is, as authors indicate, that the cases were selected from 1993 to 2008, during which time changes have taken place with

TABLE 1.—Clinicopathologic Findings at Biopsy

	Earlier HGPIN	No Earlier HGPIN	P
Age (mean, years)	60.2	58.2	0.04
Serum PSA (mean)	9.0 ng/mL	7.0 ng/mL	0.03
Single positive core	32/45 (71.1%)	2939/8622 (34.1%)	<0.0001
Maximum cancer per core (≤5%)	26/45 (57.8%)	585/8591 (6.9%)	<0.0001
Gleason score			0.5
6	38/45 (84.4%)	13,565/18,396 (73.7%)	
7 (3+4)	4/45 (8.9%)	2912/18,396 (15.8%)	
7 (4+3)	1/45 (2.2%)	1145/18,396 (6.2%)	
8-10	2/45 (4.4%)	774/18,396 (4.2%)	

TABLE 2.—Pathologic Findings at Radical Prostatectomy

	Earlier HGPIN	No Earlier HGPIN	P
Gleason score			
6	36/45 (80%)	10,907/18,346 (59.5%)	0.3
7 (3+4)	2/45 (4.4%)	4594/18,346 (25%)	
7 (4+3)	2/45 (4.4%)	1628/18,346 (8.9%)	
8-10	5/45 (11.1%)	1217/18,346 (6.6%)	
Surgical margin involvement	4/45 (8.9%)	2673/18,470 (14.5%)	0.3
Organ confined	38/45 (84.4%)	12,075/18,461 (65.4%)	0.007
Seminal vesicle involvement	0/45 (0%)	990/18,494 (5.3%)	0.1
Lymph node metastasis	0/45 (0%)	448/18,494 (2.4%)	0.6

regards to biopsy procedure and Gleason grading. Even then the study is a good revelation regarding carcinoma preceding HGPIN.

S. A. Chandrakanth, MD, FRCPC

Reference

1. Epstein JI, Herawi M. Prostate needle biopsies containing prostatic intraepithelial neoplasia or atypical foci suspicious for carcinoma: implications for patient care. *J Urol.* 2006;175:820-834.

PAX8 and PAX2 Immunostaining Facilitates the Diagnosis of Primary Epithelial Neoplasms of the Male Genital Tract

Tong G-X, Memeo L, Colarossi C, et al (Columbia Univ Med Ctr, NY; Mediterranean Inst of Oncology, Catania, Italy; et al)
Am J Surg Pathol 35:1473-1483, 2011

PAX8 and PAX2 are cell-lineage-specific transcription factors that are essential for the development of Wolffian and Müllerian ducts and have recently emerged as specific diagnostic markers for tumors of renal or Müllerian origin. Little is known about their expression in the Wolffian duct-derived human male genital tract. We report our findings of PAX8 and PAX2 expression in the epithelium of the normal male genital tract and in epithelial tumors derived therefrom using immunohistochemistry (IHC). We found that PAX8 and PAX2 were expressed in the epithelium of the male genital tract from the rete testis to the ejaculatory duct. Rare glands in the prostatic central zone, a tissue of purported Wolffian duct origin, were focally positive for PAX2, but no PAX8 was detected in this area, a finding that may warrant further study. We found diffuse expression of PAX8 and PAX2 in 1 case each of serous cystadenoma of the epididymis, carcinoma of the rete testis, Wolffian adnexal tumor of the seminal vesicle, and endometrioid carcinoma of the seminal vesicle. Neither PAX8 nor PAX2 was detected in the seminiferous tubules and interstitium of the normal testis, nor in Leydig cell tumors (n = 6), Sertoli cell tumors (n = 2), or 48 of 49 germ cell tumors. One pediatric yolk sac tumor showed focal and weak staining for PAX8. Tumors of mesothelial origin, that is,

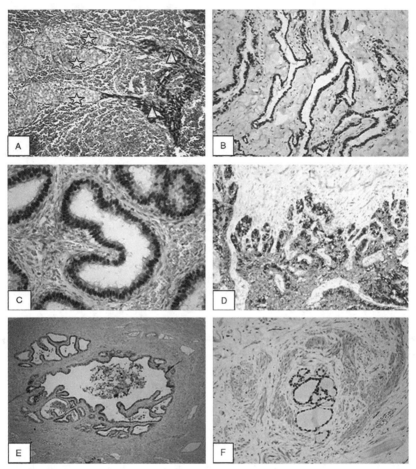

FIGURE 1.—Expression of PAX8 and PAX2 in the male genital tract (only PAX8 is depicted here; PAX2 showed a similar pattern of staining). A, Rete ductuli (▲), x100; and seminiferous tubule (*), x200. B, Rete testis, ×40. C, Epididymis, ×40. D, Seminal vesicle, ×40. E, Ejaculatory duct, ×40. F, Mesonephric remnants, ×100. (Reprinted from Tong G-X, Memeo L, Colarossi C, et al. PAX8 and PAX2 immunostaining facilitates the diagnosis of primary epithelial neoplasms of the male genital tract. *Am J Surg Pathol.* 2011;35:1473-1483, with permission from Lippincott Williams & Wilkins.)

adenomatoid tumors (n = 3) and peritoneal malignant mesotheliomas (n = 37) in men, were negative for PAX2 and PAX8. Neither PAX2 nor PAX8 was present in other areas of the prostate. Expression of PAX8 and PAX2 in these primary epithelial neoplasms of the male genital tract is due to their histogenetic relationship with Wolffian or Müllerian ducts. PAX8 and PAX2 IHC may facilitate the diagnosis of these tumors and should be included in the differential diagnostic IHC panel (Figs 1 and 2).

▶ This article highlights the use of PAX 8 and PAX 2 in the diagnosis of primary epithelial neoplasms of the male genital tract. PAX 2 and PAX 8 are novel

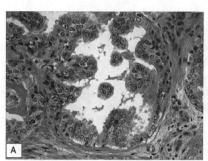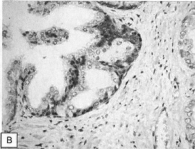

FIGURE 2.—Rare central zone glands of the prostate contained few PAX2-positive epithelial cells. No PAX8 was detected in this area. A, Central zone glands of the prostate (hematoxylin and eosin, ×100). B, PAX2 immunostain (×100). (Reprinted from Tong G-X, Memeo L, Colarossi C, et al. PAX8 and PAX2 immunostaining facilitates the diagnosis of primary epithelial neoplasms of the male genital tract. *Am J Surg Pathol.* 2011;35:1473-1483, with permission from Lippincott Williams & Wilkins.)

markers for transcription factors essential for the development of Wolffian and Müllerian ducts and specific diagnostic markers for tumors of renal or Müllerian origin. These markers help in the clinical investigation and pathologic examination to rule out the possibility of metastases or local invasion from other, more common malignant tumors such as carcinoma of the prostate, colon/rectum, lung, or urinary bladder. This article also highlights the use of PAX 8 and PAX 2 in central zone of the prostate with regard to its Wolffian duct origin (Figs 1 and 2). This study demonstrates PAX 8 and PAX 2 are expressed in Wolffian ductal normal epithelium and in primary epithelial tumors of the male genital tract. Both Wolffian type and Müllerian type epithelial tumors in the male genital tract were positive for PAX 8 and PAX 2.

S. A. Chandrakanth, MD, FRCPC

Flat urothelial carcinoma in situ of the bladder with glandular differentiation
Lopez-Beltran A, Jimenez RE, Montironi R, et al (Faculty of Medicine Cordoba Univ, Spain; Mayo Clinic, Rochester MN; Polytechnic Univ of the Marche Region, Ancona, Italy; et al)
Hum Pathol 42:1653-1659, 2011

We present the clinicopathologic and immunohistochemical features of 25 cases of flat urothelial carcinoma in situ with glandular differentiation. Previously, cases on this category have been reported as in situ adenocarcinoma (a term not currently preferred). Fourteen of 25 cases had concurrent conventional urothelial carcinoma in situ. Five of the cases were primary carcinoma in situ with glandular differentiation; twenty cases of secondary carcinoma in situ with glandular differentiation were associated with urothelial carcinoma alone (n = 11) or with glandular differentiation (n = 7), discohesive (n = 1) or micropapillary carcinoma (n = 1). The individual tumor cells were columnar. The architectural pattern of the carcinoma in situ with glandular differentiation consisted of 1 or more papillary, flat or cribriform glandular patterns. Univariate statistical analysis showed no survival differences between urothelial carcinoma in situ with glandular differentiation and conventional urothelial carcinoma in situ (log-rank 0.810; $P = .368$). Carcinoma in situ with glandular differentiation showed high ki-67 index and p53 accumulation, high nuclear and cytoplasmic p16 expression and diffuse PTEN expression, a phenotype that also characterized concurrent conventional carcinoma in situ. MUC5A, MUC2, CK20, and c-erbB2 were positive in all 25 cases of urothelial carcinoma in situ with glandular differentiation, and CDX-2 was present in 19 cases; MUC1, CK7, or 34βE12 was focally present in 21, 19, and 18 cases, respectively. MUC1core was negative in all cases. We concluded that urothelial carcinoma in situ with glandular differentiation is a variant of carcinoma in situ that follows the natural history of conventional urothelial carcinoma in situ. The immunophenotype suggests urothelial origin with the expression of MUC5A and CDX2 as signature for glandular differentiation (Figs 1 and 2, Table 2).

▶ This study shows the natural history of flat urothelial carcinoma in situ with glandular differentiation as similar to conventional urothelial carcinoma in situ. The various immunohistochemical stains also suggest toward conventional urothelial carcinoma in situ (Table 2, Fig 2). The statistical analysis shows no survival difference between urothelial carcinoma in situ with glandular differentiation and conventional urothelial carcinoma in situ. The urothelial carcinoma in situ with glandular differentiation is a rare variant of urothelial carcinoma

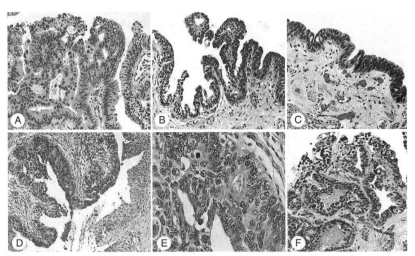

FIGURE 1.—Flat carcinoma in situ with glandular differentiation showing cribriform glandular (A), papillary (B) and flat (C) architectural patterns; CISg as compared with non-neoplastic urothelium (right) (D), high power view of a glandular structure with luminal mucin and columnar cells (E), CISg in von Brunn nests with tumor necrosis and occasional pleomorphism (F) (hematoxylin and eosin; original magnification ×200 [A-F], ×100 [D]). (Reprinted from Lopez-Beltran A, Jimenez RE, Montironi R, et al. Flat urothelial carcinoma in situ of the bladder with glandular differentiation. *Hum Pathol.* 2011;42:1653-1659, Copyright 2011, with permission from Elsevier.)

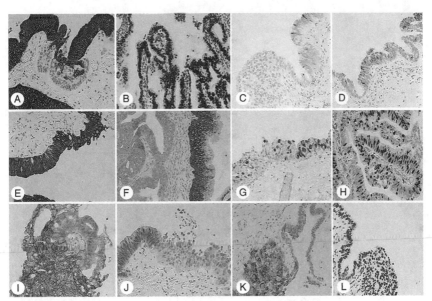

FIGURE 2.—Immunophenotype of CISg. CK20 (A), CDX2 (B), MUC5A, notice positive expression in CISg and negative in the adjacent cCIS (C), MUC2 (D), CK7 (E), 34βE12, notice the higher intensity in nonneoplastic urothelium (right) (F), p53 (G), Ki67 (H), c-erbB2, notice positive expression in both CISg and cCIS (I), p16, notice higher intensity in CISg (left) (J), MUC1 in both CISg and cCIS (K), and PTEN expression in both CISg and cCIS (L). Biotin-streptavidin immunohistochemistry (original magnification ×200 [A-L]). (Reprinted from Lopez-Beltran A, Jimenez RE, Montironi R, et al. Flat urothelial carcinoma in situ of the bladder with glandular differentiation. *Hum Pathol.* 2011;42:1653-1659, Copyright 2011, with permission from Elsevier.)

in situ, which may pose a significant differential diagnostic problem (Fig 1). In the current study, the number of patients is large, which has a statistical significance. Flat urothelial carcinoma in situ with glandular differentiation has been the subject of recent interest, and there is a large documented study comprising 19 cases by Miller and Epstein.[1] This is a vast report on a wide panel of immunohistochemical markers that attempts to define the immunophenotype of this interesting variant of carcinoma in situ but also aims at the current knowledge on the histogenesis of this entity. The article also emphasizes how to differentiate between intestinal metaplasia and carcinoma in situ with glandular differentiation.

S. A. Chandrakanth, MD, FRCPC

Reference

1. Miller JS, Epstein JI. Noninvasive urothelial carcinoma of the bladder with glandular differentiation: report of 24 cases. *Am J Surg Pathol.* 2009;33:1241-1248.

TABLE 2.—Summary of Immunohistochemical Findings in 25 Cases of Carcinoma In Situ with Glandular Differentiation Arising in the Bladder as Compared with 14 Cases of Concurrent Conventional Urothelial Carcinoma In Situ

% + Cells	CIS Type	CDX-2 + Cases (%)	PTEN + Cases (%)	P53 + Cases (%)	Ki67 + Cases (%)	P16 + Cases (%)	CK20 + Cases (%)	CK7 + Cases (%)	34BE12 + Cases (%)	c-erbB2 + Cases (%)	MUC5A + Cases (%)	MUC2 + Cases (%)	MUC1 + Cases (%)	MUC1 Core + Cases (%)
≤25%	CISg	12 (48)	0	21 (84)	0	8 (32)	0	14 (56)	0	0	0	10 (40)	10 (40)	0
	cCIS	0	0	0	0	0	11 (79)	0	2 (14)	0	0	0	0	0
26%-50%	CISg	3 (12)	0	4 (16)	6 (24)	15 (60)	0	5 (20)	12 (48)	2 (8)	9 (36)	15 (60)	11 (44)	0
	cCIS	0	0	0	4 (29)	9 (64)	3 (21)	0	5 (36)	2 (14)	0	4 (29)	6 (40)	6 (40)
51%-100%	CISg	4 (16)	25 (100)	0	19 (76)	2 (8)	0	0	6 (24)	23 (92)	16 (64)	0	0	0
	cCIS	0	14 (100)	14 (100)	10 (71)	5 (36)	0	14 (100)	7 (50)	12 (86)	0	10 (71)	8 (60)	8 (60)
Range + cells (%)	CISg	5-60	73-94	19-28	44-74	20-52	52-97	12-28	34-61	50-85	50-80	19-41	17-34	
	cCIS	0	71-89	66-84	41-83	42-61	15-36	88-98	23-58	48-89	0	44-72	40-69	38-63
Total + cases (%)	CISg	19 (76)	25 (100)	25 (100)	25 (100)	25 (100)	25 (100)	19 (76)	18 (72)	25 (100)	25 (100)	25 (100)	21 (84)	0
	cCIS	0	14 (100)	14 (100)	14 (100)	14 (100)	14 (100)	14 (100)	14 (100)	14 (100)	0	14 (100)	14 (100)	14 (100)

CD44v6, chromogranin, and MUC6 were negative in CISg and cCIS; CKAE1/AE3 diffusely stained both CISg and cCIS.

D2-40 immunoreactivity in penile squamous cell carcinoma: a marker of aggressiveness

Minardi D, d'Anzeo G, Lucarini G, et al (Polytechnic Univ of Marche Med School-United Hosps, Ancona, Italy; Polytechnic Univ of Marche Med School, Ancona, Italy; et al)
Hum Pathol 42:1596-1602, 2011

D2-40 immunohistochemical expression was investigated in tissue specimens from 39 patients with squamous cell carcinoma of the penis who underwent partial or total penectomy between 1987 and 2008. Patient age, tumor size, and grade; D2-40—positive lymphatic vessel density in intratumoral, peritumoral, and normal tissue; cell positivity for D2-40 in intratumoral and normal tissue; and D2-40 staining intensity and distribution were analyzed and correlated with disease-specific survival. Analysis of D2-40-positive lymphatics disclosed that mean lymphatic vessel density was greater in peritumoral tissue than in intratumoral and normal tissue and lower in patients with lymph node metastasis than in those without lymph node metastasis. The receiver operating characteristic curve showed that an intratumoral lymphatic vessel density greater than 2.0 had 83.3% sensitivity and 78% specificity in predicting lymph node metastasis. Analysis of cell immunoreactivity showed cytoplasmic D2-40 positivity in intratumoral and normal tissue in 89.7% and 65.5% of patients, respectively. A strong correlation emerged between grade of cell differentiation and D2-40 immunoreactivity in intratumoral tissue; in particular, 88.9% of tumors with weak podoplanin expression were G1, whereas strong cellular immunoreactivity was detected in 83.3% of G3 patients ($P = .003$; χ^2 test). A significant correlation was also noted between pattern of reactivity and tumor grade because the basal layer was positive in patients with undifferentiated tumors (100% of G3) and in 72.2% of G1 tumors ($P = .021$; χ^2 test). D2-40 seems to be a useful marker for the development of node

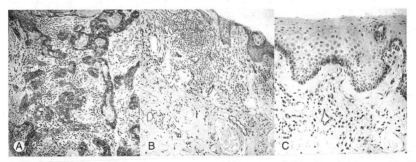

FIGURE 1.—D2-40 immunostaining in SCC of the penis. Intratumoral tissue showed immunopositive LV and high epithelial cell positivity for D2-40 (A, original magnification ×200); in peritumoral compartment, LVD was greater than in intratumoral tissue, but D2-40 expression in the epithelial cells was low (B, original magnification ×150); in normal tissue, D2-40 was weakly expressed both in LV and in epithelium, where it was found mainly at basal cell layer level (C, original magnification ×300). (Reprinted from Minardi D, d'Anzeo G, Lucarini G, et al. D2-40 immunoreactivity in penile squamous cell carcinoma: a marker of aggressiveness. *Hum Pathol* 2011;42:1596-1602, Copyright 2011, with permission from Elsevier.)

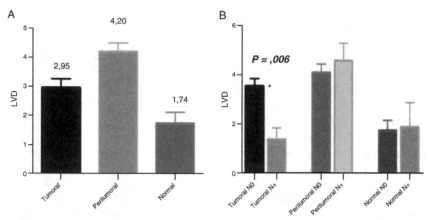

FIGURE 2.—A, LVD in intratumoral, peritumoral, and normal tissue. B, LVD in patients with and without lymph node metastasis. (Reprinted from Minardi D, d'Anzeo G, Lucarini G, et al. D2-40 immunoreactivity in penile squamous cell carcinoma: a marker of aggressiveness. *Hum Pathol* 2011;42:1596-1602, Copyright 2011, with permission from Elsevier.)

metastasis in squamous cell carcinoma of the penis, although validation in larger series is required to confirm its predictive value (Figs 1 and 2).

▶ This study demonstrates the usefulness of D2-40 immunohistochemical stain in squamous cell carcinoma of the penis and its value in recognizing the intratumoral lymphatic vessel tumor cells as in Figs 1 and 2. D2-40 can also be used to demonstrate metastatic deposits in other sites of the body. The immunoreactivity of D2-40 was evaluated in intratumoral, normal, and peritumoral squamous epithelium. The authors also noted a significant correlation between pattern of D2-40 reactivity and tumor grade, because diffuse infiltrating positivity was detected in undifferentiated tumors and basal pattern in gastrointestinal tumors. The specific biological significance of D2-40 immunopositivity is still unclear. D2-40 reactivity has been found in normal tissues, such as mesothelial cells, osteocytes, and epidermal cells as well as human tumors.[1] It is very interesting to note that the tumor stage, but not the grade of the tumor, predicted the lymph node metastasis.

S. A. Chandrakanth, MD, FRCPC

Reference

1. Wicki A, Christofori G. The potential role of podoplanin in tumour invasion. *Br J Cancer.* 2007;96:1-5.

Gleason Score 7 Prostate Cancer on Needle Biopsy: Relation of Primary Pattern 3 or 4 to Pathological Stage and Progression After Radical Prostatectomy

Amin A, Partin A, Epstein JI (The Johns Hopkins Med Inst, Baltimore, MD)
J Urol 186:1286-1290, 2011

Purpose.—There have been only a few contradictory publications assessing whether Gleason score $4 + 3 = 7$ has a worse prognosis than $3 + 4 = 7$ on biopsy material in predicting pathological stage and biochemical recurrence. Older studies predated the use of the modified Gleason grading system established in 2005.

Materials and Methods.—We retrospectively studied 1,791 cases of Gleason score 7 on prostatic biopsy to determine whether the breakdown of Gleason score 7 into $3 + 4$ vs $4 + 3$ has prognostic significance in the modern era.

Results.—There was no difference in patient age, preoperative serum prostate specific antigen, maximum tumor percent per core or the number of positive cores between Gleason score $3 + 4 = 7$ and Gleason score $4 + 3 = 7$. Gleason score $4 + 3 = 7$ showed an overall correlation with pathological stage (organ confined, focal extraprostatic extension, nonfocal extraprostatic extension, seminal vesicle invasion/lymph node metastases, $p = 0.005$). On multivariate analysis Gleason score $4 + 3 = 7$ ($p = 0.03$), number of positive cores ($p = 0.002$), maximum percent of cancer per core ($p = 0.006$) and preoperative serum prostate specific antigen ($p = 0.03$) all correlated with pathological stage. Gleason score $4 + 3 = 7$ on biopsy was also associated with an increased risk of biochemical progression after radical prostatectomy ($p = 0.0001$). On multivariate analysis Gleason score $4 + 3 = 7$ ($p = 0.001$), maximum percent of cancer per core ($p < 0.0001$) and preoperative serum prostate specific antigen ($p < 0.0001$) but not number of positive cores correlated with the risk of biochemical progression after radical prostatectomy.

Conclusions.—Our study further demonstrates that Gleason score 7 should not be considered a homogenous group for the purposes of disease management and prognosis (Tables 1 and 2).

▶ This study addresses the issue of Gleason grading 4 + 3 versus 3 + 4 and clinical outcome. The authors studied a significant number of cases retrospectively. Clinical parameters such as age, preoperative prostate-specific antigen,

TABLE 1.—Preoperative Clinicopathological Data

	Mean	Median	Range
Pt age	59.6	60	43−76
PSA (ng/ml)	6.7	6.6	1.6−62.2
No. cores sampled	12.3	12.4	1−37
Max % involvement/core	56.2	60	5−100

TABLE 2.—Relation of Biopsy Gleason Score to Pathological Stage

	No./Total No. (%)	
	Gleason Score $3 + 4 = 7$	Gleason Score $4 + 3 = 7$
Organ confined	720/1,262 (57.0)	253/519 (48.7)
Focal EPE	179/1,262 (14.2)	82/519 (16.8)
Nonfocal EPE	260/1,262 (20.6)	121/519 (23.3)
Seminal vesicle or lymph node metastases	103/1,262 (8.2)	63/519 (12.1)

tumor percent per core, and the number of positive cores were considered. Both scores have shown overall correlation with pathological stage.

The study demonstrates that a Gleason score of 7 should not be considered homogenous for disease management and prognosis. The modified Gleason score that came into effect in 2005 was used for this study. One author is a member of the International Society of Urological Pathology consensus group and a well-known uropathologist. The radical prostatectomy grade was based on the grade of the index tumor rather than the average grade for all tumors. The authors also included cribriform pattern as grade 4. This increased diagnosis of Gleason score 7. There are only a few studies demonstrating prognostic significance between 3 + 4 and 4 + 3, and this is one of them.

S. A. Chandrakanth, MD, FRCPC

11 Kidney

Role of Immunohistochemistry in the Evaluation of Needle Core Biopsies in Adult Renal Cortical Tumors: An Ex Vivo Study

Al-Ahmadie HA, Alden D, Fine SW, et al (Memorial Sloan-Kettering Cancer Ctr, NY)
Am J Surg Pathol 35:949-961, 2011

Multiple therapeutic options for renal tumors that are now available have put pathologists under increasing pressure to render diagnosis on limited material. Results on biopsies by hematoxylin and eosin (H&E) have historically not been encouraging. Currently, multiple immunohistochemical markers with differential expression in these renal tumors are available. We studied the utility of such markers on needle biopsies that were obtained ex vivo. After nephrectomy, two 18-guage cores were obtained and processed routinely. Expressions of carbonic anhydrase (CA) IX, CD117, α-methylacyl-CoA racemase (AMACR), cytokeratin 7 (CK7), and CD10 were evaluated. Results, with or without immunostaining, were compared with the final nephrectomy diagnosis. We studied 145 tumors, including 119 renal cell carcinomas (83 clear cell, 18 papillary, 14 chromophobe, and 4 type unclassified), 11 oncocytomas, and 15 miscellaneous tumors. Adequate evaluable material was present in 123 (85%) cases. In such biopsies, 81% of cases were correctly classified by H&E alone, with correct diagnosis in 90% of cases in the most common tumor subtypes (clear cell, papillary and chromophobe renal cell carcinoma, and oncocytoma). By adding immunostains, the accuracy was 90% overall and 99% among the 4 most common subtypes. The following extent and patterns of immuneexpression were highly useful in the diagnoses: diffuse, membranous CAIX expression in clear cell renal cell carcinoma, diffuse positivity for AMACR in papillary renal cell carcinoma, distinct peripheral cytoplasmic accentuation for CD117 in chromophobe renal cell carcinoma, widespread and intense positivity for CK7 in chromophobe and papillary renal cell carcinoma, and diffuse membranous reactivity in clear cell and patchy/luminal in papillary renal cell carcinoma for CD10. In conclusion, utilizing immunostains improves classification of renal tumors on needle biopsy, which may be of particular help for pathologists with limited experience. Both extent and patterns must be considered for a definitive diagnosis (Table 4).

▶ This article provides practical suggestions for a panel of immunohistochemical stains that may be useful in the evaluation of needle core biopsies of renal

TABLE 4.—Quantitative and Qualitative Analysis of IHC Markers in Common Renal Cortical Tumors

	Clear Cell RCC		Papillary RCC		Chromophobe RCC		Oncocytoma	
	N (%)	Staining Pattern	N (%)	Staining Pattern	N (%)	Staining Pattern	N (%)	Staining Pattern
CAIX	69/69 (100%)	Diffuse, membranous	10/14 (71%)	Focal, papillary tips/perinecrotic	1/11 (9%)	Perinecrotic	0/5 (0%)	Absent
CD10*	67/74 (91%)	Diffuse, membranous	13/17 (76%)	Membranous, luminal, focal or diffuse	3/13 (23%)	Cytoplasmic, focal	3/4 (75%)	Cytoplasmic, focal
AMACR*	46/68 (68%)	Cytoplasmic, focal or diffuse	17/17 (100%)	Cytoplasmic, finely granular, diffuse	5/13 (38%)	Cytoplasmic, focal	3/5 (60%)	Cytoplasmic, focal
CK7	19/74 (26%)	Cytoplasmic, focal	15/17 (88%)	Membranous, diffuse	10/11 (91%)	Membranous, diffuse	1/5 (20%)	Cytoplasmic, focal
CD117*	5/73 (7%)	Cytoplasmic, focal	1/17 (6%)	Cytoplasmic, focal (rare)	8/13 (62%)	Cytoplasmic with peripheral accentuation, diffuse	2/5 (40%)	Cytoplasmic, diffuse/focal

RCC indicates renal cell carcinoma.
*Cases of RCC urclassified type were immunoreactive with CD117 and CD10 (1 case each) and AMACR (3 cases).

masses. Strengths of the article include the number and diversity of renal lesions evaluated and the ability to compare the ex vivo biopsy results quickly to the complete mass excision. Ex vivo samples consisted of two 18-gauge needle core biopsies obtained via palpation. Surprisingly, 15% of cases did not contain sufficient diagnostic material on the ex vivo biopsy samples to make a diagnosis. This highlights the geographic variability and sampling issues associated with renal neoplasms. Another strength was the description of the qualitative features of the stains in each tumor type (Table 4). It should be noted that the correct diagnosis was obtained in more than 80% of the cases based on hematoxylin and eosin (H&E) morphology alone. In practice, only selected cases that are difficult to classify on H&E alone may need immunohistochemical analysis. Furthermore, as is described at the end of the abstract, the differential diagnosis based on histology might suggest 1 of 2 stains that may be of the highest benefit.

M. L. Smith, MD

Immunohistochemical Distinction of Primary Adrenal Cortical Lesions From Metastatic Clear Cell Renal Cell Carcinoma: A Study of 248 Cases

Sangoi AR, Fujiwara M, West RB, et al (El Camino Hosp, Mountain View, CA; Stanford Univ, CA; et al)
Am J Surg Pathol 35:678-686, 2011

The diagnosis of metastatic clear cell renal cell carcinoma (CC-RCC) can be difficult because of its morphologic heterogeneity and the increasing use of small image-guided biopsies that yield scant diagnostic material. This is further complicated by the degree of morphologic and immunophenotypic overlap with nonrenal neoplasms and tissues, such as adrenal cortex. In this study, a detailed immunoprofile of 63 adrenal cortical lesions, which included 54 cortical neoplasms, was compared with 185 metastatic CC-RCCs using traditional [anticalretinin, CD10, antichromogranin, antiepithelial membrane antigen, anti-inhibin, antimelanA, anticytokeratins (AE1/AE3 and AE1/CAM5.2), antirenal cell carcinoma marker, and antisynaptophysin)] and novel [anticarbonic anhydrase-IX, antihepatocyte nuclear factor-1b, antihuman kidney injury molecule-1 (hKIM-1), anti-PAX-2, anti-PAX-8, antisteroidogenic factor-1 (SF-1), and anti-T-cell immunoglobulin mucin-1] antibodies. Tissue microarray methodology was used to

TABLE 2.—Immunohistochemical Staining Results* for Metastatic CC-RCC Versus ACL With Adrenocortical Markers

	Calretinin (C, N)	Inhibin (C)	MelanA (C)	SF-1 (N)	Synaptophysin (C)
CC-RCC (overall)	18/184 (10%)	17/184 (9%)	18/184 (10%)	0/184 (0%)	3/184 (2%)
CC-RCC (WD)	13/133 (10%)	11/133 (8%)	11/133 (8%)	0/133 (0%)	2/133 (2%)
CC-RCC (PD)	5/51 (10%)	6/51 (12%)	7/51 (14%)	0/51 (0%)	1/51 (2%)
ACL	56/63 (89%)	54/63 (86%)	54/63 (86%)	54/63 (86%)	37/63 (59%)

ACL indicates adrenal cortical lesion; C, cytoplasmic; N, nuclear; PD, poorly differentiated; WD, well differentiated.
*≥2+ staining intensity considered positive.

TABLE 3.—Immunohistochemical Staining Results* for Metastatic CC-RCC Versus ACLs With Renal Epithelial Markers

	AE1/AE3 (M/C)	CAM5.2/AE1 (M/C)	CD10 (M/C)	EMA (M/C)	RCC (M/C)	CAIX (M/C)	hKIM-1 (M/C)	HNF-1b (N)	PAX-2 (N)	PAX-8 (N)	TIM-1 (M/C)
CC-RCC (overall)	101/184 (55%)	110/184 (60%)	142/185 (77%)	144/185 (78%)	33/185 (18%)	160/184 (87%)	153/185 (83%)	139/184 (76%)	91/185 (49%)	152/184 (83%)	68/184 (37%)
CC-RCC (WD)	64/133 (48%)	72/133 (54%)	103/133 (77%)	108/133 (81%)	28/133 (21%)	119/133 (89%)	110/133 (83%)	98/133 (74%)	70/133 (53%)	108/133 (81%)	50/131 (38%)
CC-RCC (PD)	37/51 (73%)	38/51 (75%)	39/52 (75%)	36/52 (69%)	5/52 (10%)	41/51 (80%)	43/52 (83%)	41/51 (80%)	21/52 (40%)	44/51 (86%)	18/53 (34%)
ACL	6/63 (10%)	5/63 (8%)	6/63 (10%)	0/63 (0%)	0/63 (0%)	2/63 (3%)	0/63 (0%)	0/63 (0%)	0/63 (0%)	0/63 (0%)	0/63 (0%)

ACL indicates adrenal cortical lesion; C, cytoplasmic; M, membranous; N, nuclear; PD, poorly differentiated; WD, well differentiated.
*≥2+ staining intensity considered positive.

simulate small image-guided biopsies. Staining extent and intensity were scored semiquantitatively for each antibody. In comparing different intensity thresholds required for a "positive" result, a value of ≥2+ was identified as optimal for diagnostic sensitivity/specificity. For the distinction of adrenal cortical lesions from metastatic CC-RCCs, immunoreactivity for the adrenal cortical antigens SF-1 (86% adrenal; 0% CC-RCC), calretinin (89% adrenal; 10% CC-RCC), inhibin (86% adrenal; 9% CC-RCC), and melanA (86% adrenal; 10% CC-RCC) and for the renal epithelial antigens hKIM-1 (0% adrenal; 83% CC-RCC), PAX-8 (0% adrenal; 83% CC-RCC), hepatocyte nuclear factor-1b (0% adrenal; 76% CC-RCC), epithelial membrane antigen (0% adrenal; 78% CC-RCC), and carbonic anhydrase-IX (3% adrenal; 87% CC-RCC) had the most potential use. Use of novel renal epithelial markers hKIM-1 (clone AKG7) and/or PAX-8 and the adrenocortical marker SF-1 in an immunohistochemical panel for distinguishing adrenal cortical lesions from metastatic CC-RCC offers improved diagnostic sensitivity and specificity (Tables 2 and 3).

▶ This article addresses our current lack of sensitive and specific markers for the differentiation of metastatic renal cell carcinoma from primary adrenal cortical lesions, such as adrenal cortical carcinoma. Tables 2 and 3 show the results of the study and percentages of reactivity for both traditional and novel markers. As the authors indicate, SF-1, PAX-8, and hKIM-1 show the greatest promise. hKIM-1 is not available commercially, so PAX-8 and SF-1 may be more immediately useful. The results also highlight the need for a panel approach to staining, as there is not one gold standard. The authors also bring up the difficult question of how much staining is required for a "positive" interpretation. The 2 + cutoff the authors used was defined as 2+ or greater intensity in greater than 10% of tumor cells. This allows for a lot of staining (1 +, less than 10%) that is still interpreted as negative. The staining was done on simulated needle core biopsies using tissue microarray methodologies. While this allowed for simulated biopsies, it did not allow for detailed studies of pattern of staining in larger tissue sections.

M. L. Smith, MD

Handling and reporting of nephrectomy specimens for adult renal tumours: a survey by the European Network of Uropathology
Algaba F, Delahunt B, Berney DM, et al (Fundacion Puigvert-University Autonomous, Barcelona, Spain; Univ of Otago, Wellington, New Zealand; Barts Cancer Inst, London, UK; et al)
J Clin Pathol 2011 [Epub ahead of print]

Aim.—To collect information on current practices of European pathologists for the handling and reporting of nephrectomy specimens with renal tumours.

Methods and Results.—A questionnaire was circulated to the members of the European Network of Uropathology, which consists of 343 pathologists in 15 European countries. Replies were received from 48% of members.

These replies indicated that nephrectomy specimens are most often received in formalin. Lymph nodes are found in less than 5% of nephrectomy specimens. All respondents give an objective measure of tumour size, most commonly in three diameters. The most common method to search for capsule penetration is to slice tissue outside the tumour perpendicularly into the tumour. The most common sampling algorithm from tumours greater than 2 cm is one section for every centimetre of maximum tumour diameter. Most respondents use the 2004 WHO renal tumour classification although only slightly over half consider small papillary tumours malignant if the diameter is greater than 5 mm. The Fuhrman grading system is widely used. Almost all use immunohistochemistry for histological typing in some cases, while only 7% always use it. The most utilised special stains are CK7 (95%), CD10 (93%), vimentin (86%), HMB45 (68%), c-kit (61%) and Hale's colloidal iron (52%). Only 18% use other ancillary techniques for diagnosis in difficult cases.

Conclusions.—While most pathologists appear to follow published guidelines for reporting renal carcinoma, there is still a need for the development of consensus and further standardisation of practice for contentious areas of specimen handling and reporting.

▶ This is an interesting retrospective survey-based study on the practice of grossing and reporting renal tumors in Europe. The most important aspect of practice that this article highlights is the lack of overall standardization in gross handling and reporting of renal tumor specimens. As the physician responsible for definitive reporting, classification, and pathologic staging, pathologists owe it to patients to standardize their practice. One of the more surprising findings was that only 75% of respondents looked for nonneoplastic renal disease in the uninvolved renal parenchyma. In patients who have just had their glomerular filtration rate decreased by 50%, the search and identification of nonneoplastic disease is of great importance. It should also be noted that there is little consensus on how to report small (< 10 mm) papillary neoplasms. Strengths of the article include the large number of participants (175) from a range of practice settings, including academic institutions (55%) and community hospitals (41%). Weaknesses include selection bias based on survey response and overall response rate (47.5%).

M. L. Smith, MD

Pure Epithelioid PEComas (So-Called Epithelioid Angiomyolipoma) of the Kidney: A Clinicopathologic Study of 41 Cases: Detailed Assessment of Morphology and Risk Stratification
Nese N, Martignoni G, Fletcher CD, et al (Cedars-Sinai Med Ctr, Los Angeles, CA; Universita'di Verona, Italy; Brigham and Women's Hosp and Dana-Farber/ Harvard Med School, Boston, MA; et al)
Am J Surg Pathol 35:161-176, 2011

Epithelioid angiomyolipomas (perivascular epithelioid cell tumors) of the kidney are defined as potentially malignant mesenchymal lesions that are closely related to classic angiomyolipoma. Although approximately 120 cases are published, mostly as case reports with variably used diagnostic criteria, the pathologic prognostic predictors of outcome are unknown. We analyzed the clinicopathologic parameters in a large series of 41 cases of pure epithelioid angiomyolipomas of the kidney, which we designate as pure (monotypic) epithelioid PEComas to contrast them from classic angiomyolipomas that are regarded by some as PEComas. We use the terminology "pure" to separate these cases from those that may have variable epithelioid components. The mean age of the patients was 40.7 years (range, 14 to 68 y). The male-to-female ratio was 1:1. Seventy-nine percent of patients were symptomatic at presentation with metastatic disease at onset in 12 cases. Follow-up and/or disease progression information were available for 33 of 41 cases (mean, 44.5 mo and median, 24.5 mo; range, 4 to 240); 9 patients had a history of associated tuberous sclerosis. Recurrence and metastasis were seen in 17% and 49%of patients; 33%of patients died of disease. Lymph node involvement was seen in 24% of patients; the liver (63%), lung (25%), and mesentery (18.8%) were the most common metastatic sites. Clinicopathologic parameters associated with disease progression (recurrence, metastasis, or death due to disease) in univariate analysis included associated tuberous sclerosis complex or concurrent angiomyolipoma (any metastasis, $P = 0.046$), necrosis (metastasis at diagnosis, $P = 0.012$), tumor size >7 cm (progression, $P = 0.021$), extrarenal extension and/or renal vein involvement (progression, $P = 0.023$), and carcinoma-like growth pattern (progression, $P = 0.040$) (the 5 adverse prognostic parameters for pure epithelioid PEComas). Tumors with <2 adverse prognostic parameters (13 cases) were considered to be low risk for progression tumor, with 15% having disease progression. Tumors with 2 to 3 adverse prognostic parameters (14 cases) were considered to be "intermediate risk," with 64% having disease progression. Tumors with more than 4 or more adverse prognostic parameters (6 cases) were considered to be high risk, with all patients having disease progression. Of tumors with 3 or more adverse prognostic parameters, 80% had disease progression. An exact logistic regression analytic model showed that only carcinoma-like growth pattern and extrarenal extension and/or renal vein involvement were significant predictors of outcome ($P = 0.009$ and 0.033, respectively). Our data of a large series with uniform definitional criteria confirm the malignant potential for pure epithelioid PEComas and provide adverse prognostic parameters for risk stratification in these patients (Table 3).

▶ Epithelial PEComas (EP) can be challenging lesions from a diagnostic and prognostic perspective. This is an excellent article that summarizes the histologic features and patterns of EP with precise inclusion and exclusion details. Immunohistochemical inclusion criteria included negative reactions for epithelial markers, such as pan-cytokeratin, EMA, and Cam 5.2 as well as positive reactions for both melanocytic differentiation (melan-A and HMB45) and actins. The goal of the authors was to create a homogenous set of cases to study. Two major patterns were observed, a carcinomalike growth pattern (pattern A) and a diffuse

TABLE 3.—Risk Stratification in 33 Cases

Risk Stratification	Cases With Progression, N (%)	Cases Without Progression, N (%)	Total
Low-risk group (0-1 adverse parameters)	2 (15.4)	11 (84.6)	13 (39.4)
Intermediate-risk group (2-3 adverse parameters)	9 (64.3)	5 (35.7)	14 (42.4)
High-risk group (4-5 adverse parameters)	6 (100)	0 (0)	6 (18.2)
Total	17 (51.5)	16 (48.5)	33 (100)

growth pattern (pattern B). Table 3 shows the risk stratification in cases based on parameters associated with progression listed in the abstract. This is important prognostic information that has not been previously available. Strengths of this article include the strict inclusion criteria, detailed clinical histories, and large number of cases of a relatively rare entity. The biggest weakness is the retrospective nature of the design and the possibility of selection bias.

M. L. Smith, MD

Immunohistochemical markers of tissue injury in biopsies with transplant glomerulitis
Batal I, Azzi J, El-Haddad N, et al (Univ of Pittsburgh Med Ctr, PA; Brigham and Women's Hosp, Boston, MA)
Hum Pathol 2011 [Epub ahead of print]

Transplant glomerulitis is associated with suboptimal graft function. To understand its pathogenesis and to assess the parameters of potential prognostic value, we immunostained 25 paraffin-embedded allograft biopsies showing glomerulitis for markers of complement activation (C4d), cytotoxicity (Granzyme-B), apoptosis (Bcl-XL, Bcl-2, and Fas-L), and endothelial injury (von Willebrand factor). Staining was semiquantitatively assessed in different anatomical compartments, and comparison was made with 40 control allograft biopsies without glomerulitis. Biopsies with glomerulitis had more frequent incidence of "mixed" T-cell and antibody-mediated rejection compared with controls [8/25 (32%) versus 4/40 (10%), $P = .046$]. Furthermore, they had higher glomerular capillary-C4d scores (1.9 ± 1.1 versus 1.2 ± 1.2, $P = .015$), which tended to persist when biopsies showing transplant glomerulopathy were excluded. Higher glomerular capillary-C4d scores were observed in samples with versus without donor-specific antibody (2.5 ± 0.9 versus 1.2 ± 1.2, $P = .01$). Compared with controls, biopsies with glomerulitis had more intraglomerular (4.8 ± 4.5 versus 0.9 ± 0.8 cells/glomerulus, $P < .001$) and interstitial mainly peritubular capillary (6.1 ± 4.1 versus 3.2 ± 3.4 cells/hpf, $P = .002$) Granzyme-B+ leukocytes. Higher mesangial—von Willebrand factor scores were noted in the glomerulitis group (1.8 ± 1.0 versus 0.8 ± 0.8, $P = .003$) and correlated with the percentage of inflamed glomeruli ($r = 0.54$, $P < .001$). Interstitial—von Willebrand factor was associated with a higher peritubular

TABLE 1.—Histologic Assessment, Detection of Circulating DSA, and Follow-up Information for Cases Studied

	No Glomerulitis (n = 40)	Glomerulitis (n = 25)
Mixed rejection (TCMR and AMR)[a]	4/40 (10%)	8/25 (32%)
TCMR	17/40 (43%)	7/25 (28%)
AMR (diagnostic/ suspicious)	6/40 (15%)	2/25 (8%)
Borderline changes suspicious for TCMR	13/40 (32%)	8/25 (32%)
Tubulitis (t)	1.8 ± 0.8	2.0 ± 0.9
Interstitial inflammation (i)	1.7 ± 0.7	1.9 ± 0.8
Intimal arteritis (v)	0.1 ± 0.4	0.1 ± 0.4
Peritubular capillaritis[b]	0.5 ± 0.8	1.2 ± 1.0
TGP (cg)	0.03 ± 0.16	0.36 ± 0.76
Mesangial matrix expansion (mm)	0.2 ± 0.5	0.7 ± 0.9
Interstitial fibrosis (ci)	1.0 ± 0.6	1.2 ± 0.6
Tubular atrophy (ct)	1.1 ± 0.5	1.2 ± 0.5
Arteriolar hyalinosis (ah)	0.9 ± 0.7	0.8 ± 0.8
Arterial fibrointimal thickening (cv)	0.9 ± 0.7	1.1 ± 0.8
DSA at the biopsy	4/32 (13%)	4/18 (22%)
DSA at anytime during the transplantation course	11/40 (28%)	9/25 (36%)
Development of TGP[c]	1/28 (4%; 682 d postbiopsy)	4/16 (25%; 256 ± 160 d postbiopsy)
2-y postbiopsy graft failure[d]	5/28 (18%)	11/16 (69%)

NOTE. Information on DSA at the time of biopsy was available on 50 occasions (18 with and 32 without glomerulitis). Follow-up information on development of TGP and 2-year postbiopsy graft failure was available for 44 patients (16 with and 28 without glomerulitis).
[a]Mixed rejection: $P = .046$ (glomerulitis vs no glomerulitis; Fisher exact test).
[b]Peritubular capillaritis: $P = .02$ (glomerulitis *vs* no glomerulitis; Mann-Whitney test).
[c]Development of TGP: $P = .05$ (glomerulitis *vs* no glomerulitis; Fisher exact test).
[d]Two-year postbiopsy graft failure: $P = .001$ (glomerulitis vs no glomerulitis; Fisher exact test).

capillaritis score (interstitial—von Willebrand factor: 1.6 ± 1.2 versus no interstitial—von Willebrand factor: 0.6 ± 0.9, $P = .02$). Glomerular capillary—Bcl-XLwas not associated with accommodation. Finally, no difference in Bcl-2 or Fas-L was observed upon comparing glomerulitis to controls. In conclusion, glomerular injury in transplant glomerulitis appears to be mediated by complement activation and cellular cytotoxicity. Mesangial— or interstitial—von Willebrand factor identified cases with more severe microcirculation injury (Table 1).

▶ This interesting retrospective case-control study sought to immunohisto-chemically characterize cases of transplant glomerulitis (TG) in an effort to provide clues to its pathogenesis. TG is only used in the Banff schema for allograft rejection in the antibody-mediated changes category. However, TG is often seen isolated from other features of antibody-mediated rejection and in cases of acute cellular rejection. Cases of TG more often showed C4d in the glomerular capillaries and an increase in Granzyme B positive cells, which suggest both antibody- and cellular rejection—mediated components, respectively. In this series, TG was strongly associated with transplant glomerulopathy and 2-year graft failure (Table 1). Von Willebrand factor is unlikely to be of clinical use because strong staining was mostly seen in cases with high PTC and G scores. These data should be correlated with the molecular expression profiles of antibody- and cellular-mediated rejection. Weaknesses of this study include the smaller sample size and short follow-up time period, and a strength includes the broad array of immunohistochemical markers used in the analysis. For further reading on microcirculation injury in the renal allograft, I recommend Einecke et al.[1]

M. L. Smith, MD

Reference

1. Einecke G, Sis B, Reeve J, et al. Antibody-mediated microcirculation injury is the major cause of late kidney transplant failure. *Am J Transplant.* 2009;9:2520-2531.

The Nature of Biopsies with "Borderline Rejection" and Prospects for Eliminating This Category

de Freitas DG, Sellarés J, Mengel M, et al (Univ of Alberta, Edmonton, Canada; et al)
Am J Transplant 2011 [Epub ahead of print]

In kidney transplantation, many inflamed biopsies with changes insufficient to be called T-cell-mediated rejection (TCMR) are labeled "borderline", leaving management uncertain. This study examined the nature of borderline biopsies as a step toward eventual elimination of this category. We compared 40 borderline, 35 TCMR and 116 nonrejection biopsies. TCMR biopsies had more inflammation than borderline but similar degrees of tubulitis and scarring. Surprisingly, recovery of function after biopsy was similar in all categories, indicating that response to treatment is unreliable for defining TCMR. We studied the molecular changes in TCMR, borderline and nonrejection using microarrays, measuring four published features: T-cell burden; a rejection classifier; a canonical TCMR classifier; and risk score. These reassigned borderline biopsies as TCMR like 13/40 (33%) or nonrejection-like 27/40 (67%). A major reason that histology diagnosed molecularly defined TCMR as borderline was atrophy-scarring, which interfered with assessment of inflammation and tubulitis. Decision tree analysis showed that i-total >27% and tubulitis extent >3% match the molecular diagnosis of TCMR in 85% of cases. In summary, most cases designated borderline by histopathology are found to be nonrejection by molecular phenotyping. Both molecular measurements and histopathology offer opportunities for more precise assignment of these cases after clinical validation (Fig 7).

▶ This is a fascinating article that uses the molecular phenotype of renal allograft cell-mediated rejection cases and nonrejection cases to help solve the frustrating dilemma of borderline changes in renal allograft biopsies. This category is challenging to both pathologists and clinicians, as no clear treatment direction is given, and the changes may be nonspecific changes or represent rejection. Fig 7 shows the decision tree analysis that was developed based on the findings in the study. Two features in addition to traditional Banff criteria

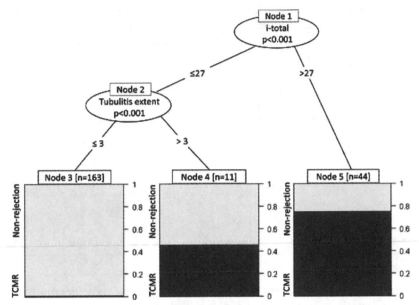

FIGURE 7.—Decision tree analysis. The i-total and t-extent lesions are the closest histological approximation of the molecular method of eliminating borderline. (Reprinted from de Freitas DG, Sellarés J, Mengel M, et al. The nature of biopsies with "Borderline Rejection" and prospects for eliminating this category. *Am J Transplant*. 2011 [Epub ahead of print], with permission from The American Society of Transplantation and the American Society of Transplant Surgeons.)

proved useful in the subclassification, total inflammation, and tubulitis extent. These represent the percentage of renal cortex or tubules involved with inflammation or tubulitis, respectively. The importance of these scores in this study highlights the need to evaluate atrophic and scarred tubules and areas for active inflammatory cell infiltrates. Finally, while molecular array studies suffer from sampling bias similar to that of light microscopy, it must be remembered that molecular data are based on the entire core of tissue rather than just several thin sections. Further validation of both molecular and pathologic methods to reclassify borderline changes is needed.

M. L. Smith, MD

Overlapping pathways to transplant glomerulopathy: chronic humoral rejection, hepatitis C infection, and thrombotic microangiopathy

Baid-Agrawal S, Farris AB III, Pascual M, et al (Charite Universitatsmedizin Berlin, Germany; Emory Univ, Atlanta, GA; Univ Hosp of Lausanne (CHUV), Switzerland; et al)
Kidney Int 80:879-885, 2011

Transplant glomerulopathy (TG) has received much attention in recent years as a symptom of chronic humoral rejection; however, many cases lack C4d deposition and/or circulating donor-specific antibodies (DSAs).

TABLE 1.—Pathological Features of Patients with TG According to HCV and C4d Status

	HCV⁻TG (n=16; %)	HCV⁺TG (n=9; %)	C4d⁻TG (n=13)	C4d⁺TG (n=12)
GBM duplication (both LM+EM)	16 (100%)	9 (100%)	13 (100%)	12 (100%)
Mesangial hypercellularity	11 (69%)[a]	2 (22%)[a]	8 (62%)	5 (42%)
Mononuclear cells in glomeruli[b] (≥10 cells/glomerulus)	10/14 (71%)	5/7 (71%)	10/13 (77%)	5/8 (63%)
Mononuclear cells in PTC[c] (in >10% PTC)	3/13 (23%)	2/7 (29%)	1/12 (8%)	4/8 (50%)
PTCBMML (≥3 layers)[d]	4/8 (50%)	4/4 (100%)	1/3 (33%)	7/9 (78%)
Additional features of TMA (n=8)	3 (19%)	5 (56%)	6 (46%)	2 (17%)
Complement C4d deposits in PTC (n=12)	9 (56%)	3 (33%)	0	12
HCV positivity	0	9	6/13 (46%)	3/12 (25%)

Abbreviations: EM, electron microscopy; GBM, glomerular basement membrane; HCV, hepatitis C virus; LM, light microscopy; PTC, peritubular capillary; PTCBMML, peritubular capillary basement membrane multilayering; TG, transplant glomerulopathy; TMA, thrombotic microangiopathy.
[a]$P=0.04$.
[b]Data could be analyzed in 21/25 cases.
[c]Data could be analyzed in 20/25 cases.
[d]Data could be analyzed in 12/25 cases.

To determine the contribution of other causes, we studied 209 consecutive renal allograft indication biopsies for chronic allograft dysfunction, of which 25 met the pathological criteria of TG. Three partially overlapping etiologies accounted for 21 (84%) cases: C4d-positive (48%), hepatitis C-positive (36%), and thrombotic microangiopathy (TMA)-positive (32%) TG. The majority of patients with confirmed TMA were also hepatitis C-positive, and the majority of hepatitis C-positive patients had TMA. DSAs were significantly associated with C4d-positive but not with hepatitis C-positive TG. The prevalence of hepatitis C was significantly higher in the TG group than in 29 control patients. Within the TG cohort, those who were hepatitis C-positive developed allograft failure significantly earlier than hepatitis C-negative patients. Thus, TG is not a specific diagnosis but a pattern of pathological injury involving three major overlapping pathways. It is important to distinguish these mechanisms, as they may have different prognostic and therapeutic implications (Table 1).

▶ This excellent article reminds us that not all cases of transplant glomerulopathy (TG), namely, double contour formation or glomerular basement membrane duplication with or without mesangial expansion, are uniquely related to chronic humoral rejection. As pathologists, we should investigate individual cases showing features of TG to look for causes other than rejection, such as thrombotic microangiopathy (TMA) and hepatitis C virus (HCV) infection. Table 1 shows the histologic findings in the 25 cases of TG, stratified by HCV and C4d positivity. There is broad overlap in the histologic findings, and all categories showed at least 17% of cases with additional features of TMA such as thrombi, mucoid intimal thickening, and red blood cell fragments. This broad overlap highlights the fact that these diagnoses are mutually exclusive, and there may be etiologic overlap in many of these cases. Weaknesses of this study include the small number of cases and lack of donor specific antibody data on 13 of the 25 total cases.

M. L. Smith, MD

Low glomerular density is a risk factor for progression in idiopathic membranous nephropathy
Tsuboi N, Kawamura T, Miyazaki Y, et al (The Jikei Univ School of Medicine, Tokyo, Japan)
Nephrol Dial Transplant 26:3555-3560, 2011

Background.—The adverse histological features predicting a progressive loss of renal function in idiopathic membranous nephropathy (IMN), before the establishment of impaired renal function with advanced glomerulosclerosis and/or interstitial fibrosis, are still poorly understood. The present study examined the relationship between the glomerular density (GD; non-sclerotic glomerular number/renal cortical area of biopsy) and the renal prognosis in IMN patients, especially in those without any apparent renal dysfunction at the time of diagnosis.

Methods.—The predictive value of the factors at biopsy, including the GD, on the renal outcome was retrospectively analyzed in the 65 IMN patients with an estimated glomerular filtration rate (eGFR) of ≥60 mL/min/1.73m² (mean, 80 mL/min/1.73m²) at biopsy.

Results.—The individual values for GD ranged from 1.6 to 6.5/mm² with 4-fold variation. A lower GD was associated with progression based on a ≥50% reduction in eGFR or reaching to end-stage renal disease. An association between a lower GD and progression was observed, especially in patients with persistent proteinuria of ≥1 g/day at follow-up. In contrast, any patients who achieved proteinuria of <1 g/day at follow-up did not show progression regardless of their GD levels. In addition, among the various clinicopathological factors observed, the GD was the only factor at biopsy that independently predicted the slope of the renal function during the observation periods.

Conclusion.—These results suggest that low GD is a plausible risk factor for progression in IMN patients, especially in those that do not achieve a remission of proteinuria during the follow-up (Fig 1).

▶ Several points from this morphologic study of glomerular density (GD) in patients with membranous nephropathy deserve mention. First, the authors identified a higher rate of progression in patients with decreased GD, but only in patients without a good clinical response to treatment and ongoing proteinuria (Fig 1). Therefore, continued proteinuria is the primary case of progression. Second, there was no mention of the variation of glomerular density based on which level was used for evaluation. Many renal pathologists have experienced a wide variation in the number glomeruli seen per section depending on what level is being evaluated. GD does not take overall renal cortical volume into account. Perhaps a future study may be to correlate GD

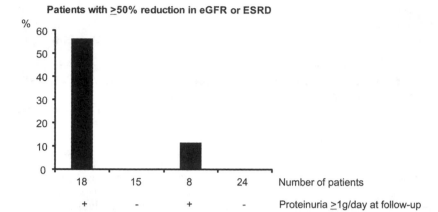

Patients with ≥50% reduction in eGFR or ESRD

FIGURE 1.—Effects of persistent proteinuria on the progression of IMN in relation to the GD levels. The patients were divided into four groups according to the presence or absence of persistent proteinuria (≥1 g/day) at follow-up and the lower (<3.1/mm²) or higher GD (≥3.1/mm²). The indices give the rate of the patients with progression, which was defined as ≥50% reduction in eGFR or ESRD, in each group. The progression was enhanced by the presence of persistent proteinuria, especially in the cases with a lower GD. (Reprinted from Tsuboi N, Kawamura T, Miyazaki Y, et al. Low glomerular density is a risk factor for progression in idiopathic membranous nephropathy. *Nephrol Dial Transplant.* 2011;26:3555-3560, with permission from The Author.)

with renal cortical volume and assess for predictive outcomes. Finally, it should also be noted that globally sclerotic glomeruli were excluded from the calculation of GD. This may lead to lower GD in patents who have more significant prior renal cortical injury from etiologies other than membranous nephropathy, such as hypertension.

M. L. Smith, MD

Postinfectious Glomerulonephritis in the Elderly
Nasr SH, Fidler ME, Valeri AM, et al (Mayo Clinic, Rochester, MN; Columbia Univ, NY)
J Am Soc Nephrol 22:187-195, 2011

Postinfectious glomerulonephritis (PIGN) is primarily a childhood disease that occurs after an upper respiratory tract infection or impetigo; its occurrence in older patients is not well characterized. Here, we report 109 cases of PIGN in patients ≥65 years old diagnosed by renal biopsy. The male to female ratio was 2.8:1. An immunocompromised background was present in 61%, most commonly diabetes or malignancy. The most common site of infection was skin, followed by pneumonia and urinary tract infection. The most common causative agent was staphylococcus (46%) followed by streptococcus (16%) and unusual gram-negative organisms. Hypocomplementemia was present in 72%. The mean peak serum creatinine was

TABLE 5.—Light Microscopic Findings

Pathologic Findings	No. of Patients	Percentage of Patients
Mean number of glomeruli	17	
Percentage of globally sclerotic glomeruli	22%	
Number of cases with cellular crescents (<20% of glomeruli, ≥20% of glomeruli)	40 (26/14)	37 (65/35)
Number of cases with necrosis (<20% of glomeruli, ≥20% of glomeruli)	21 (17, 4)	19 (81, 19)
Interstitial inflammation: none/focal/diffuse	5/93/11	5/85/10
Acute tubular injury: none/focal/diffuse	13/54/42	12/50/39
Tubular atrophy and interstitial fibrosis: none/mild/moderate/severe	13/71/21/4	12/65/19/4
Arteriosclerosis and arteriolar hyalinosis: none/mild/moderate/severe	3/34/64/8	3/31/59/7

5.1 mg/dl, and 46% of patients required acute dialysis. The most common light microscopic patterns were diffuse (53%), focal (28%), and mesangial (13%) proliferative glomerulonephritis. IgA-dominant PIGN occurred in 17%. Of the 72 patients with ≥3 months of follow-up (mean, 29 months), 22% achieved complete recovery, 44% had persistent renal dysfunction, and 33% progressed to ESRD. The presence of diabetes, higher creatinine at biopsy, dialysis at presentation, the presence of diabetic glomerulosclerosis, and greater tubular atrophy and interstitial fibrosis predicted ESRD. In summary, the epidemiology of PIGN is shifting as the population ages. Older men and patients with diabetes or malignancy are particularly at risk, and the sites of infection and causative organisms differ from the typical childhood disease. Prognosis for these older patients is poor, with fewer than 25% recovering full renal function (Table 5).

▶ This is an excellent and comprehensive retrospective review of the clinicopathologic features of postinfectious glomerulonephritis in the elderly population. The large number of cases (109) of this relatively rare diagnosis in elderly patients is a strength of the study. The light-microscopic findings are presented in Table 5. Not surprisingly, elderly patients showed significant evidence of chronic disease, such as glomerulosclerosis, interstitial fibrosis, tubular atrophy, and hyaline arteriolosclerosis. Obviously, patients with more advanced chronic disease were less likely to recover renal function. Immunoglobulin (Ig) A—predominant disease accounted for 17% of cases. This diagnosis should be considered in patients with C3 and IgA alone or predominant reactivity by immunofluorescence. Diabetes and a staphylococcal infection are the major risk factors for IgA-predominant postinfectious disease. Approximately 5% of the cases from the study showed a concurrent positive antineutrophil cytoplasmic antibody (ANCA), suggesting that one should not assume that positive ANCA and acute renal failure means pauci-immune glomerulonephritis.

M. L. Smith, MD

A composite urine biomarker reflects interstitial inflammation in lupus nephritis kidney biopsies
Zhang X, Nagaraja HN, Nadasdy T, et al (The Ohio State Univ College of Medicine, Columbus)
Kidney Int 2011 [Epub ahead of print]

The initial treatment of lupus nephritis is usually based on a renal biopsy. Subsequent disease flares, however, are often treated without the benefit of kidney pathology because repeat biopsies are infrequent. A noninvasive, real-time method to assess renal pathology would be useful to adjust treatment and improve outcome. To develop such a method we collected urine samples at or close to the time of 64 biopsies from 61 patients with lupus nephritis to identify potential biomarkers of tubulointerstitial inflammation and correlated these to biopsy parameters scored by a renal pathologist using a semiquantitative scale. Linear discriminant analysis was used to weight variables and derive composite biomarkers that identified the level of tubulointerstitial inflammation based on urine concentrations of monocyte chemotactic protein-1, hepcidin (a marker of active lupus), and liver fatty acid—binding protein. The discriminant function that described the most accurate composite biomarkers included urine monocyte chemotactic protein-1 and serum creatinine as the independent variables. This composite had sensitivity, specificity, positive predictive value, and negative predictive value of 100, 81, 67, and 100%, respectively. Only 14% of the biopsies were misclassified. Thus, specific renal pathologic lesions can be

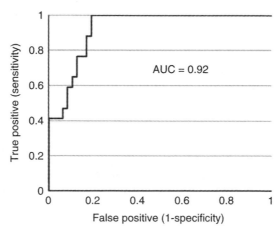

FIGURE 1.—Receiver operating characteristic (ROC) curve for a composite biomarker of renal interstitial inflammation. This ROC curve is based on Equation (1) that combines urine monocyte chemoattractant protein-1 (uMCP-1) and serum creatinine (SCr) to differentiate biopsies with none—mild interstitial inflammation from moderate—severe interstitial inflammation. The area under the curve (AUC) is 0.92. (Reprinted from Zhang X, Nagaraja HN, Nadasdy T, et al. A composite urine biomarker reflects interstitial inflammation in lupus nephritis kidney biopsies. *Kidney Int.* 2011;[Epub ahead of print], with permission from Macmillan Publishers Ltd: Kidney International.)

TABLE 2.—Comparison of Patients with Different Levels of Interstitial Inflammation

Demographic/Clinical Feature/ Biomarker Level	None—Mild Inflammation	Moderate—Severe Inflammation
Caucasian (%)	25 (53)	4 (24)
African American (%)	16 (34)	11 (64)[a]
Other (%)	6 (13)	2 (12)[a]
Age	30±1.1	32±2.1
Mean SCr[b] (mg/dl)	1.09±0.10	2.61±0.37
Mean uPCR	2.80±0.42	5.33±1.23[c]
Class II (%)	6 (13%)	0
Class III, III+V (%)	11 (23%)	4 (23.5%)
Class IV, IV+V (%)	25 (53%)	12 (70.5%)
Class V (%)	5 (11%)	1 (6%)
uMCP-1 (ng per mg Cr)	1.22±0.15	5.21±1.18[d]
uHepcidin (ng per mg Cr)	235±55	658±229[e]
uLFABP (ng per mg Cr)	71±10	152±31[f]

Abbreviations: Cr, creatinine; SCr, serum creatinine; uHepcidin, urine hepcidin; uLFABP, urine liver-type fatty acid—binding protein; uMCP-1, urine monocyte chemoattractant protein-1; uPCR, urine protein/creatinine ratio.
[a]African Americans plus other races/ethnicities were significantly overrepresented in the moderate—severe interstitial inflammation group (P=0.048, Fisher's exact test).
[b]SCr ± s.e.m.
[c]P<0.0001 versus none—mild inflammation (Mann—Whitney test).
[d]Biomarker levels are mean ± s.e.m.; P<0.0001 versus none—mild inflammation (Mann—Whitney test).
[e]P<0.003 versus none—mild inflammation (Mann—Whitney test).
[f]P<0.002 versus none—mild inflammation (Mann—Whitney test).

modeled by composite biomarkers to noninvasively follow and adjust the treatment of lupus nephritis reflecting renal injury (Fig 1, Table 2).

▶ This study describes the development of a urine-based assay for the prediction of interstitial inflammation, specifically in cases of lupus nephritis. Fig 1 shows impressive receiver operating characteristics for the composite biomarker, with an area under the curve of 0.92. It should be noted that the composite biomarker was only designed to predict interstitial inflammation, not glomerular lesions that may very well lead to kidney damage and fibrosis. Table 2 presents several cases with very active lupus nephritis (23% had World Health Organization class III, and 53% class IV) and nonmild interstitial inflammation. Nevertheless, this preliminary study demonstrates possibilities for urine based noninvasive surveillance of not only lupus nephritis, but also of other renal diseases associated with interstitial inflammation. It would be interesting to study the ability to predict glomerular disease as well. The weaknesses of this study include the relatively small sample size and restriction to associations with interstitial inflammation.

M. L. Smith, MD

Immunohistochemical evaluation of podocalyxin expression in glomerulopathies associated with nephrotic syndrome

Kavoura E, Gakiopoulou H, Paraskevakou H, et al (Natl and Kapodistrian Univ of Athens, Greece; et al)

Hum Pathol 42:227-235, 2011

It is now well established that morphological change of podocytes is closely correlated to the development of proteinuria. The aim of this study was to investigate the role of podocalyxin, a major podocyte protein, in the pathogenesis of glomerulopathies primarily associated with the nephrotic syndrome. Immunohistochemical expression of podocalyxin has been evaluated in 51 renal samples, including healthy controls, patients with podocytopathies (minimal change disease [MCD], focal segmental glomerulosclerosis [FSGS]) and membranous glomerulopathy (MG). A computerized image analysis program has been used. Statistical analysis was performed using analysis of variance and Bonferroni tests. Immunohistochemical expression of podocalyxin has been observed within the podocytes of healthy controls. In MCD, podocalyxin expression was globally reduced despite the normal appearance of the glomeruli. In FSGS, podocalyxin loss was observed in both the segmental sclerotic and the nonsclerotic areas being significantly more prominent in the former. Reduction of podocalyxin in MG was demonstrated for the first time immunohistochemically. The percentage of the

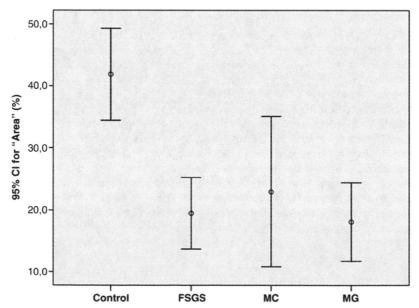

FIGURE 6.—Histogram showing the mean value and the 95% confidence interval (95% CI) for the 3 groups (MC indicates minimal change disease). (Reprinted from Kavoura E, Gakiopoulou H, Paraskevakou H, et al. Immunohistochemical evaluation of podocalyxin expression in glomerulopathies associated with nephrotic syndrome. *Hum Pathol.* 2011;42:227-235, Copyright 2011, with permission from Elsevier.)

stained area was statistical significantly higher in the controls than in each pathologic group. However, among pathologic groups (FSGS, MCD, MG), there was no statistically significant difference. This is one of the few studies investigating podocalyxin immunohistochemical expression in glomerulopathies associated with nephrotic syndrome. The observed reduction in podocalyxin expression suggests that it constitutes a target molecule in nephrotic syndrome pathogenesis regardless of the underlying cause (Fig 6).

▶ This study furthers our understanding of the pathophysiology of nephrotic syndrome and suggests a similar process in all types of nephrotic syndromes. The main findings are demonstrated in Fig 6, which highlights the decrease in podocalyxin expression, as measured by surface area of staining, in all cases of membranous compared with normal control samples. The finding of decreased staining in the areas of segmental scarring in cases of focal segmental glomerulonephritis is interesting and raises the question of whether decreased podocalyxin is a cause or an effect of the segmental sclerosis. One may hypothesize that because other diseases also show decreased podocalyxin, it is a key protein in the development of proteinuria. Strengths of the study include the use of image analysis software for the stain scoring and study of a variety of causes of nephrotic syndrome. It would have been nice to have all glomeruli from each case evaluated instead of only 7 to 10, which allows for selection bias. I would be interested to see how podocalyxin expression varies in other disease processes, such as proliferative glomerulonephritis, menbranoproliferative glomerulonephritis, and crescentic glomerulonephritis.

M. L. Smith, MD

The Relevance of Periglomerular Fibrosis in the Evaluation of Routine Needle Core Renal Biopsies
Jenkins J, Brodsky SV, Satoskar AA, et al (The Ohio State Univ, Columbus)
Arch Pathol Lab Med 135:117-122, 2011

Context.—Renal interstitial fibrosis and, to a lesser extent, sclerotic glomeruli correlate with poor renal function. However, not all nonfunctional glomeruli are sclerotic. Many or most glomeruli with periglomerular fibrosis, while retaining blood flow, probably do not filter; therefore, they may not contribute to renal function.

Objective.—To examine the relationship of periglomerular fibrosis and the sum of globally sclerotic glomeruli and glomeruli with periglomerular fibrosis (GSG+PF) with interstitial fibrosis and renal function.

Design.—Native kidney biopsies from 177 patients with chronic renal injury were assessed for interstitial fibrosis, glomerular sclerosis, and GSG+PF. Renal biopsies with active or acute lesions were not included. The percentage of globally sclerotic glomeruli and GSG+PF was correlated with the degree of interstitial fibrosis and serum creatinine levels.

Results.—The percentage of GSG+PF correlates better with the degree of interstitial fibrosis and renal function than does the percentage of globally sclerotic glomeruli alone. This appears particularly true in chronic renal diseases of patients without diabetes. The number of globally sclerotic glomeruli correlates better with interstitial fibrosis and renal function than does the sum of globally and segmentally sclerotic glomeruli.

Conclusions.—The percentage of GSG+PF in a renal biopsy specimen provides a better estimate of chronic renal injury than does the percentage of sclerotic glomeruli alone, probably because many or most glomeruli with periglomerular fibrosis are nonfunctional. Therefore, we recommend that the number of glomeruli with periglomerular fibrosis also be provided in the renal biopsy report.

▶ This retrospective morphologic study is simple in design but suggests a change in clinical practice that is worth considering based on the findings. Although the reporting of globally sclerotic and segmentally sclerotic glomeruli is nearly universal, few pathologists recognize or report the number of glomeruli with periglomerular fibrosis. In this study, periglomerular fibrosis was defined as glomeruli with open capillary loops and lamellated, frequently wrinkled, Bowman capsular basement membrane and circumferential layers of interstitial type collagen around, within, or between the Bowman capsule basement membrane (Fig 2 in the original article). It is interesting that the effect is less prominent in patients with diabetes compared with nondiabetic chronic renal disease. This may have been due to more advanced fibrosis in the diabetic cohort. A weakness of the study was the use of creatinine instead of a calculated glomerular filtration rate. One must remember, however, that the amount of interstitial fibrosis correlates best with creatinine and glomerular filtration. Nevertheless, renal pathologists should recognize and report periglomerular fibrosis, especially in nondiabetic renal disease.

M. L. Smith, MD

12 Head and Neck

Salivary gland carcinoma in Denmark 1990–2005: A national study of incidence, site and histology. Results of the Danish Head and Neck Cancer Group (DAHANCA)
Bjørndal K, Krogdahl A, Therkildsen MH, et al (Odense Univ Hosp, Denmark; Copenhagen University Hospital/Rigshospitalet, Denmark; et al)
Oral Oncol 47:677-682, 2011

To describe the incidence, site and histology (WHO 2005) of salivary gland carcinomas in Denmark. Nine hundred and eighty-three patients diagnosed from 1990 to 2005 were identified from three nation-wide registries. The associated clinical data were retrospectively retrieved from patient medical records. Histological revision was performed in 886 cases (90%). Based on histological revision, 31 patients (3%) were excluded from the study leaving 952 for epidemiological analysis. The mean crude incidence in Denmark was 1.1/100,000/year. The male vs. female ratio was 0.97 and the median age was 62 years. The parotid gland was the most common site (52.5%) followed by the minor salivary glands of the oral cavity (26.3%). The most frequent histological subtypes were adenoid cystic carcinoma (25.2%), mucoepidermoid carcinoma (16.9%), adenocarcinoma NOS (12.2%) and acinic cell carcinoma (10.2%). The revision process changed the histological diagnosis in 121 out of 886 cases (14%). The incidence of salivary gland carcinoma in Denmark is higher than previously reported. More than half of salivary gland carcinomas are located in the parotid gland with adenoid cystic carcinoma being the most frequent subtype. Histological classification of salivary gland carcinomas is difficult and evaluation by dedicated pathology specialists might be essential for optimal diagnosis and treatment (Table 3).

▶ The World Health Organization Classification of Tumors: Pathology and Genetics of Head and Neck Tumors, 2005 review of salivary gland tumors mentions mucoepidermoid carcinoma as the most common malignant salivary gland tumor both in adults and children.[1] This fact has been long standing and unchallenged in most head and neck pathology reference books to date and taught by most of us to our medical students and trainees. It is a fact based on previously well-documented studies. While this may still be the case in many parts of the world, it may not be the case in other parts. I came across this very interesting epidemiological study from Denmark that lists adenoid cystic carcinoma as the most common malignant salivary gland neoplasm in Denmark after reviewing and revising the diagnosis of 886 malignant salivary gland tumors over a 15-year

TABLE 3.—Histological Distribution According to Gender and Age

Histological Type	N (%)	Males n (%)	Females n (%)	p-Value*	Median age
Adenoid cystic carcinoma	240 (25.2)	107 (11.2)	133 (14.0)	n.s.	59
Mucoepidermoid carcinoma	161 (16.9)	84 (8.8)	77 (8.1)	n.s.	51
Adenocarcinoma NOS	116 (12.2)	72 (7.6)	44 (4.6)	p = 0.004	70
Acinic cell carcinoma	97 (10.2)	34 (3.6)	63 (6.6)	p = 0.004	55
Carcinoma ex pleomorphic adenoma	79 (8.3)	41 (4.3)	38 (4.0)	n.s.	63
Polymorphous low-grade adenocarcinoma	73 (7.7)	26 (2.7)	47 (4.9)	p = 0.02	58
Squamous cell carcinoma	52 (5.5)	35 (3.7)	17 (1.8)	p = 0.01	74
Salivary duct carcinoma	34 (3.6)	21 (2.2)	13 (1.4)	n.s.	63
Epithelial-myoepithelial carcinoma	27 (2.8)	16 (1.7)	11 (1.2)	n.s.	67
Lymphoepithelial carcinoma	25 (2.6)	9 (0.9)	16 (1.7)	n.s.	59
Basal cell adenocarcinoma	14 (1.5)	7 (0.7)	7 (0.7)	n.s.	65
Oncocytic carcinoma	15 (1.6)	7 (0.7)	8 (0.8)	n.s.	70
Cystadenocarcinoma	4 (0.4)	2 (0.2)	2 (0.2)		
Mucinous adenocarcinoma	3 (0.3)	2 (0.2)	1 (0.1)		
Myoepithelial carcinoma	2 (0.2)	1 (0.1)	1 (0.1)		
Carcinosarcoma	1 (0.1)	0	1 (0.1)		
Clear cell adenocarcinoma NOS	1 (0.1)	0	1 (0.1)		
Not possible to classify — besides carcinoma	8 (0.8)	5 (0.5)	3 (0.3)		
TOTAL	952 (22)	469 (11)	483 (51)		

n.s. = Not significant.

period from 1990 to 2005 (Table 3) and also mentions the increased incidence of salivary gland tumors to what was thought before. These facts in themselves are interesting in showing the difference to the prevailing view in most pathology textbooks and may denote a regional variation in that part of Europe. However, the more important question that comes to mind is what other global variations may be encountered about salivary gland tumors if similarly conducted national studies were available from other parts of the world, particularly those regions where the diagnosis and documentation of salivary gland tumors may be hampered by lack of adequate health care, and how much these variations, if available, may help our understanding of the etiological factors, racial origin, or gender variations, for example, that may contribute to the prevalence of these or certain subtype of these sometimes quite aggressive tumors.

M. S. Said, MD, PhD

Reference

1. Barnes L, Eveson JW, Reichart P, Sideransky D, eds. World Health Organization Classification of Tumors: Pathology and Genetics: Head and Neck Tumors. IARC Press; 2005:219-220.

Cribriform Adenocarcinoma of Minor Salivary Gland Origin Principally Affecting the Tongue: Characterization of New Entity

Skalova A, Sima R, Kaspirkova-Nemcova J, et al (Charles Univ Prague, Pilsen, Czech Republic; Med Faculty Hosp, Pilsen, Czech Republic; et al)
Am J Surg Pathol 35:1168-1176, 2011

We present a series of 23 cases of a distinctive, hitherto poorly recognized low-grade adenocarcinoma, with several histologic features reminiscent of papillary carcinoma of the thyroid, and which mostly but not exclusively occurs in the tongue. All the tumors were unencapsulated and were divided into lobules that were composed mainly of cribriform and solid growth patterns. Therefore, we propose the name "cribriform adenocarcinoma of minor salivary gland origin (CAMSG)." All the patients were adults with a mean age at diagnosis of 55.8 years (range, 25 to 85 y). Fourteen of the 23 tumors were localized in the tongue, 3 in the soft palate, 2 in the retromolar buccal mucosa, 3 in the lingual tonsils, and 1 in the upper lip. Fifteen patients of 23 had synchronous metastases in the cervical lymph nodes at the time of diagnosis, bilateral in 3 cases. In 3 patients, the nodal metastasis was the first evidence of disease, later investigation revealing primary neoplasms in the base of tongue and tonsil, respectively. In addition, 1 patient developed a cervical lymph node metastasis 8 years after excision of a primary tumor of the tongue. Data on treatment and follow-up were available in 14 cases. The patients were treated by radical excision with clear margins (12 cases) or by simple excision (2 cases). Neck dissection was performed in 10 patients; 9 received radiotherapy, but none were treated by chemotherapy. Clinical follow-up ranged from 2 months to 13 years (mean, 6 y and 5 mo). Twelve patients are alive with no evidence of recurrent or metastatic disease after treatment, 1 patient died 2 years after surgery without evidence of tumor, and 1 patient is alive with recurrent tumor of the palate (Figs 2-5).

▶ This is an interesting multi-institutional study characterizing a new salivary gland entity "cribriform adenocarcinoma of minor salivary glands" (CAMSG) in a series of 23 cases selected from the authors' collective registry of approximately 5000 salivary gland tumors. Although described principally in the tongue in 1999,[1] it was vaguely characterized by the World Health Organization in 2005 and not distinctly removed from polymorphous low grade adenocarcinoma (PLGA) as a new entity.

This articles affirms its independent nature, describes it in sites other than the tongue (palate, tonsils, lip, and retromolar trigone), and recounts its histopathologic (Figs 2 and 3), immunohistochemical (Fig 4), ultrastructural (Fig 5), molecular, treatment, and follow-up features. Perhaps one of the important features that clinically differentiate this tumor from PLGA is its propensity for cervical lymph node metastasis; however, the patients' prognosis remains good after follow-up periods up to 13 years. From the histological point of view, the monomorphous (in contrast to PLGA) dual secretory and myoepithelial nature of the tumor is among the distinct features that should be considered

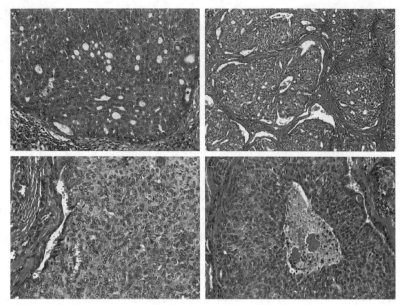

FIGURE 2.—A, The tumors are composed predominantly of solid and cribriform growth structures in variable proportions (hematoxylin and eosin). B, They are divided by fibrous septa into irregular nodules composed of solid, cribriform, and microcystic structures (hematoxylin and eosin). C, In the solid areas, the tumor nests are detached from the adjacent fibrous stroma by artificial clefting (hematoxylin and eosin). D, The peripheral layer of such solid tumors nests display hyperchromatic nuclei in a vaguely palisading pattern (hematoxylin and eosin). (Reprinted from Skalova A, Sima R, Kaspirkova-Nemcova J, et al. Cribriform adenocarcinoma of minor salivary gland origin principally affecting the tongue: characterization of new entity. *Am J Surg Pathol*. 2011;35:1168-1176, with permission from Lippincott Williams & Wilkins.)

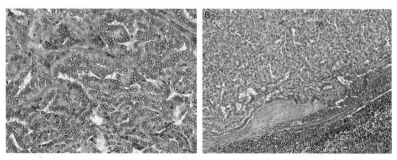

FIGURE 3.—A, The nuclei, which often overlap one with another, were pale, optically clear, and vesicular with a ground-glass appearance, so that the tumors cytologically strongly resemble papillary carcinoma of the thyroid gland. B, The cervical lymph node metastases has identical appearances to the primary tumors. (Reprinted from Skalova A, Sima R, Kaspirkova-Nemcova J, et al. Cribriform adenocarcinoma of minor salivary gland origin principally affecting the tongue: characterization of new entity. *Am J Surg Pathol*. 2011;35:1168-1176, with permission from Lippincott Williams & Wilkins.)

in its differential diagnosis (expression of pancytokeratin, S100 protein, and smooth muscle actin). The authors proposed the name *secretory myoepithlium* for these cells in other sites.[2]

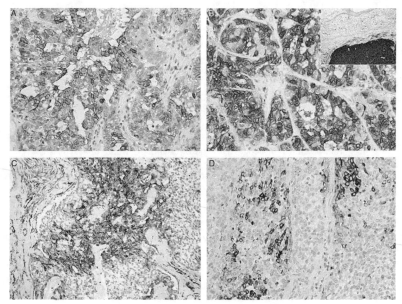

FIGURE 4.—A, Positivity for c-kit (range of positive cells 20% to 80%) with strong cytoplasmic and membranous expression (immunohistochemical staining CD117). B, The immunostaining for p16 protein has a typical patchy pattern with variable amount of positive cells (range, 50% to 100%). The staining for p16 protein was strong cytoplasmic/nuclear and diffuse in the whole tumor in 3 cases (inset). C, Peripheral layer of solid and cribriform tumor nests often displayed myoepithelial differentiation (immunohistochemical staining smooth muscle actin). D, Expression of CK19 was variable with mild-to-moderate staining of membranes and cytoplasm in up to 5% of cells (immunohistochemical staining CK19). (Reprinted from Skalova A, Sima R, Kaspirkova-Nemcova J, et al. Cribriform adenocarcinoma of minor salivary gland origin principally affecting the tongue: characterization of new entity. *Am J Surg Pathol.* 2011;35: 1168-1176, with permission from Lippincott Williams & Wilkins.)

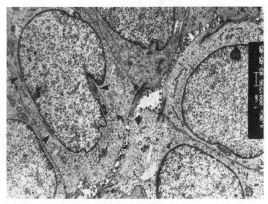

FIGURE 5.—Secretory myoepithelias. The secretory cells bearing microvilli on the apical border also contain groups of microfilaments (arrowheads). (Reprinted from Skalova A, Sima R, Kaspirkova-Nemcova J, et al. Cribriform adenocarcinoma of minor salivary gland origin principally affecting the tongue: characterization of new entity. *Am J Surg Pathol.* 2011;35:1168-1176, with permission from Lippincott Williams & Wilkins.)

Perhaps one of the most characteristic features of CAMSG is the remarkable resemblance of its tumor cells to those of more commonly encountered papillary thyroid carcinoma as their main differential diagnosis, particularly in nodal disease. However, thyroid markers (TTF1 and thyroglobulins) are negative. No significant mutations were found in these cases.

M. S. Said, MD, PhD

References

1. Michael M, Skálová A, Simpson RH, et al. Cribriform adenocarcinoma of the tongue: a hitherto unrecognized type of adenocarcinoma characteristically occurring in the tongue. *Histopathology.* 1999;35:495-501.
2. Del Vecchio M, Foschini MP, Peterse JL, Eusebi V. Lobular carcinoma of the breast with Hybrid myoepithelial and secretory ("myosecretory") cell differentiation. *Am J Surg Pathol.* 2005;29:1530-1536.

Lymphadenoma of the salivary gland: clinicopathological and immunohistochemical analysis of 33 tumors
Seethala RR, Thompson LDR, Gnepp DR, et al (Presbyterian Univ Hosp, Pittsburgh, PA; Woodland Hills Med Ctr, CA; Rhode Island Hosp of Brown Univ, Providence; et al)
Mod Pathol 1-10, 2011

Lymphadenomas (LADs) are rare salivary gland tumors. Their clinicopathologic characteristics and etiopathogenesis are poorly understood. We examined 33 LADs in 31 patients (17 women and 14 men) aged 11–79 years (median 65 years). There were 22 sebaceous LADs in 21 patients (9 women and 12 men) and 11 nonsebaceous LADs in 10 patients (8 women and 2 men). Two patients had synchronous double tumors. Twentysix tumors (79%) arose in parotid, three in the neck, and two each in submandibular gland and oral cavity. Extraparotid tumors were seen in 2 of 21 (10%) patients with sebaceous and 4 of 10 (40%) patients with nonsebaceous LADs. Seven of twenty-three (30%) patients had immunosuppressive therapy for unrelated diseases. The tumors were well circumscribed, encapsulated ($n = 28$, 84%) painless masses, varying in size from 0.6 to 6 cm (median 2.2). The cut surfaces were gray-tan to yellow, homogeneous and multicystic ($n = 24$, 72%). The epithelial cells were basaloid, squamous and glandular, forming solid nests, cords, tubules, and cysts. Sebaceous differentiation was restricted to sebaceous lymphadenoma. The epithelial cells expressed basal cell markers (p63, 34BE12, and/or CK5/6, 18/18, 100%) and the luminal glandular cells expressed CK7 (12/12, 100%). Myoepithelial cells were absent ($n = 10/16$, 63%) or focal. The lymphoid stroma was reactive, with germinal centers in 28 (84%). There was no evidence of HPV (0/11), EBV (0/7), and HHV-8 (0/8). Malignant transformation to sebaceous and basal cell adenocarcinoma was seen in one patient each. None of the 11 patients with follow-up (1–8 years)

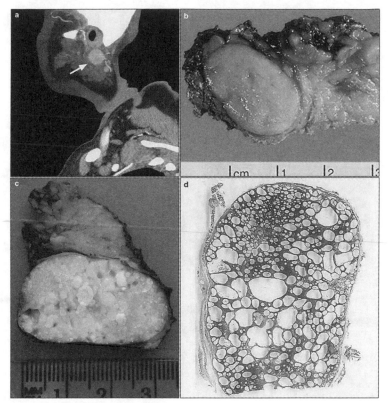

FIGURE 1.—Sebaceous lymphadenoma. (**a, b**) Sixty-four-year-old woman (SL19): contrast enhanced computerized tomography shows a well-defined mass (arrow) in the right preauricular area (**a**). The tumor was firm and well circumscribed, measured 2.2 cm in size and had a tan, homogeneous cut surface (**b**). (**c, d**) Seventy-nine-year-old man with a 3.5-cm encapsulated mass in the right parotid (SL20). The cut surface is tan yellow and multicystic (**c**) with cysts measuring up to 5 mm (**d**). (Reprinted from Seethala RR, Thompson LDR, Gnepp DR, et al. Lymphadenoma of the salivary gland: clinicopathological and immunohistochemical analysis of 33 tumors. *Mod Pathol.* 2011;1-10, with permission from Macmillan Publishers Ltd: Modern Pathology, Copyright 2010.)

recurred. In summary, sebaceous and non-sebaceous LADs are benign, encapsulated, solid and cystic tumors affecting older adults. Non-sebaceous LADs affect women and extraparotid sites more frequently than sebaceous LADs. Altered immune status may have a role in their etio-pathogenesis. Multiple synchronous tumors, origin in buccal mucosa, and malignant transformation may rarely occur (Figs 1, 2, 4 and 5).

▶ This is a large multi-institutional series study of 33 collected cases describing the little-known and benign salivary gland entity of lymphadenomas (LADs). As the authors mention, the largest reported series of these tumors contained only 3 cases.[1] The study is well illustrated (Figs 1, 2, 4, and 5) and confirms the prevailing belief from the previous literature that sebaceous LADs are more common than nonsebaceous ones. Following are the interesting clinical

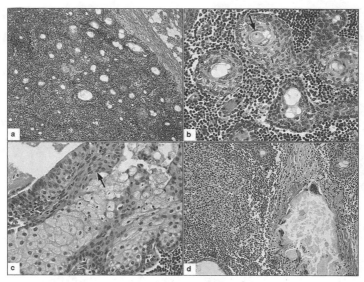

FIGURE 2.—Sebaceous lymphadenoma (**a, b** from SL19, same case as in Figures 1a and b). The tumor is biphasic with epithelial and lymphoid components, and is separated from the adjacent uninvolved parotid gland by a thin fibrous capsule (**a**, ×10). Solid and microcystic clusters with squamous and sebaceous differentiation on the inside and basal cells on the outside. Focal keratinization (arrow) is seen (**b**, ×40). Sebaceous lymphadenoma (SL17) showing a cyst lined by columnar cells, large foamy sebaceous cells, a small area of squamous cells (arrow) and basal cells at the periphery (**c**, ×40). Foreign body type giant cell reaction to ruptured cyst contents is seen adjacent to a lymphoid follicle with germinal center (**d**, ×20). (Reprinted from Seethala RR, Thompson LDR, Gnepp DR, et al. Lymphadenoma of the salivary gland: clinicopathological and immunohistochemical analysis of 33 tumors. *Mod Pathol.* 2011;1-10, with permission from Macmillan Publishers Ltd: Modern Pathology, Copyright 2010.)

findings concluded from this study, which allow a better clinical understanding of these tumors: first, the absence of clear viral etiology (human papilloma virus, Epstein-Barr virus, or human herpes virus-8) in the described cases; second, that 7 of the patients had altered immune status for different reasons; third that although malignant transformation in LADs is rare and may affect both the epithelial or the lymphoid component, 7 patients had an association with other metachronus or synchronous salivary or nonsalivary malignant tumors; and lastly, the even rarer presence of these tumors in children. The study also raises the importance of that group of mostly benign tumors in the differential diagnosis of nodal metastasis and perhaps also in fine needle aspirations interpretations to avoid unnecessary extensive surgeries and morbidities.

M. S. Said, MD, PhD

Reference

1. Ma J, Chan JK, Chow CW, Orell SR. Lymphadenoma: a report of three cases of uncommon salivary gland neoplasm. *Histopathology.* 2002;41:342-350.

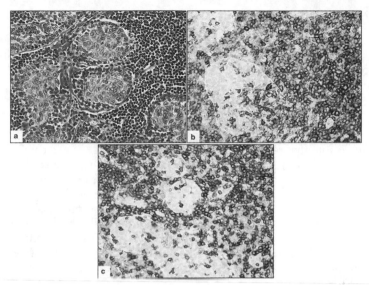

FIGURE 4.—(a–c) Non-sebaceous lymphadenoma in a 70-year-old man with chronic lymphocytic leukemia (NSL8). The basaloid epithelial cells are arranged in solid clusters and cords with intraepithelial and stromal malignant small B lymphocytes (a, ×40) that are positive for CD20 (b, ×40) and CD5 (c, ×40). (Reprinted from Seethala RR, Thompson LDR, Gnepp DR, et al. Lymphadenoma of the salivary gland: clinicopathological and immunohistochemical analysis of 33 tumors. *Mod Pathol*. 2011;1-10, with permission from Macmillan Publishers Ltd: Modern Pathology, Copyright 2010.)

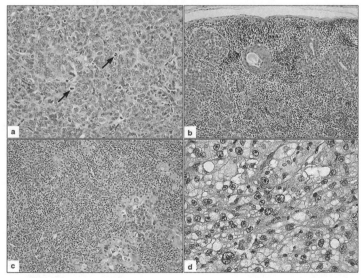

FIGURE 5.—Malignant transformation in lymphadenoma. (a–b) Seventy-four-year-old man with 1.5 cm sebaceous lymphadenoma in the right parotid gland. Tumor shows an area of basal cell adenocarcinoma comprising sheets of monomorphic basaloid cells with frequent mitoses (arrows, a, ×40). The capsule is intact and benign areas consistent with lymphadenoma are present within the tumor (b, ×40). (c, d) Sebaceous carcinoma arising in a sebaceous lymphadenoma with area of transition between benign (upper left) and malignant (lower right) epithelial cells (c, ×40). Tumor cells show significant cytologic atypia with abundant foamy cytoplasm, large pleomorphic vesicular nuclei, and prominent nucleoli (d, ×40). (Reprinted from Seethala RR, Thompson LDR, Gnepp DR, et al. Lymphadenoma of the salivary gland: clinicopathological and immunohistochemical analysis of 33 tumors. *Mod Pathol*. 2011;1-10, with permission from Macmillan Publishers Ltd: Modern Pathology, Copyright 2010.)

Salivary Gland Anlage Tumor: A Clinicopathological Study of Two Cases

Gauchotte G, Coffinet L, Schmitt E, et al (Central Univ Hosp (CHU) Nancy, France)

Fetal Pediatr Pathol 30:116-123, 2011

We report two cases of salivary gland anlage tumor (SGAT), a nasopharyngeal lesion that affects newborns. The first case concerned a male newborn, presenting respiratory distress secondary to a nasopharyngeal mass. The second case was diagnosed in a 6-week-old girl, suffering from respiratory difficulties due to a nasal cavity mass. A magnetic resonance imaging (MRI) in the second case revealed the presence of several small round and linear fluid-like areas. Histologically, both lesions were suggestive of SGAT, characterized by epithelial structures that blended with spindlecells, drawing highly cellular nodules. Connective tissue between nodules contained squamous cystic nests and ducts (Fig 2, Table 1).

▶ This is a nice case report of the very rare salivary gland anlage tumors, and is included as a reminder of the rarity of these cases and because of its inclusion of a record/review of the previous cases encountered in the English-language literature (Table 1). Most cases from the review seen (Table 1) occurred in the nasopharynx, with male predominance, and exhibited similar biphasic structure of squamous nests and spindle cells (Fig 2). Awareness of this entity is important, as its differential diagnosis is rather large and includes both benign and malignant lesions, particularly when seeing from this review that once these lesions are correctly identified and removed, they do not recur and that the surgical procedures to remove them are rather simple in principle.

M. S. Said, MD, PhD

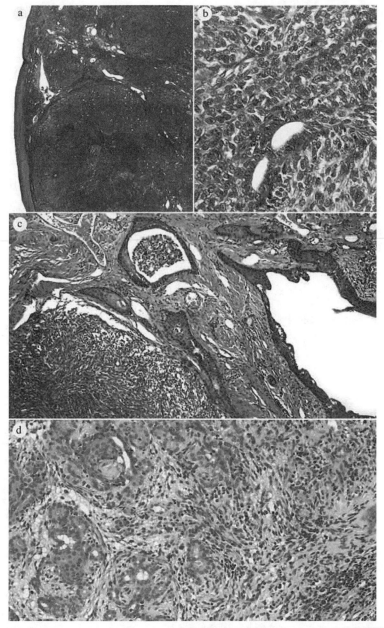

FIGURE 2.—Haematoxylin, eosin, and saffron stained tissue sections (a) Case no. 1. Multiple highly cellular nodules (×25). (b) Case no. 1. Nodules are composed of spindle cells interspersed with acinar structures (×400). (c) Case no. 1. Connective tissue between nodules contains duct-like or cystic squamous nests (×100). (d) Case no. 2. Bi-phasic pattern: epithelial structures (solid squamous cells nests and acini) interspersed with mesenchymal spindle cells (×200). (Reprinted from Gauchotte G, Coffinet L, Schmitt E, et al. Salivary gland anlage tumor: a clinicopathological study of two cases. *Fetal Pediatr Pathol* 2011;30:116-123, with permission from Informa Healthcare USA, Inc.)

TABLE 1.—Clinical Features of SGAT

No.	Reference	Age	Sex	Clinical Presentation	Localization	Size (cm)	Procedure	Outcome
1	Present case	1 day	M	Respiratory distress	Nasopharynx	3×1.7×1	Excision	NED at 30 mo
2	Present case	6 wk	F	Respiratory difficulty	Left nasal cavitymass	1.6×1.5×0.9	Excision	NED at 18 mo
3	[1]	NB	M	Nasal obstruction, feeding difficulty	Nasopharynx	2×1.5	Excision	NED at 1½ yr
4	[2]	7 day	M	Nasal obstruction	Naso- and oropharynx	3×2.5×1.5	Excision	Death from sepsis at 6mo, NED
5	[3]	6 wk	M	Respiratory difficulty	Posterior pharynx	1.5	Excision	NED at 5 yr
6	[3]	1 wk	M	Respiratory difficulty with nasal obstruction	Posterior septum and nasopharynx	2.5×1.9×1.2	Excision	NED at 4 yr
7	[3]	6 day	M	Upper respiratory obstruction	Nasopharynx	2.5×1.5×1.5	Excision	NED at 2 yr
8	[3]	1 wk	M	Upper respiratory obstruction	Nasopharynx	3×1.8	Excision	NED at 6 yr
9	[3]	NB	F	Respiratory difficulty at birth, bleeding at 4 d	Nasopharynx	—	Expulsion during resuscitation	No follow up
10	[3]	3.5 mo	F	Intermittent respiratory and feeding difficulties	Nasopharynx	1.5×1×0.5	Excision	NED at 1 yr
11	[3]	NB	M	Facial plethora, sonorous breathing and progressive respiratory distress	Nasopharynx	1.3×1×0.5	Excision	NED at 3.5 yr
12	[4]	8 day	M	Progressive respiratory distress	Pharynx, protruding to oesophagus	3×2	Excision	NED at 3 yr
13	[4]	1 day	M	Respiratory distress	Pharynx	2×2	Excision	NED at 8 mo
14	[4]	2 day	M	Nasal obstruction, feeding difficulty	Pharynx	2×2	Excision	NED at 2 yr
15	[5]	1 wk	M	—	Nasopharynx	3×2×2	Excision	NED at 2 yr
16	[6]	1 day	M	Respiratory distress	Nasopharynx	1.4×1.4×0.8	Excision	NED at 1 mo

		Age	Sex	Symptoms	Location	Size	Treatment	Outcome
17	[6]	1 day	M	Stridor	—	—	Expelled	NED at 10 yr
18	[6]	8 wk	F	Respiratory distress, nasal obstruction	—	—	Excision	NED at 8 yr
19	[6]	10 wk	M	Respiratory distress	—	—	Excision	NED at 6 yr
20	[6]	8 wk	F	Respiratory distress	—	—	Excision	NED at 3 yr
21	[6]	4 day	M	Respiratory distress	—	—	Excision	NED at 3 yr
22	[6]	1 day	—	Respiratory distress	—	—	Excision	NED at 2 yr
23	[7]	11 day	M	Nasal obstruction, feeding difficulty	Nasopharynx	1.5	Expelled during cannulation	NED at 1.5 yr
24	[8]	NB	M	Respiratory and feeding difficulties	Nasopharynx	4×3×2	Excision	NED at 5 yr
25	[9]	2 day	M	Stridor, feeding difficulty	Nasopharynx	1.4×1.2×1	Excision	NED at 12 mo
26	[10]	2 wk	—	Nasal breathing difficulty	Left nasal cavity	3×2.3×0.8	Excision	—
27	[11]	12 mo	M	Intermittent airway obstruction, otitis media	Nasopharynx	1.7×1×0.6	Excision	—

Abbreviations: NB: newborn; M: male; F: female; NED: no evidence of disease; wk: week; yr: year; mo: month.
Editor's Note: Please refer to original journal article for full references.

A Histologic and Immunohistochemical Study Describing the Diversity of Tumors Classified as Sinonasal High-grade Nonintestinal Adenocarcinomas

Stelow EB, Jo VY, Mills SE, et al (Univ of Virginia, Charlottesville; et al)
Am J Surg Pathol 35:971-980, 2011

Nonintestinal sinonasal adenocarcinomas (SNACs) are somewhat poorly characterized and high-grade nonintestinal SNACs have been only rarely reported. Here, we review our experience with these tumors. Twenty-seven cases of high-grade nonintestinal SNACs were identified

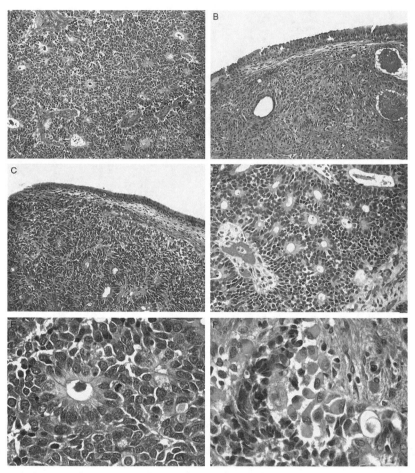

FIGURE 1.—High-grade nonintestinal adenocarcinoma. Nine tumors in our study were composed of trabecula and ribbons of neoplastic cells with interspersed rosette-like glands (A—F). Focally, the neoplastic cells had a more spindled appearance (B). In 2 cases, possible stromal components such as rhabdomyoblastic differentiation were identified (F). However, other features of teratocarcinosarcoma were not seen. (Reprinted from Stelow EB, Jo VY, Mills SE, et al. A histologic and immunohistochemical study describing the diversity of tumors classified as sinonasal high-grade nonintestinal adenocarcinomas. *Am J Surg Pathol.* 2011;35:971-980, with permission from Lippincott Williams & Wilkins.)

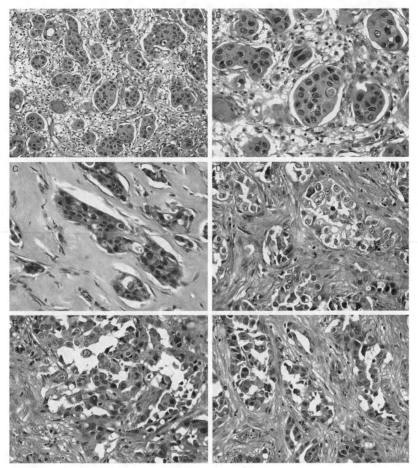

FIGURE 2.—High-grade nonintestinal adenocarcinoma. Six of our tumors were composed of infiltrating glands with a somewhat apocrine phenotype (A—F). (Reprinted from Stelow EB, Jo VY, Mills SE, et al. A histologic and immunohistochemical study describing the diversity of tumors classified as sinonasal high-grade nonintestinal adenocarcinomas. *Am J Surg Pathol*. 2011;35:971-980, with permission from Lippincott Williams & Wilkins.)

from 22 men and 5 women. Ages ranged from 22 to 83 years (mean ± 1 standard deviation = 54.7 ± 18.6 y; median = 60 y). Thirteen cases involved the nasal cavity and sinuses, 10 involved the nasal cavity only, and 4 involved sinuses only. Most cases had marked cytologic and nuclear pleomorphism, abundant mitotic activity, and necrosis; however, these features were not uniform. Although histologically heterogeneous, recurrent growth patterns were seen that resembled other neoplasms of the area. Tumors lacked CDX2 and CK20 immunoreactivity (aside from rare CK20 immunoreactive cells). High-grade nonintestinal SNACs are more common in men and, although they occur over a wide age range,

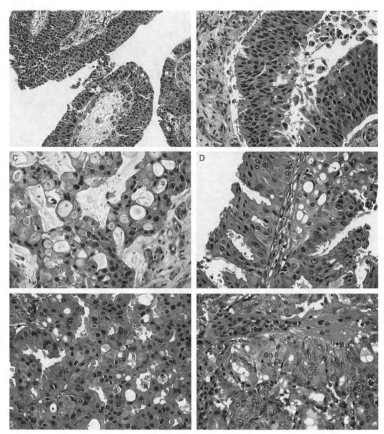

FIGURE 3.—High-grade nonintestinal adenocarcinoma. Three cases were associated with oncocytic Schneiderian papillomas (A, B, and D). Tumors were composed of admixed oncocytic and mucinous cells, sometimes growing as solid sheets and other times associated with extracellular mucus (C, E, and F). (Reprinted from Stelow EB, Jo VY, Mills SE, et al. A histologic and immunohistochemical study describing the diversity of tumors classified as sinonasal high-grade nonintestinal adenocarcinomas. *Am J Surg Pathol.* 2011;35: 971-980, with permission from Lippincott Williams & Wilkins.)

they are much more common in older individuals. Histologically, they show a great deal of heterogeneity (Figs 1-5).

▶ This is a well-illustrated (Figs 1-5) study of 27 high-grade nonintestinal sinonasal adenocarcinomas that adds a good reference article to these entities. The morphological classification into blastomatous, apocrine, oncocytic/ mucinous, poorly differentiated/undifferentiated, and also other occasional patterns (clear cells and spindle cells) that the authors used provides a means of reference comparison to readers that can be applied to researching an individual case, compared with the latest World Health Organization classification, which does not provide comparable details of the high-grade nonintestinal adenocarcinomas. At the end of the article, the authors describe an additional

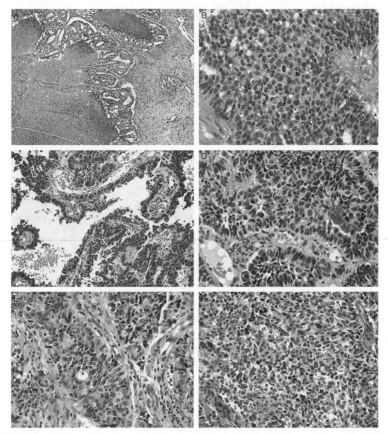

FIGURE 4.—High-grade nonintestinal adenocarcinoma. Six cases were poorly differentiated with solid and undifferentiated foci (A—F). Glandular differentiation was present in all cases (A, B, D, and E). Surface involvement was sometimes seen (C). (Reprinted from Stelow EB, Jo VY, Mills SE, et al. A histologic and immunohistochemical study describing the diversity of tumors classified as sinonasal high-grade nonintestinal adenocarcinomas. *Am J Surg Pathol.* 2011;35:971-980, with permission from Lippincott Williams & Wilkins.)

high-grade case that was positive for high-risk human papilloma virus (HPV), observed after the submission of their article. They note that 4 other previous cases from their series were negative for HPV. It is unfortunate that such a good study was not complemented with a study of HPV on all the available study tumors because HPV seems to play an important role in the etiology of head and neck cancers, particularly squamous cell carcinoma. Documenting the percentage of the 27 cases that are HPV-positive may have been an additional important contribution to the article, which deals with adenocarcinomas. For additional reading on the subject, please refer to earlier articles.[1,2]

M. S. Said, MD, PhD

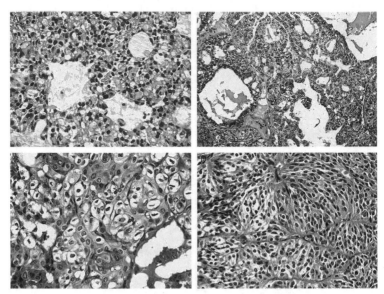

FIGURE 5.—High-grade nonintestinal adenocarcinoma. Other histologic patterns included a predominately clear cell phenotype (A). Another tumor showed predominately microcystic growth (B). A single case was composed of nested clear (C) and spindled cells (D) and had an appearance reminiscent of a paraganglioma. (Reprinted from Stelow EB, Jo VY, Mills SE, et al. A histologic and immunohistochemical study describing the diversity of tumors classified as sinonasal high-grade nonintestinal adenocarcinomas. *Am J Surg Pathol.* 2011;35:971-980, with permission from Lippincott Williams & Wilkins.)

References

1. Heffner DK, Hyams VJ, Hauck KW, Lingeman C. Low-grade adenocarcinoma of the nasal cavity and paranasal sinuses. *Cancer.* 1982;50:312-322.
2. Orvidas LJ, Lewis JE, Weaver AL, Bagniewski SM, Olsen KD. Adenocarcinoma of the nose and paranasal sinuses: a retrospective study of diagnosis, histologic characteristics, and outcomes in 24 patients. *Head Neck.* 2005;27:370-375.

Sinonasal neuroendocrine carcinoma: impact of differentiation status on response and outcome

Likhacheva A, Rosenthal DI, Hanna E, et al (The Univ of Texas MD Anderson Cancer Ctr, Houston)
Head Neck Oncol 3:32, 2011

Background.—The impact of tumor differentiation on the behavior and response of sinonasal neuroendocrine carcinoma is unknown.

Methods.—We performed a retrospective review of the patients treated for neuroendocrine carcinoma (NEC) of the nasal cavity or paranasal sinuses from 1992 to 2008 at MDACC.

Results.—The results of our study suggest that pathologic differentiation may not be a critical factor in the clinical management of patients with NEC

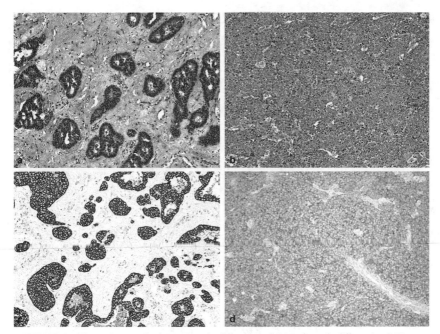

FIGURE 1.—Photomicrograph of a moderately differentiated (A) and poorly differentiated (B) neuroendocrine carcinomas of the sinonasal tract. Figure 1C shows a chromogranin positivity in the cytoplasm of tumor cells of a MDNEC and Figure 1D displays synaptophysin positive PDNEC. (Reprinted from Likhacheva A, Rosenthal DI, Hanna E, et al. Sinonasal neuroendocrine carcinoma: impact of differentiation status on response and outcome. *Head Neck Oncol.* 2011;3:32, with permission from Likhacheva et al; licensee BioMed Central Ltd.)

of the sinonasal tract. This is in contrast to laryngeal and lung NEC for which pathological differentiation has traditionally guided clinical management.

Conclusion.—Mutlimodality approach should be the cornerstone of treating sinonasal NEC regardless of their differentiation. Specifically, RT may provide durable local control for patients with moderately differentiated NEC if resection is not feasible or desirable, while surgical resection can benefit patients with chemo-resistant or radio-resistant disease (Fig 1, Tables 1 and 2).

▶ Neuroendocrine carcinomas in different body sites are a prolific group of tumors that have, in more recent times, undergone revisions for classification into well, moderately, and poorly differentiated entities, depending on their architecture, mitotic/proliferative indices, and presence or absence of necrosis. In many cases the tumors were correlated to the prognostic impacts of such classifications and their response to different treatment modalities (Fig 1, Tables 1 and 2). In this context, it was found in this study of 20 patients with neuroendocrine nasal/paranasal carcinomas that moderately differentiated neuroendocrine carcinomas were treated successfully with radiation therapy in contrast to other sites, like the larynx, where they seem to be, at least in some cases, resistant to

TABLE 1.—Patient Demographics and Outcome

Pt	Sex/age	Differentiation	TNM (stage)	Surgical Resection	Chemotherapy	Radiotherapy	Failure (mo)	Definitive Treatment of recurrence	Follow-up (mo)
1	M/22	mod	T4aN0M0 (IVA)	ND, MM, mandibulectomy	none	AdRT	none	none	NED (166)
2	F/67	mod	T4aN2bM0 (IVA)	CFR, R ND (I-III)	NAC	AdRT	dural metastases (21)	none	DOD (56.2)
3	F/43	mod	T1N0M0 (I)	SPH, ETH	none	AdRT	none	none	NED (31.3)
4	M/46	mod	T4bN1M0 (IVb)	none	NAC	CRT	none	none	NED (16.6)
5	M/54	mod	T4N0M0 (IV)	STR ES	Concurrent	AdCRT	Bilateral cervical LN (46)	ND, AdRT	NED (107)
6	M/47	mod	T4bN0M0 (IVB)	STR CFR	none	AdRT	Ipsilateral level I (125)	ND, AdCRT	NED (172)
7	M/54	mod	TxN0M0	S	AdC	AdRT	local (80)	NAC/RT/AdC, CFR	DOD (119)
8	M/78	poorly	T4bN0M0 (IVB)	S	none	none	none	none	NED/Dead (77)
9	F/24	poorly	T4bN0M0 (IVB)	none	NAC; AdC	RT	none	none	NED (136)
10	F/47	poorly	T4bN1M0 (IVB)	none	NAC	RT	leptomeningeal dz (4.1)	none	DOD (13)
11	F/38	poorly	T4bN0M0 (IVB)	CFR	none	AdRT	none	none	NED (47.5)
12	M/53	poorly	TxN0M0	STR ETH	AdC; concurrent	AdCRT	none	none	NED (17.8)
13	M/51	poorly	T3N0M0 (III)	none	NAC; AdC	RT	persistent (0)	none	DOD (17)
14	F/57	poorly	T4aN0M0 (IVA)	CFR, SPH	NAC	none	none	persistent (0)	DOC (16)
15	M/70	poorly	T4bN0M0 (IVB)	STR ETH	AdC	none	persistent (0)	CFR/RT	DOD (16)
16	F/33	poorly	T2N0M0 (II)	CFR	none	AdRT	Ipsilateral levels I-V (5)	ND, AdRT	NED (149)
17	M/38	poorly	T2N0M0 (II)	none	NAC	RT	local (11)	ETH/MM/SPH, AdCRT	DOD (37.5)
18	F/60	poorly	T4bN0M0 (IVB)	STR CFR	AdC	AdRT	persistent (0)	AdC	NED/Dead (112)
19	F/38	poorly	T4aN0M0 (IVA)	CFR	none	AdRT	none	none	NED (168)
20	M/64	poorly	T4bN0M0 (IVB)	STR CFR	Concurrent	AdCRT	none	none	NED (63)

AWD = alive with disease; NED = no evidence of disease; DOD = dead of disease; DOC = dead of treatment complications. S = resection of unknown type, RT = radiation therapy, AdRT = adjuvant radiation therapy, NAC = neoadjuvant chemotherapy, AdC = adjuvant chemotherapy, AdCRT = adjuvant chemoradiation. CFR = Craniofacial Resection, ETH = Ethmoidectomy, SPH = Sphenoidectomy, MM = Medial Maxillectomy, STR = Subtotal Resection.

TABLE 2.—Characteristics, Presentations, and Outcome of Patients With Sinonasal Moderately Differentiated (MDNEC) and Poorly Differentiated (PDNEC) Neuroendocrine Carcinoma

Characteristic	MDNEC	PDNEC
Demographics		
Age at presentation	47.6 (22-67)	50 (24-78)
M:F ratio	5:2	6:7
Major Presenting Symptoms		
Congestion/Sinusitis	3 (43%)	7 (54%)
Epistaxis	3 (43%)	3 (23%)
Hearing loss	1 (14%)	0
Neck mass	0	2 (15%)
Stage		
I	1 (14%)	0
II	0	2 (15%)
III	0	1 (8%)
IV	5 (71%)	9 (69%)
DFS		
Ch + RT	11 (mon)	7.6 (mon)
RT + Surgery	63 (mon)	16.0 (mon)

- Ch: Chemotherapy.
- MDNEC: Moderately differentiated.
- PDNEC: Poorly differentiated.
- RT: Radiotherapy.

radiation, while poorly differentiated neuroendocrine carcinomas traditionally have been treated with chemoradiation therapy. Such studies highlight the further uniqueness of the nasal cavity when discussing the many particular types of tumors that can afflict this region of the head and neck.

M. S. Said, MD, PhD

Basal cell carcinoma on the ear is more likely to be of an aggressive phenotype in both men and women

Jarell AD, Mully TW (Univ of California, San Francisco)
J Am Acad Dermatol 2011 [Epub ahead of print]

Background.—We observed that basal cell carcinoma (BCC) on the ear demonstrates a more aggressive phenotype compared with other body sites.

Objective.—We sought to determine if it is statistically significant that BCC on the ear is more aggressive.

Methods.—We queried our 2009 database for all BCCs biopsied from the ear. Multiple data points, including tumor subtype and risk level, were analyzed for 100 BCCs on the ear and 100 BCCs on the cheek.

Results.—BCC on the ear was diagnosed 471 times. Of the first 100 occurrences of BCC on the ear, 57% were high risk compared with 38% on the cheek (odds ratio 2.16, 95% confidence interval 1.23-3.81, $P = .01$). Men were more likely to have BCC on the ear: 79% male on

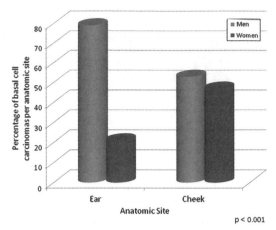

FIGURE 1.—Basal cell carcinoma on ear (but not cheek) is much more common in men. (Reprinted from Jarell AD, Mully TW. Basal cell carcinoma on the ear is more likely to be of an aggressive phenotype in both men and women. *J Am Acad Dermatol*. 2011 [Epub ahead of print], Copyright 2011, with permission from the American Academy of Dermatology, Inc.)

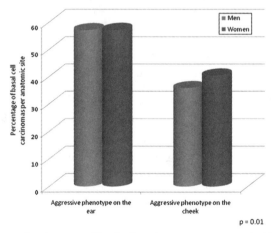

FIGURE 2.—Aggressive phenotype of basal cell carcinoma on ear compared with cheek. (Reprinted from Jarell AD, Mully TW. Basal cell carcinoma on the ear is more likely to be of an aggressive phenotype in both men and women. *J Am Acad Dermatol*. 2011 [Epub ahead of print], Copyright 2011, with permission from the American Academy of Dermatology, Inc.)

the ear and 53% male on the cheek ($P < .001$). However, BCC on the ear in women is also more likely to be aggressive (57%, 12 of 21).

Limitations.—The data were retrieved from a single year at our institution, and there could potentially be regional bias given that the population of data is from a single institution. Many of the specimens we evaluate are reviewed in consultation and may thus represent a selection bias.

Conclusion.—BCC on the ear presents as an aggressive phenotype in the majority of cases for both men and women, and it occurs much more

TABLE 1.—Patient Demographics and Summary of Results, First 100 Basal Cell Carcinomas on Ear

	N	Average Age, y	Left Side	Right Side	Aggressive Phenotype	Nonaggressive Phenotype
Men	79	70.1	42	37	45	34
Women	21	72.7	13	8	12	9
Total	100	70.5	55	45	57	43

TABLE 2.—Patient Demographics and Summary of Results, First 100 Basal Cell Carcinomas on Cheek

	N	Average Age, y	Left Side	Right Side	Aggressive Phenotype	Nonaggressive Phenotype
Men	53	69.9	26	27	19	34
Women	47	67.6	32	15	19	28
Total	100	68.8	58	42	38	62

frequently in men. Knowledge of this information can help guide physicians and ensure that these tumors are adequately biopsied and treated (Figs 1 and 2, Tables 1 and 2).

▶ Basal cell carcinoma (BCC) of the head and neck is a very commonly encountered skin malignancy. It can be particularly problematic in the head region, where it occurs most commonly, if it reached regions in which the anatomy is rather complex and intricate, like the ear with its associated mastoid bony compartments, which translates into more extensive and probably repeated surgeries. This article explores an observation that is probably encountered by many clinicians and pathologists diagnosing these tumors in the ear, which is the prevalence of the more aggressive variants of BCC in the ear, and contrasts that to the BBC types occurring in the nearby head and neck region, namely the cheek (Tables 1 and 2 and Figs 1 and 2). In both men and women, more aggressive phenotypes of BCC were seen (morphealike, infiltrative, and micronodular) than in the cheek region. The authors also mention that a deeper biopsy may be recommended in those sites more than the superficial skin biopsies encountered in practice to ensure the proper classification of the BCC type. These findings, in the light of previous findings also by Betti et al,[1] of the prevalence of nodular or morphoeic/infiltrative subtype being higher among BCCs on the head and neck than other body locations may also mean, if we extrapolate from both articles, that the ear may be a site with a higher prevalence of the more aggressive BCC subtypes than all other body parts, including the other head and neck regions.

M. S. Said, MD, PhD

Reference

1. Betti R, Radaelli G, Bombonato C, Crosti C, Cerri A, Menni S. Anatomic location of Basal cell carcinomas may favor certain histologic subtypes. *J Cutan Med Surg.* 2010;14:298-302.

A Combined Molecular-Pathologic Score Improves Risk Stratification of Thyroid Papillary Microcarcinoma

Niemeier LA, Kuffner Akatsu H, Song C, et al (Univ of Pittsburgh School of Medicine, PA; Univ of Pittsburgh Graduate School of Public Health, PA)
Cancer 2011 [Epub ahead of print]

Background.—Thyroid papillary microcarcinoma (TPMC) is an incidentally discovered papillary carcinoma that measures ≤1.0 cm in size. Most TPMCs are indolent, whereas some behave aggressively. The objective of the study was to evaluate whether the combination of v-raf murine sarcoma viral oncogene homolog B1 (*BRAF*) mutation and specific histopathologic features allows risk stratification of TPMC.

Methods.—A group aggressive TPMCs was selected based on the presence of lymph node metastasis or tumor recurrence. Another group of nonaggressive tumors included TPMCs matched with the first group for age, sex, and tumor size, but with no extrathyroid spread. A molecular analysis was performed, and histologic slides were scored for multiple histopathologic criteria. A separate validation cohort of 40 TPMCs was evaluated.

Results.—*BRAF* mutations were detected in 77% of aggressive TPMCs and in 32% of nonaggressive tumors (*P* = .001). Several histopathologic features differed significantly between the groups. By using multivariate regression analysis, a molecular-pathologic (MP) score was developed that included *BRAF* status and 3 histopathologic features: superficial tumor location, intraglandular tumor spread/multifocality, and tumor

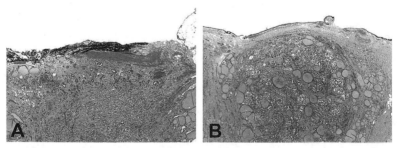

FIGURE 2.—Superficial tumor location as a histologic feature contributing to the molecular-pathologic score included tumor location immediately at the surface of the thyroid either (A) with extrathyroid extension or (B) without extrathyroid extension. (Reprinted from Niemeier LA, Kuffner Akatsu H, Song C, et al. A combined molecular-pathologic score improves risk stratification of thyroid papillary microcarcinoma. *Cancer.* 2011;[Epub ahead of print], Copyright 2011 American Cancer Society, with permission of Wiley-Liss, Inc., a subsidiary of John Wiley & Sons, Inc.)

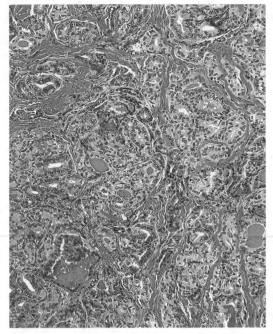

FIGURE 3.—This photomicrograph illustrates significant (2+) sclerotic-type tumor fibrosis that contributed to the molecular-pathologic score. (Reprinted from Niemeier LA, Kuffner Akatsu H, Song C, et al. A combined molecular-pathologic score improves risk stratification of thyroid papillary microcarcinoma. *Cancer.* 2011;[Epub ahead of print], Copyright 2011, American Cancer Society, with permission of Wiley-Liss, Inc., a subsidiary of John Wiley & Sons, Inc.)

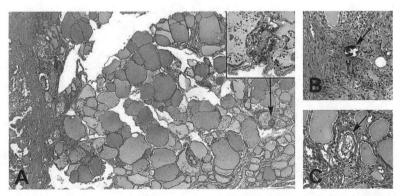

FIGURE 4.—Criteria for intraglandular tumor spread (IGS) included (A) small tumor focus separated from the main tumor mass by a layer of benign thyroid parenchyma (arrow and *inset*), (B) isolated psammoma bodies in the thyroid stroma (arrow), or (C) tumor aggregates within the lymphatic channel (arrow). (Reprinted from Niemeier LA, Kuffner Akatsu H, Song C, et al. A combined molecular-pathologic score improves risk stratification of thyroid papillary microcarcinoma. *Cancer.* 2011;[Epub ahead of print], Copyright 2011, American Cancer Society, with permission of Wiley-Liss, Inc., a subsidiary of John Wiley & Sons, Inc.)

TABLE 3.—Molecular-Pathologic Scores in the Validation Cohort of Thyroid Papillary Microcarcinomas and the Risk of More Aggressive Tumor Behavior[a]

		Risk Groups	
Variable	Low	Intermediate	High
MP_U score	0-2	3	4
MP_W score	0-7	8-10	12
Probability of extrathyroid spread or recurrence, %	0	20	60

Abbreviations: MP_U, unweighted molecular-pathologic score; MP_W, weighted molecular-pathologic score; TPMCs, thyroid papillary microcarcinomas.
[a]The MP score included v-raf murine sarcoma viral oncogene homolog B1 BRAF status and 3 histopathologic features (superficial tumor location, intraglandular tumor spread/multifocality, and tumor fibrosis).

fibrosis. By adding the histologic criteria to BRAF status, sensitivity was increased from 77% to 96%, and specificity was increased from 68% to 80%. In the independent validation cohort, the MP score stratified tumors into low-risk, moderate-risk, and high-risk groups with the probability of lymph node metastases or tumor recurrence in 0%, 20%, and 60% of patients, respectively.

Conclusions.—BRAF status together with several histopathologic features allowed clinical risk stratification of TPMCs. The combined MP risk stratification model was a better predictor of extrathyroid tumor spread than either mutation or histopathologic findings alone (Figs 2-4 and Table 3).

▶ Papillary microcarcinomas are quite common incidental findings when assessing a thyroidectomy specimen for other more sizeable lesions. It is informative for the endocrinologists/oncologists to be supplied with the pathology reports when there is a molecular-pathologic (MP) score of microcarcinomas (Figs 2—4 and Table 3), which may help guide the ultimate follow-up treatment for their patients in cases in which the consequences of that finding are not clear. It is significant to know that it is the combined score of both the molecular (BRAF status) and histologic parameters that is of significance, rather than consideration of either on its own merit. Probably also one of the significant clinical findings in this series is that there was no distant metastasis or tumor-related deaths, as is already observed with papillary microcarcinomas, and, as mentioned, the measure of aggressiveness was defined as the presence of lymph node metastasis. What perhaps would have been interesting to add to the study is a comment on the size of the metastatic disease. Was it microscopic to the lymph node, or did it involve the whole node? Also, was there extracapsular lymph node spread? This may have enabled more insight into the burden of metastatic disease when compared with aggressive papillary carcinomas > 1 cm in size.

M. S. Said, MD, PhD

Adenomatous tumors of the middle ear and temporal bone: clinical, morphological and tumor biological characteristics of challenging neoplastic lesions

Duderstadt M, Förster C, Welkoborsky H-J, et al (Academic Hosp, Hannover, Germany)
Eur Arch Otorhinolaryngol 2011 [Epub ahead of print]

Adenomatous tumors of the middle ear and temporal bone are rare tumors. In this retrospective study, we examined nine patients who underwent surgery for an adenomatous tumor of the middle ear, mastoid cavity or eustachian tube. In seven patients, a middle ear adenoma (MEA) and in two patients an aggressive papillary tumor (APT) was diagnosed. We report the clinical, radiologic, morphologic, immunohistochemical and DNA image cytometrical characteristics that can help to correctly classify these tumors. Therapy consisted of surgical excision of the tumors in eight cases. In one

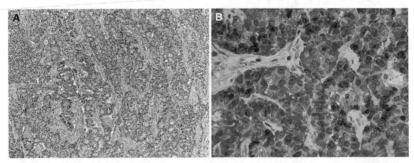

FIGURE 1.—a MEA with typical glandular growth pattern (H&E staining, ×40); b chromogranin A expression in a MEA (×100). (Reprinted from Duderstadt M, Förster C, Welkoborsky H-J, et al. Adenomatous tumors of the middle ear and temporal bone: clinical, morphological and tumor biological characteristics of challenging neoplastic lesions. *Eur Arch Otorhinolaryngol.* 2011;[Epub ahead of print], with permission from Springer-Verlag.)

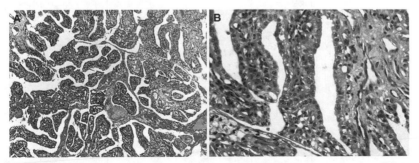

FIGURE 2.—a Histology of APT: typical papillary formation of an APT (H&E staining, ×40), b Same tumor (H&E, ×100). (Reprinted from Duderstadt M, Förster C, Welkoborsky H-J, et al. Adenomatous tumors of the middle ear and temporal bone: clinical, morphological and tumor biological characteristics of challenging neoplastic lesions. *Eur Arch Otorhinolaryngol.* 2011;[Epub ahead of print], with permission from Springer-Verlag.)

TABLE 1.—Clinical Data of Patients with Adenomatous Tumors of the Middle Ear and Temporal Bone

Case	Age and Sex	Initial Clinical Symptoms	Primary Site	Number of Surgical Procedures	Regional Metastasis	Local Recurrence	Interval to Recurrence	Disease Free Time
1 MEA	61 F	Hearing loss	Sinus tympani, hypotympanon	2	—	—	—	6 years
2 MEA	54 M	Otorrhea	Sinus tympani, hypotympanon	3	—	1	12 months	5 years
3 MEA	37 M	Hearing loss	Attic, mesotympanon	3	—	—	—	4 years
4 MEA	36 F	Hearing loss, Tinnitus	Epi-, meso-, hypotympanon	3	—	—	—	3 years
5 MEA	48 F	Hearing loss	Nasopharynx/ eustachian tube	1	—	—	—	2 years
6 MEA	83 F	Hearing loss	Epi-, meso-, hypotympanon	1	—	—	—	4 years
7 MEA	34 F	Hearing loss, middle ear effusion	Epi-, mesotympanon	3	—	1	10 months	13 years
8 APT	93 F	Middle ear effusion	Nasopharynx	1	—	—	—	6 years
9 APT	55 M	Hearing loss	Middle ear cleft, temporal bone	2	—	1	8 years	n.a.

MEA middle ear adenoma, APT aggressive papillary tumor, n.a. not accessible.

elderly patient, only a large biopsy was taken, because this patient suffered from cardial and kidney disorders and was not suitable for an extended surgical approach. This patient received stereotactic radiotherapy. Seven patients underwent planned second look operation. Recurrences occurred in three patients (one with APT, two with MEA), whereas in two of these cases rather a residual tumor due to initial incomplete tumor resection occurred. By image analysis, DNA cytometry MEA were considered benign, whereas the appearance of aneuploid tumor cells in APT confirmed these tumors as low grade malignant lesions. The proliferation rates were equally low in both entities. APT and MEA are tumor entities which can only be correctly classified by a synopsis of histopathology, immunohistochemistry and DNA image cytometry. The recommended therapy is the complete tumor excision. In cases of APT, von Hippel—Lindau syndrome has to be excluded (Figs 1 and 2, Tables 1-3).

▶ This is an interesting study of 9 cases of the rare entity of adenomatous middle ear and temporal bone tumors from Germany that includes diagnostic features of these sometimes unfamiliar tumors (Figs 1 and 2, Tables 1 and 2). Most of what is reported in the article is in line with the findings and previous writings about these tumors. The DNA cytometry studies presented in this study were interesting and confirmed the benign nature of middle ear adenoma (MEA) (diploid DNA content), while confirming the previously observed aggressive behavior of aggressive papillary tumor (APT) as low-grade malignant tumors (aneuploid DNA content) (Table 3). Probably one of the more interesting aspects of this study is what they offer in observation of the site of origin of the APTs, which are thought to arise in the endolymphatic sac. While this may be the case in many of them, the observed origin in one of these tumors in this study was from the eustachian tube and not the endolymphatic sac region. Thus, the authors confirm that a middle ear origin for these tumors cannot be discounted based on their observation in this case, a fact

TABLE 2.—Microscopic and Immunohistochemical Features of Adenomatous Tumors of the Middle Ear and Temporal Bone

Case	Age and Sex	Growth Pattern	Epithelial Markers	Neuroendocrine Markers	Mitosis	Anaplasia	MIB1 (%)
1 MEA	61 F	Glandular, trabecular	+	+	−	−	1
2 MEA	54 M	Glandular	+	−	−	−	<1
3 MEA	37 M	Trabecular, glandular	+	+	−	−	5
4 MEA	36 F	Glandular	+	+	−	−	1−2
5 MEA	48 F	Glandular, trabecular, solid	+	+	−	−	5
6 MEA	83 F	Glandular	+	−	−	−	<1
7 MEA	34 F	Adenoid, solid	+	+	−	−	<1
8 APT	93 F	Tubular, papillary	+	−	−	−	1
9 APT	55 M	Papillary	+	n.a.	−	−	1

Epithelial markers = CK 5/6, CK 7, CK AE1/AE3. Neuroendocrine markers = chromogranin A, synaptophysin, neuron-specific enolase.
MEA middle ear adenoma, *APT* aggressive papillary tumor, *n.a.* not accessible.

TABLE 3.—Results of Quantitative DNA Cytometry

Case	Age and Sex	2cDI	5cER	DNA MG	DNA-SL
MEA 1	61 F	0.45	0	0.29	1.97
MEA 2	54 M	0.15	0	0.11	2.05
MEA 3	37 M	0.64	0.3	0.38	1.95
MEA 4	36 F	0.72	0.34	0.42	1.95
MEA 5	48 F	0.25	0	0.17	1.85
MEA 6	83 F	0.66	0.8	0.38	1.95
MEA 7	34 F	0.37	0	0.24	2.21
Mean MEA		0.46285714	0.20571429	0.28428571	1.99
STA MEA		0.21921939	0.30259198	0.11702666	0.11313708
APT 1	93 F	0.87	1.94	0.48	2.44
APT 2	55 M	0.98	2	0.59	2.32
Mean APT		0.925	1.97	0.535	2.38
STA APT		0.07778175	0.04242641	0.07778175	0.08485281

MEA middle ear adenoma, *APT* aggressive papillary tumor, *STA* standard deviation, *2cDI* 2c deviation index, *5cER* 5c exceeding rate, *DNA MG* DNA malignancy grade, *DNA SL* ploidy of stem cell line in the tumor.

that contributes to the current debate about the origin of these tumors. Additional previous cases have also suggested that possibility in the literature.[1-3]

M. S. Said, MD, PhD

References

1. Schick B, Kronsbein H, Kahle G, Prescher A, Draf W. Papillary tumor of the temporal bone. *Skull Base.* 2001;11:25-33.
2. Tysome JR, Harcourt J, Patel MC, Sandison A, Michaels L. Aggressive papillary tumor of the middle ear: a true entity or an endolymphatic sac neoplasm? *Ear Nose Throat J.* 2008;87:378-393.
3. Muller M, Zammit-Maempel I, Hill J, Wilkins B. An unusual middle-ear mass. *J Laryngol Otol.* 2010;124:108-110.

The Chernobyl Thyroid Cancer Experience: Pathology

LiVolsi VA, Abrosimov AA, Bogdanova T, et al (Univ of Pennsylvania, Philadelphia; Med Radiological Res Ctr, Obninsk, Kaluga Region, Russia; Academy of Med Sciences of Ukraine, Kiev; et al)
Clin Oncol 23:261-267, 2011

The Chernobyl accident was followed by a large increase in the incidence of thyroid carcinoma in the areas exposed to high levels of fallout. The Chernobyl Tumor Bank was set up in 1998 to make tumours available for study internationally, and a pathology panel reviewed all the tumours and established an agreed diagnosis. The thyroid tumours that were discovered after the Chernobyl nuclear accident were virtually all (95%) of the papillary carcinoma type. Rare examples of other tumour types were identified. Within the papillary group, several subtypes were noted, including classical or usual type, follicular variant, solid variant and mixed patterns

Diffuse sclerosis variant, cribriform/morular type and Warthin-like variant were rare. No tall cell or columnar cell variants were identified. The tumours examined by the Pathology Panel of the Chernobyl Tumor Bank constitute a large representative sample (estimated at about 50%) of the tumours that developed in this population. This overview describes the method adopted by the panel and the different diagnostic categories adopted; illustrates the pathology of these neoplasms; compares the pathological characteristics of the early lesions with those identified after long latency periods and the institution of screening programmes and outlines the possible associated causes for the various morphological patterns seen (Tables 1-5).

▶ This is one article in a series of articles in a special edition of *Clinical Oncology* (2011) that dealt with the thyroid cancer following the Chernobyl nuclear power plant disaster in north Ukraine in April 1986.[1-6] These articles are an excellent effort to inform and educate the medical profession in particular, and the public at large in general, about this particular cancer type seen commonly after radiation exposure. This particular article dealt with the pathologic/morphologic aspects of these thyroid tumors (Tables 2—5 and above abstract) and offered very interesting findings. More than 95% of the thyroid cancers after the Chernobyl exposure were Papillary Thyroid Carcinoma (PTC). The tumors identified in the first decade after the accident were the solid variant of PTC, while those in the second decade were the classic or follicular variant PTC. As noted by the authors, although the solid variant showed morphologically aggressive features and occurred mostly in the younger/pediatric age group, the clinical prognosis of these patients with treatment was excellent. The predominance of the solid pattern was also correlated to low iodine content in the diet of the people in the area around Chernobyl.

Of interest is that the dose of exposure to radiation received also does not seem to have influenced the morphology of the tumors.

A final note by the authors also alluded to an apparent increase in follicular thyroid carcinoma with angioinvasion in children born in the post-Chernobyl era (nonexposed population). Does that mean that radiation exposure is showing evidence that it also can predispose to follicular thyroid cancer, a fact that was not shown before? That remains to be seen in future studies

TABLE 1.—The Chernobyl Pathology Panel Diagnostic Terms

PTC	Papillary Thyroid Carcinoma
FTC	Follicular thyroid carcinoma
MTC	Medullary thyroid carcinoma
FTUMP	Follicular tumour of uncertain malignant potential
WDTUMP	Well-differentiated tumour of uncertain malignant potential
WDCaNOS	Well-differentiated carcinoma (not otherwise specified)
PDC	Poorly differentiated carcinoma
FA	Follicular adenoma

TABLE 2.—Main Subtypes and Invasive Properties of the Papillary Thyroid Carcinomas (PTC; 1144 Chernobyl Tumor Bank Cases from Ukraine)

Histological Subtype of PTC	n	%	Multifocality		Exrathyroidal Spreading		Blood Invasion		Lymphatic Invasion		Lymph Nodes Metastases	
			n	%	n	%	n	%	n	%	n	%
Typical papillary	329	28.8	53/329	16.1	61/329	18.5	70/329	21.2	168/329	51.1	103/329	31.3
Follicular	179	15.6	25/179	14.0	41/179	22.9	51/179	28.5	86/179	48.0	57/179	31.8
Solid	71	6.2	12/71	16.9	31/71	43.7	42/71	59.2	40/71	56.3	25/71	35.2
Mixed	559	48.9	101/559	18.1	176/559	31.5	151/559	27.0	288/559	51.5	202/559	36.1
Diffuse sclerosing	6	0.5	6/6	100	4/6	66.7	—	—	6/6	100	5/6	83.3
Total	1144		197/1144	17.2	313/1144	27.4	314/1144	27.4	588/1144	51.4	392/1144	34.3

TABLE 3.—Mixed Variant of Papillary Thyroid Carcinomas: Structural Components and Invasive Properties (490 Chernobyl Tumor Bank Cases from Ukraine)

Structural Combination	n	%	Multifocality		Exrathyroidal Spreading		Blood Invasion		Lymphatic Invasion		Lymph nodes Metastases	
			n	%	n	%	n	%	n	%	n	%
Papillary follicular	192	34.3	34/192	17.7	63/192	32.8	50/192	26.0	111/192	57.8	76/192	39.6
Papillary solid	125	22.4	23/125	18.4	37/125	29.6	29/125	23.2	69/125	55.2	42/125	33.6
Papillary solid follicular	30	5.4	5/30	16.7	12/30	40.0	11/30	36.7	17/30	56.7	11/30	36.7
Solid follicular	212	37.9	39/212	18.4	64/212	30.2	61/212	28.8	91/212	42.9	73/212	34.4
Total	559		101/559	18.1	176/559	31.5	151/559	27.0	288/559	51.5	202/559	36.1

TABLE 4.—Main Types of Thyroid carcinomas in children and adolescents born before and after the Chernobyl accident (277 Chernobyl Tumor Bank cases from Ukraine)

Histological Type of Thyroid Carcinomas	Children Born before 26 April 1986		Children Born in 1987 and Later		Adolescents Born before 26 April 1986		Adolescents Born in 1987 and Later		Children and Adolescents Born before 26 April 1986		Children and Adolescents Born in 1987 and later	
	n	%	n	%	n	%	n	%	n	%	n	%
Papillary carciroma	22	95.7	54	73.0	100	90.9	62	88.6	122	91.7	116	80.5
Follicular carcinoma	–	–	12	16/2	7	6.4	5	7.1	7	5.3	17	11.8
Medullary carcinoma	–	–	4	5.4	1	0.9	2	2.9	1	0.8	6	4.2
Poorly differentiated carcinoma	–	–	1	1.4	–	–	1	1.4	–	–	1	0.7
Well-differentiated carcinoma, not otherwise specified	1	4.3	3	4.0	2	1.8	1	1.4	3	2.2	4	2.8
Total	23		74		110		70		133		144	

TABLE 5.—Age and Gender of Children and Adolescents with Papillary Thyroid Carcinoma Born before and after the Chernobyl Accident (238 Chernobyl Tumor Bank Cases from Ukraine)

	Children Born before 26 April 1986	Born in 1987 and Later	Adolescents Born before 26 April 1986	Born in 1987 and Later	Children and adolescents born before 26 April 1986	Born in 1987 and later
Mean age	13.5	11.8	16.5	16.4	15.9	14.2
Range of age	13–14	5–14	15–18	15–18	13–18	15–18
Females	15	41	63	47	78	88
Mean age	7	13	37	15	44	28
Female:Males	2.1:1	3.2:1	1.7:1	3.1:1	1.8:1	3.1:1

and only to add to the multitude of unknowns currently about radiation exposure. For more detailed readings, I suggest the referenced articles.[1-6]

M. S. Said, MD, PhD

References

1. Tuttle RM, Vaisman F, Tronko MD. Clinical presentation and clinical outcomes in Chernobyl-related paediatric thyroid cancers: what do we know now? What can we expect in the future. *Clin Oncol (R Coll Radiol).* 2011;23:268-275.
2. Maenhaut C, Detours V, Dom G, Handkiewicz-Junak D, Oczko-Wojciechowska M, Jarzab B. Gene expression profiles for radiation-induced thyroid cancer. *Clin Oncol (R Coll Radiol).* 2011;23:282-288.
3. Zitzelsberger H, Unger K. DNA copy number alterations in radiation-induced thyroid cancer. *Clin Oncol (R Coll Radiol).* 2011;23:289-296.
4. Schofield SJ, Lee C, Berrington de González A. Medical exposure to radiation and thyroid cancer. *Clin Oncol (R Coll Radiol).* 2011;23:244-250.
5. Bromel EJ, Havenaar JM, Guey LT. A 25 year retrospective review of the psychological consequences of the Chernobyl accident. *Clin Oncol (R Coll Radiol).* 2011; 23:297-305.
6. Saenko V, Ivanov V, Tsyb A, et al. The chernobyl accident and its consequences. *Clin Oncol (R Coll Radiol).* 2011;23:234-243.

Molecular, Morphologic, and Outcome Analysis of Thyroid Carcinomas According to Degree of Extrathyroid Extension
Rivera M, Ricarte-Filho J, Tuttle RM, et al (Memorial Sloan-Kettering Cancer Ctr, NY)
Thyroid 20:1085-1093, 2010

Background.—The impact of varying degrees of extrathyroid extension (ETE), especially microscopic ETE (METE), on survival in thyroid carcinomas (TC) has not been well established. Our objective was to analyze ETE at the molecular and histologic levels and assess the effect of its extent on outcome.

Methods.—All cases of TC with ETE but without nodal metastases at presentation (NMP) were identified over a 20-year period and grouped into gross and METE. Twelve papillary thyroid carcinomas (PTCs) without ETE and NMP were also analyzed. Cases with paraffin tissues were subjected to mass spectrometry genotyping encompassing the most significant oncogenes in TC: 111 mutations in *RET, BRAF, NRAS, HRAS, KRAS, PIK3CA*, and *AKT1*, and other related genes were surveyed.

Results.—Eighty-one (10%) of 829 patients in the database had ETE and no NMP. There was a much higher frequency of poorly differentiated and anaplastic carcinomas (12/29, 41%) in patients with gross ETE than in those with METE (3/52, 6%) ($p < 0.01$). There was a higher disease-specific survival (DSS) in patients with METE than in those with gross ETE ($p < 0.0001$). Except for an anaplastic case, no recurrences were detected in 45 patients with METE, including 23 PTC patients followed up for a median of 10 years without radioactive iodine therapy. Within patients with gross invasion into trachea/esophagus, tumors with high mitotic activity and/or tumor necrosis correlated with worse DSS ($p < 0.05$). Fifty-six cases with ETE were genotyped as follows: *BRAFV600E*, 39 (70%); *BRAFV600E-AKT1*, 1 (1.8%); *NRAS*, 1 (1.8%); *KRAS*, 1 (1.8%); *RET/PTC*, 3 (5%); wild type, 11 (19.6%). Within PTCs, BRAF positivity rate increased the risk of ETE ($p = 0.01$). If PTC follicular variants are excluded, *BRAF* positivity does not correlate with ETE status within classical/tall cell PTC.

Conclusion.—(i) PTCs with METE without NMP have an extremely low recurrence rate in contrast to tumors with gross ETE. (ii) High mitotic activity and/or tumor necrosis confers worse DSS even in patients stratified for gross ETE in trachea/esophagus. (iii) *BRAF* positivity correlates with the presence of ETE in PTC, but this relationship is lost within classical/tall cell PTC if follicular variants are excluded from the analysis (Tables 1-5).

▶ This is a well-executed study that refutes the long-held view that all extra-thyroid tumor extensions (ETE) of follicular cell origin are poor prognostic factors and enforces the idea of previous reports (eg, Ito et al)[1] that ETE should be classified according to its extent (microscopic vs. gross) and that recurrence and indeed further management (mostly radioactive iodine adjuvant [RAI] treatment) is dependent on careful assessment of the degree of extension as microscopic or gross. The authors classified ETE as such: Microscopic (1−2 microscopic foci of ETE measuring ≤1 mm), Microscopic Established (> 2 foci of ETE ≤1 mm), and Gross ETE (grossly observed by surgeon).

TABLE 1.—Histopathologic Classification According to Degree of Extrathyroid Extension

Characteristic	Micro Focal ETE ($n = 21$ patients)	Micro Established ETE ($n = 31$ patients)	Gross ETE ($n = 29$ patients)
Papillary microcarcinoma	3 (14.2%)	4 (13%)	0
Classical PTC	10 (47.6%)	14 (45.2%)	10 (34.5%)
FVPTC, infiltrative	1 (4.8%)	1 (3.2%)	1 (3.5%)
Solid variant PTC	0	1 (3.2%)	0
Tall cell variant PTC	6 (28.6%)	9 (29%)	6 (20.7%)
PD	1 (4.8%)	1 (3.2%)	9 (31%)
Anaplastic	0	1 (3.2%)	3 (10.3%)

ETE, extrathyroid extension; FVPTC, follicular variant papillary thyroid carcinoma; micro, microscopic; PD, poorly differentiated thyroid carcinoma; PTC, papillary thyroid carcinoma.

TABLE 2.—Clinicopathologic Features According to Degree of Extrathyroid Extension

Characteristic	Micro focal ETE (n = 21 patients)	Micro established ETE (n = 31 patients)	Gross ETE (n = 29 patients)	Micro (focal+established) vs. gross p^a
Age, years				0.0016
Median	49	49	68	
<45	8 (38%)	13 (42%)	2 (7%)	
>45	13 (62%)	18 (58%)	27 (93%)	
Gender				0.44
Female	17 (81%)	22 (71%)	19 (66%)	
Male	4 (19%)	9 (29%)	10 (34%)	
Tumor size (cm)				0.003
Median	1.5	1.8	3	
<4	21 (100%)	31 (100%)	21 (81%)^b	
>4	0	0	5 (19%)	
Significant VI^c				0.0009
Absent	21 (100%)	30 (97%)	21 (72%)	
Present	0	1 (3%)	8 (28%)	
Complete encapsulation				1
Absent	20 (95%)	31 (100%)	29 (100%)	
Present	1 (5%)	0	0	
Proliferative grade				0.0002
Low	20 (95%)	29 (94%)	17 (59%)	
High	1 (5%)	2 (6%)	12 (41%)	
Margins				<0.0001
Negative	20 (100%)^d	28 (90%)	12 (41%)	
Positive	0	3 (10%)	17 (59%)	
Thyroid surgery				0.33
Less than TT	6 (29%)	16 (52%)	8 (29%)^e	
TT	15 (71%)	15 (48%)	20 (71%)	
RAI therapy^f				0.004
No	11 (55%)	16 (55%)	6 (21%)	
Yes	9 (45%)	13 (45%)	22 (79%)	
Adverse outcome^g				<0.0001
Present	0	1 (4%)	16 (59%)	
None	18 (100%)	27 (96%)	11 (41%)	
Follow-up				—
Median (years)	9	10	5.99	

RAI, radioactive iodine; TT, total thyroidectomy; VI, vascular invasion.
[a]Fisher exact test, two-tailed values.
[b]Exact tumor size was available in 26 patients with gross ETE.
[c]Significant VI defined as extensive VI or angioinvasion of extrathyroid vessel.
[d]Margin status unavailable in one patient with microscopic focal ETE.
[e]The exact nature of the surgery could not be determined in one case with gross ETE.
[f]RAI status was available in 20 cases with focal microscopic ETE, 29 with microscopic established ETE, and 28 with gross ETE.
[g]Adverse outcome was defined as the presence of disease at last follow-up. Adequate follow-up data were available on 18 cases with focal microscopic ETE, 28 with microscopic established ETE, and 27 with gross ETE.

The pertinent findings of this paper (as shown in Tables 1-5) supports that fact and adds informative studies on its molecular aspects. A statistically significant finding between *BRAF* mutation and the nonencapsulated infiltrative papillary thyroid carcinomas (PTC; Table 5), suggesting that it has an important role in local invasion and that it probably is not independent of the tumor subtype.

TABLE 3.—Outcome of 46 Cases with Microscopic Extrathyroid Extension and Adequate
Follow-Up

Adverse outcome	1/46[a] (2%)
Age (median)	49.5 years
Gender	12 M:34 F
Follow-up (median)	8.7 years
Site of ETE invasion	Muscle ($n = 5$); fibroadipose tissue ($n = 41$)
Adverse outcome in patients without RAI therapy	0/24 (median follow-up: 9.7 years)

[a]The only patient with adverse outcome had anaplastic carcinoma. All other cases did not recur.

TABLE 4.—Genotyping According to Histologic Subtype in 56 Carcinomas with
Extrathyroid Extension

Characteristic	BRAFV600E	BRAFV600E-AKT1	K, N RAS	RET/PTC	Wild type
Papillary microcarcinoma ($n = 3$)	2 (66.6%)	0	0	0	1 (33.33%)
Classical PTC ($n = 26$)	18 (69%)	1 (4%)	1 (4%)	1 (4%)	5 (19%)
FVPTC, infiltrative ($n = 3$)	2 (66.66%)	0	0	0	1 (33.33%)
Solid variant PTC ($n = 1$)	0	0	0	1 (100%)	0
Tall cell variant PTC ($n = 16$)	15 (94%)	0	0	0	1 (6%)
PD ($n = 7$)	2 (29%)	0	1 (14%)	1 (14%)	3 (43%)
All cases	39 (70%)	1 (1.8%)	2 (3.6%)	3 (5%)	11 (19.6%)

TABLE 5.—Genotyping According to Histologic Subtype in 12 Papillary Thyroid Carcinoma
Cases Without Extrathyroid Extension

Characteristic	BRAFV600E	BRAFV600E-AKT1	K, N RAS	RET/PTC	Wild Type
Papillary microcarcinoma ($n = 1$)	0	0	0	0	1 (100%)
Classical PTC ($n = 4$)	4 (100%)	0	0	0	0
FVPTC, encapsulated ($n = 6$)	0	0	0	0	6 (100%)
Tall cell variant PTC ($n = 1$)	1 (100%)	0	0	0	0
All cases	5 (42%)	0	0	0	7 (58%)

The authors finally suggest, supporting the findings of Ito et al,[1] that PTC
(< 4 cm) with METE should be reclassified as T2 rather than T3 and that
these patients could be spared the RAI adjuvant therapy and its side effects.

M. S. Said, MD, PhD

Reference

1. Ito Y, Tomoda C, Uruno T, et al. Prognostic significance of extrathyroid extension
of papillary thyroid carcinoma: massive but not minimal extension affects the
relapse-free survival. *World J Surg.* 2006;30:780-786.

13 Neuropathology

TDP-43 Proteinopathy and Motor Neuron Disease in Chronic Traumatic Encephalopathy
McKee AC, Gavett BE, Stern RA, et al (Bedford Veterans Administration Hosp, MA; Boston Univ School of Medicine, MA; et al)
J Neuropathol Exp Neurol 69:918-929, 2010

Epidemiological evidence suggests that the incidence of amyotrophic lateral sclerosis is increased in association with head injury. Repetitive head injury is also associated with the development of chronic traumatic encephalopathy (CTE), a tauopathy characterized by neurofibrillary tangles throughout the brain in the relative absence of β-amyloid deposits. We examined 12 cases of CTE and, in 10, found a widespread TAR DNA-binding protein of approximately 43 kd (TDP-43) proteinopathy affecting the frontal and temporal cortices, medial temporal lobe, basal ganglia, diencephalon, and brainstem. Three athletes with CTE also developed a progressive motor neuron disease with profound weakness, atrophy, spasticity, and fasciculations several years before death. In these 3 cases, there were abundant TDP-43—positive inclusions and neurites in the spinal cord in addition to tau neurofibrillary changes, motor neuron loss, and corticospinal tract degeneration. The TDP-43 proteinopathy associated with CTE is similar to that found in frontotemporal lobar degeneration with TDP-43 inclusions, in that widespread regions of the brain are affected. Akin to frontotemporal lobar degeneration with TDP-43 inclusions, in some individuals with CTE, the TDP-43 proteinopathy extends to involve the spinal cord and is associated with motor neuron disease. This is the first pathological evidence that repetitive head trauma experienced in collision sports might be associated with the development of a motor neuron disease.

► This article provides the first evidence for an association between repetitive traumatic injury in athletes and the subsequent development of degenerative motor neuron disease (MND) and chronic traumatic encephalopathy (CTE). CTE is becoming a subject of intense interest, not only for its implications related to the neurologic risks associated with some types of professional sports, but also for its public health and policy implications.

The authors provide a comprehensive and excellent summary of the current evidence linking MND, as seen in amyotrophic lateral sclerosis (ALS), and repetitive central nervous system (CNS) trauma, including that sustained by professional athletes. In addition, they summarize earlier neuropathologic evidence showing that TDP-43 immunopositivity may be demonstrated in tissue from patients with sporadic ALS in areas with motor neuron degeneration. TDP-43 is a nucleic acid—binding protein that is thought to have widespread gene regulation effects. Patients with CTE have a TDP-43 and tau proteinopathy, with immunoreactivity for these proteins present in multiple areas of the brain, including the cortex, diencephalon, basal ganglia, and brainstem.

The seminal results that this study reports are that the spinal cords of 3 patients with CTE who also demonstrated clinical motor neuron disease before their deaths showed not only the expected neurogenerative changes in anterior horn cells, medullary pyramids, lateral corticospinal tracts, and ventral roots, but also frequent immunopositivity for TDP-43 in these areas, similar to that seen in ALS. Also similar to ALS but unlike CTE brain pathology, tau protein immunoreactivity was not seen in the spinal cords of these patients.

In addition to its unique findings, this study emphasizes the critical need for specialized brain banking,[1] without which this study could not have been performed.

D. M. Grzybicki, MD, PhD

Reference

1. Stone K. Researchers take on a preventable dementia: brain bank is giving researchers new understanding of chronic traumatic encephalopathy. *Ann Neurol.* 2011: A11-A14.

Altered microRNA expression in frontotemporal lobar degeneration with TDP-43 pathology caused by progranulin mutations
Kocerha J, Kouri N, Baker M, et al (Mayo Clinic College of Medicine, Jacksonville, FL; et al)
BMC Genomics 12:527, 2011

Background.—Frontotemporal lobar degeneration (FTLD) is a progressive neurodegenerative disorder that can be triggered through genetic or sporadic mechanisms. MicroRNAs (miRNAs) have become a major therapeutic focus as their pervasive expression and powerful regulatory roles in disease pathogenesis become increasingly apparent. Here we examine the role of miRNAs in FTLD patients with TAR DNA-binding protein 43 pathology (FTLD-TDP) caused by genetic mutations in the progranulin (*PGRN*) gene.

Results.—Using miRNA array profiling, we identified the 20 miRNAs that showed greatest evidence (unadjusted P<0.05) of dysregulation in frontal cortex of eight FTLD-TDP patients carrying *PGRN* mutations when compared to 32 FTLD-TDP patients with no apparent genetic abnormalities. Quantitative real-time PCR (qRT-PCR) analyses provided technical validation of the differential expression for 9 of the 20 miRNAs in frontal cortex. Additional qRT-PCR analyses showed that 5 out of 9 miRNAs (miR-922, miR-516a-3p, miR-571, miR-548b-5p, and miR-548c-5p) were also significantly dysregulated (unadjusted P<0.05) in cerebellar tissue samples of *PGRN* mutation carriers, consistent with a systemic reduction in

PGRN levels. We developed a list of gene targets for the 5 candidate miR-NAs and found 18 genes dysregulated in a reported FTLD mRNA study to exhibit anti-correlated miRNA-mRNA patterns in affected cortex and cerebellar tissue. Among the targets is brain-specific angiogenesis inhibitor 3, which was recently identified as an important player in synapse biology.

Conclusions.—Our study suggests that miRNAs may contribute to the pathogenesis of FTLD-TDP caused by *PGRN* mutations and provides new insight into potential future therapeutic options.

▶ As a large body of evidence regarding the clinical, cellular, and molecular changes underpinning the development of Alzheimer disease, the most frequent cause of dementia, has become available, an increasing amount of investigation has been directed toward the second leading cause of dementia, frontotemporal lobar degeneration (FTLD). Although the neuropathologic changes seen in the brains of patients with this disease have been well defined, the molecular pathway abnormalities that lead to the development of both the genetic and the sporadic forms of FTLD are unclear.

The clinical importance of defining these pathways lies in the potential for this information to drive the development of effective therapies for this disorder. The results reported by these authors contribute significantly to this goal. However, this article also serves as an elegant illustration of the importance of investigation into the role of noncoding RNAs in the development and progression of neuro-degenerative disease and neuropathologic disease in general.

D. M. Grzybicki, MD, PhD

Subtypes of medulloblastoma have distinct developmental origins
Gibson P, Tong Y, Robinson G, et al (St Jude Children's Res Hosp, Memphis, TN; et al)
Nature 468:1095-1099, 2010

Medulloblastoma encompasses a collection of clinically and molecularly diverse tumor subtypes that together comprise the most common malignant childhood brain tumor. These tumors are thought to arise within the cerebellum, with approximately 25% originating from granule neuron precursor cells (GNPCs) following aberrant activation of the Sonic Hedgehog pathway (hereafter, SHH-subtype). The pathological processes that drive heterogeneity among the other medulloblastoma subtypes are not known, hindering the development of much needed new therapies. Here, we provide evidence that a discrete subtype of medulloblastoma that contains activating mutations in the WNT pathway effector *CTNNB1* (hereafter, WNT-subtype), arises outside the cerebellum from cells of the dorsal brainstem. We found that genes marking human WNT-subtype medulloblastomas are more frequently expressed in the lower rhombic lip (LRL) and embryonic dorsal brainstem than in the upper rhombic lip (URL) and developing cerebellum. Magnetic resonance imaging (MRI) and intra-operative reports showed that human WNT-subtype tumors infiltrate the dorsal brainstem, while

SHH-subtype tumors are located within the cerebellar hemispheres. Activating mutations in *Ctnnb1* had little impact on progenitor cell populations in the cerebellum, but caused the abnormal accumulation of cells on the embryonic dorsal brainstem that included aberrantly proliferating $Zic1^+$ precursor cells. These lesions persisted in all mutant adult mice and in 15% of cases in which *Tp53* was concurrently deleted, progressed to form medulloblastomas that recapitulated the anatomy and gene expression profiles of human WNT-subtype medulloblastoma. We provide the first evidence that subtypes of medulloblastoma have distinct cellular origins. Our data provide an explanation for the marked molecular and clinical differences between SHH and WNT-subtype medulloblastomas and have profound implications for future research and treatment of this important childhood cancer.

▶ Historically, virtually all types of brain tumors have been prognostically subtyped using histologic and/or cytologic features. In many cases, the accuracy and clinical effectiveness of subtyping based on these features has been lacking. This article is an exquisite example of current investigations aimed at subtyping central nervous system (CNS) tumors based on molecular characteristics. This report, focused on medulloblastoma, correlates a subtype of this tumor that uses the Wnt signaling pathway with its development outside the cerebellum and a worse prognosis. A related article from a separate group of investigators[1] provides additional information about this subtype of medulloblastoma related to noncoding RNAs that are important for expression of its specific phenotype. It is expected that the synthesis of molecular information generated from these types of investigations will provide information that may be useful for the development of specific subtype therapies.

D. M. Grzybicki, MD, PhD

Reference

1. Gokhale A, Kunder R, Goel A, et al. Distinctive microRNA signature of medulloblastomas associated with the WNT signaling pathway. *J Cancer Res Ther*. 2010;6: 521-529.

Amyloid Triggers Extensive Cerebral Angiogenesis Causing Blood Brain Barrier Permeability and Hypervascularity in Alzheimer's Disease
Biron KE, Dickstein DL, Gopaul R, et al (Univ of British Columbia, Vancouver, Canada; Mount Sinai School of Medicine, NY)
PLoS One 6:e23789, 2011

Evidence of reduced blood-brain barrier (BBB) integrity preceding other Alzheimer's disease (AD) pathology provides a strong link between cerebrovascular angiopathy and AD. However, the "Vascular hypothesis", holds that BBB leakiness in AD is likely due to hypoxia and neuroinflammation leading to vascular deterioration and apoptosis. We propose an alternative hypothesis: amyloidogenesis promotes extensive neoangiogenesis leading to increased vascular permeability and subsequent hypervascularization in AD. Cerebrovascular integrity was characterized in Tg2576 AD model mice that overexpress the human amyloid precursor protein (APP) containing the double missense mutations, APPsw, found in a Swedish family, that causes early-onset AD. The expression of tight junction (TJ) proteins, occludin and ZO-1, were examined in conjunction with markers of apoptosis and angiogenesis. In aged Tg2576 AD mice, a significant increase in the incidence of disrupted TJs, compared to age matched wild-type littermates and young mice of both genotypes, was directly linked to an increased microvascular density but not apoptosis, which strongly supports amyloidogenic triggered hypervascularity as the basis for BBB disruption. Hypervascularity in human patients was corroborated in a comparison of postmortem brain tissues from AD and controls. Our results demonstrate that amylodogenesis mediates BBB disruption and leakiness through promoting neoangiogenesis and hypervascularity, resulting in the redistribution of TJs that maintain the barrier and thus, provides a new paradigm for integrating vascular remodeling with the pathophysiology observed in AD. Thus the extensive angiogenesis identified in AD brain, exhibits parallels to the neovascularity evident in the pathophysiology of other diseases such as age-related macular degeneration.

▶ Until recently, the potential direct role of neurovascular abnormalities for the development of Alzheimer's disease (AD) went essentially unexplored. This lack of emphasis on a primary role for the cerebral microvasculature has been supported by the observations that essentially all individuals eventually develop cerebral amyloid angiopathy (CAA) with aging and that many individuals with CAA suffer intracerebral hemorrhages without having any other neuropathological changes consistent with AD. These observations support the "vascular hypothesis" for the pathogenesis of blood brain barrier (BBB) dysfunction in AD (ie, hypoxia and inflammation lead to endothelial cell apoptosis and consequently to leaking BBB microvasculature). The alternative hypothesis these investigators support is that amyloid deposition in cerebral microvessels causes pathologic changes in endothelial cell tight junction proteins that stimulate angiogenesis, thus generating new BBB microvessels that are highly permeable. The significance of this alternative hypothesis lies in its implications for the potential utility of antiangiogenic factors for prevention and treatment of AD. Although the authors provide some convincing evidence supporting the alternative hypothesis (eg, their Western blot data), their confocal microscopy data, which is meant to provide a major portion of their evidence, is highly limited by the unconvincing nature of many of the captured images. In fact, a critical flaw of the study is in the use of confocal microscopy as the method of choice for the demonstration of the presence and localization of tight junction proteins, given the highly subjective nature of this microscopic method. This article provides information to support further examination of the alternative hypothesis regarding the role of the cerebral microvasculature in the development of AD, but future studies should be performed using alternative, less subjective methods for demonstration of the location and expression of tight junction cellular proteins.

D. M. Grzybicki, MD, PhD

Toward Brain Tumor Gene Therapy Using Multipotent Mesenchymal Stromal Cell Vectors

Bexell D, Scheding S, Bengzon J (Lund Univ, Sweden)
Mol Ther 18:1067-1075, 2010

Gene therapy of solid cancers has been severely restricted by the limited distribution of vectors within tumors. However, cellular vectors have emerged as an effective migratory system for gene delivery to invasive cancers. Implanted and injected multipotent mesenchymal stromal cells (MSCs) have shown tropism for several types of primary tumors and metastases. This capacity of MSCs forms the basis for their use as a gene vector system in neoplasms. Here, we review the tumor-directed migratory potential of MSCs, mechanisms of the migration, and the choice of therapeutic transgenes, with a focus on malignant gliomas as a model system for invasive and highly vascularized tumors. We examine recent findings demonstrating that MSCs share many characteristics with pericytes and that implanted MSCs localize primarily to perivascular niches within tumors, which might have therapeutic implications. The use of MSC vectors in cancer gene therapy raises concerns, however, including a possible MSC contribution to tumor stroma and vasculature, MSC-mediated antitumor immune suppression, and the potential malignant transformation of cultured MSCs. Nonetheless, we highlight the novel prospects of MSC-based tumor therapy, which appears to be a promising approach.

▶ The current research focus on molecular neuropathology holds the promise of providing critical information for the development of specific and effective gene therapies for malignant tumors. A separate but related area of study involves the elucidation of effective and safe methods for gene therapy using various vectors. This review is an excellent resource for all anatomic pathologists and neuroscientists interested in learning in detail about one specific type of vector, multipotent mesenchymal stromal cells, with a focus on their therapeutic usefulness for malignant gliomas.

The authors give a highly interesting, easy-to-read, and comprehensive review that includes not only a consideration of the positive findings and aspects of this type of vector but also of the potential limitations of this method. Perhaps the greatest strength of this review is that it presents information supporting the eventual effective role of gene therapy for solid brain tumors.

D. M. Grzybicki, MD, PhD

Enhanced invasion *in vitro* and the distribution patterns *in vivo* of CD133[+] glioma stem cells

Yu S-P, Yang X-J, Zhang B, et al (Tianjin Med Univ General Hosp, China)
Chin Med J 124:2599-2604, 2011

Background.—Recent studies have suggested that cancer stem cells cause tumor recurrence based on their resistance to radiotherapy and chemotherapy. Although the highly invasive nature of glioblastoma cells is also implicated in the failure of current therapies, it is not clear whether cancer stem cells are involved in invasiveness. This study aimed to assess invasive ability of glioma stem cells (GSCs) derived from C6 glioma cell line and the distribution patterns of GSCs in Sprague-Dawley (SD) rat brain tumor.

Methods.—Serum-free medium culture and magnetic isolation were used to gain purely CD133$^+$ GSCs. The invasive ability of CD133$^+$ and CD133$^-$ C6 cells were determined using matrigel invasion assay. Immunohistochemical staining for stem cell markers and luxol fast blue staining for white matter tracts were performed to show the distribution patterns of GSCs in brain tumor of rats and the relationship among GSCs, vessels, and white matter tracts. The results of matrigel invasion assay were estimated using the Student's *t* test and the analysis of Western blotting was performed using the one-way analysis of variance (ANOVA) test.

Results.—CD133$^+$ GSCs (number: 85.3 ± 4.0) were significantly more invasive *in vitro* than matched CD133$^-$ cells (number: 25.9 ± 3.1) (*t*=14.5, *P* <0.005). GSCs invaded into the brain diffusely and located in perivascular niche of tumor-brain interface or resided within perivascular niche next to white fiber tracts. The polarity of glioma cells containing GSCs was parallel to the white matter tracts.

Conclusions.—Our data suggest that CD133$^+$ GSCs exhibit more aggressive invasion *in vitro* and GSCs *in vivo* probably disseminate along the long axis of blood vessels and transit through the white matter tracts. The therapies targeting GSCs invasion combined with traditional glioblastoma multiforme therapeutic paradigms might be a new approach for avoiding malignant glioma recurrence.

▶ The microinvasiveness of glioblastoma multiforme (GBM) is one of its biologic characteristics that prevents complete tumor debulking and, therefore, ensures recurrence in essentially all patients. Previous studies have provided evidence that glioma stem cells exist in malignant tumors that appear to confer resistance to ancillary radio- and chemotherapy.[1,2] The interesting and important question examined by these investigators is whether glioma stem cells are involved in microinvasion. They address this question of glioma stem cell invasive ability using a rat model and glioma stem cells prepared in vitro.

Their experiment is performed using Sprague-Dawley rats that have received intracranial injections of glioma cells from a C6 glioma cell line that contains a small subpopulation of glioma stem cells that are differentiated from non—stem cells by their immunopositivity for the cell surface marker CD133. In addition, the authors perform an in vitro invasiveness assay comparing the invasiveness of CD133$^+$ C6 glioma cells and CD133$^-$ C6 glioma cells.

The in vivo findings are presented in excellent images that show the increased propensity for CD133$^+$ cells in the brains of rats with tumors to be localized around vessels and along white matter tracts, similar to the anatomic distribution of human GBM cells. In addition, the in vitro invasiveness assay clearly demonstrates the increased ability of CD133$^+$ stem cells to invade, compared with CD133$^-$ cells.

The evidence provided by these investigators provides strong and clinically significant evidence for the potential utility of anti–stem cell therapies for improving outcomes in patients with this currently uniformly and rapidly fatal tumor.

D. M. Grzybicki, MD, PhD

References

1. Nagano N, Sasaki H, Aoyagi M, Hirakawa K. Invasion of experimental rat brain tumor: early morphological changes following microinjection of C6 glioma cells. *Acta Neuropathol.* 1993;86:117-125.
2. Sanai N, Alvarez-Buylla A, Berger MS. Neural stem cells and the origin of gliomas. *N Engl J Med.* 2005;353:811-822.

Inducible nitric oxide synthase is present in motor neuron mitochondria and Schwann cells and contributes to disease mechanisms in ALS mice
Chen K, Northington FJ, Martin LJ (Johns Hopkins Univ School of Medicine, Baltimore, MA)
Brain Struct Funct 214:219-234, 2010

Amyotrophic lateral sclerosis (ALS) is a fatal neurodegenerative disease of motor neurons (MNs). The molecular pathogenesis of ALS is not understood, thus effective therapies for this disease are lacking. Some forms of ALS are inherited by mutations in the *superoxide dismutase-1* (SOD1) gene. Transgenic mice expressing human Gly93 → Ala (G93A) mutant SOD1 (mSOD1) develop severe MN disease, oxidative and nitrative damage, and mitochondrial pathology that appears to involve nitric oxide-mediated mechanisms. We used G93A-mSOD1 mice to test the hypothesis that the degeneration of MNs is associated with an aberrant up-regulation of the inducible form of nitric oxide synthase (iNOS or NOS2) activity within MNs. Western blotting and immunoprecipitation showed that iNOS protein levels in mitochondrial-enriched membrane fractions of spinal cord are increased significantly in mSOD1 mice at pre-symptomatic stages of disease. The catalytic activity of iNOS was also increased significantly in mitochondrial-enriched membrane fractions of mSOD1 mouse spinal cord at pre-symptomatic stages of disease. Reverse transcription-PCR showed that iNOS mRNA was present in the spinal cord and brainstem MN regions in mice and was increased in pre-symptomatic and early symptomatic mice. Immunohistochemistry showed that iNOS immunoreactivty was up-regulated first in spinal cord and brainstem MNs in pre-symptomatic and early symptomatic mice and then later in the course of disease in numerous microglia and few astrocytes. iNOS accumulated in the mitochondria in mSOD1 mouse MNs. iNOS immunoreactivity was also up-regulated in Schwann cells of peripheral nerves and was enriched particularly at the paranodal regions of the nodes of Ranvier. Drug inhibitors of iNOS delayed disease onset and significantly extended the lifespan of G93A-mSOD1 mice. This work identifies two new potential early mechanisms for MN degeneration in mouse ALS involving iNOS at MN mitochondria and Schwann cells and suggests that therapies targeting iNOS might be beneficial in treating human ALS.

▶ This article is of interest primarily because it provides current and strong evidence for the critical role of free radical damage involving the free radical nitric oxide (NO) in the pathogenesis of the inherited form of amyotrophic lateral sclerosis (ALS). The fact that the inherited form of this disease involves a mutation in superoxide dismutase-1 (SOD1) is not new; however, the authors demonstrate that this mutation results in the upregulation of NOS2, one form of the NO synthase enzyme, in both motor neurons and Schwann cells in transgenic mice lacking the *SOD1* gene. In addition to showing localization in the expected cell types for development and progression of this disease, these authors also describe a baseline upregulation of NOS2 in these cells prior to development of disease, a finding that may be interpreted as the manifestation of a genetic propensity for free radical damage in these mice. The clinical outcomes experiment described at the end of this report may be of particular interest. In that experiment, the authors show that administration of a NOS inhibitor significantly slows onset of disease and extends the lifespan of the affected mice. A limitation of the outcomes experiment is that to date, clinical therapeutic use of NOS inhibitors for other diseases in humans has not been as effective as hypothesized from animal experiments; however, these findings support the continued investigation into the molecular pathways and potential therapies for this disease.

S. S. Raab, MD

14 Cytopathology

Randomized healthservices study of human papillomavirus-based management of low-grade cytological abnormalities
Dillner L, Kemetli L, Elfgren K, et al (Lund Univ, Malmö, Sweden; Regional Oncologic Centre, Stockholm, Sweden; Karolinska Univ Hosp Huddinge and Solna, Stockholm, Sweden; et al)
Int J Cancer 129:151-159, 2011

Human papillomavirus (HPV)-based management of women with borderline atypical squamous cells of undetermined significance (ASCUS) or mildly abnormal cervical intraepithelial neoplasia (CINI) cervical cytology has been extensively studied in the research setting. We wished to assess safety and health care resource use of a real-life health care policy using HPV triaging. All 15 outpatient clinics involved in the organized population-based screening program in Stockholm, Sweden screening program were randomized to either continue with prior policy (colposcopy of all women with ASCUS/CINI) or to implement a policy with HPV triaging and colposcopy only of HPV-positive women. The trial enrolled the 3,319 women who were diagnosed with ASCUS ($n = 1,335$) or CINI ($n = 1,984$) in Stockholm during 17th March 2003 to 16th January 2006. Detection of high-grade cervical lesions (CINII+) and health care cost consumption was studied by registry linkages. The proportion of histopathology-verified CINII+ was similar for the two policies (395 of 1,752 women (22.5%; 95% Confidence interval [CI]: 20.6–24.6%) had CINII+ diagnosed with HPV triaging policy, 318 of 1,567 women (20.3%; 95%CI: 18.3–22.4%) had CINII+ with colposcopy policy). Sixty-four percent of women with ASCUS and 77% of women with CINI were HPV positive. HPV-positivity was age-dependent, with 81% of women below 35 years of age and 44% of women above 45 years of age testing HPV-positive. HPV triaging was cost-effective only above 35 years of age. In conclusion, a real-life randomized healthservices study of HPV triaging of women with ASCUS/CINI demonstrated similar detection of CINII+ as colposcopy of all women.

▶ Dillner at al report on a Swedish study that randomly assigned women who had atypical squamous cells of undetermined significance (ASCUS)/cervical intraepithelial neoplasia (CIN 1) to 2 groups: (1) colposcopic examination and (2) high-risk human papillomavirus (HPV) testing triage with only high-risk HPV-positive women undergoing colposcopic examination. This paradigm is different from the paradigm in the United States in which women who have ASCUS receive the high-risk HPV test. It would have been useful for the US audience if the ASCUS and CIN 1 had at least been split out for the analysis. The results of the detection frequency are not surprising (detection of high-grade squamous intraepithelial lesions + was equal). From the cost point of view, high-risk HPV triage was only beneficial in women 35+ years of age, perhaps again reflecting the high prevalence in the younger age group. For the US health care leaders, this study supports the rationale for ASCUS HPV testing triage from a cost standpoint. The movement to use high-risk HPV testing as the primary screening modality (replacing Pap tests) was not evaluated. For additional reading, please see reference section.[1,2]

S. S. Raab, MD

References

1. Arbyn M, Paraskevaidis E, Martin-Hirsch P, Prendiville W, Dillner J. Clinical utility of HPV-DNA detection: triage of minor cervical lesions, follow-up of women treated for high-grade CIN: an update of pooled evidence. *Gynecol Oncol*. 2005; 99:S7-S11.
2. Scott DR, Hagmar B, Maddox P, et al. Use of human papillomavirus DNA testing to compare equivocal cervical cytologic interpretations in the United States, Scandinavia, and the United Kingdom. *Cancer*. 2002;96:14-20.

---

p16/Ki-67 Dual-Stain Cytology in the Triage of ASCUS and LSIL Papanicolaou Cytology: Results From the European Equivocal or Mildly Abnormal Papanicolaou Cytology Study
Schmidt D, for the European CINtec Cytology Study Group (Inst of Pathology, Mannheim, Germany; et al)
Cancer Cytopathol 119:158-166, 2011

Background.—The objective of this study was to analyze the diagnostic performance of a newly established immunocytochemical dual-stain protocol, which simultaneously detects p16^{INK4a} and Ki-67 expression in cervical cytology samples, for identifying high-grade cervical intraepithelial neoplasia (CIN2+) in women with Papanicolaou (Pap) cytology results categorized as atypical squamous cells of undetermined significance (ASCUS) or low-grade squamous intraepithelial lesions (LSIL).

Methods.—Residual liquidbased cytology material from 776 retrospectively collected ASCUS/LSIL cases that were available from a recent study evaluating p16 cytology and HPV testing were subjected to p16/Ki-67 dual staining. The presence of 1 or more double-immunoreactive cell(s) was regarded as a positive test outcome, irrespective of morphology. Test results were correlated to histology follow-up.

Results.—Sensitivity of p16/Ki-67 dualstain cytology for biopsy-confirmed CIN2+ was 92.2% (ASCUS) and 94.2% (LSIL), while specificity rates were 80.6% (ASCUS) and 68.0% (LSIL), respectively. Similar sensitivity/specificity profiles were found for both age groups of women aged <30 years versus women aged ≥30 years. Dual-stain cytology showed comparable sensitivity, but significantly higher specificity, when compared with human papillomavirus (HPV) testing.

Conclusions.—The results of this study show that p16/Ki-67 dual-stain cytology provided a high sensitivity for the detection of underlying CIN2+ in women with ASCUS or LSIL Pap cytology results, comparable to the rates previously reported for HPV testing and p16 single-stain cytology. However, the specificity of this morphology-independent interpretation of p16/Ki-67 dual-stain cytology testing was further improved compared with the earlier p16 single-stain cytology approach, which required morphology interpretation, and it is significantly higher when compared with HPV testing.

▶ The introduction of the Pap smear resulted in the global reduction of cervical cancer. However, concerns regarding the low sensitivity of the Pap test in detecting cervical intraepithelial neoplasia (CIN) lesions prompted a search for newer methods to either supplement or possibly replace it. The addition of human papillomoa virus (HPV) testing for triage in mildly abnormal Pap tests (eg, atypical squamous cells of undetermined significance [ASCUS]) significantly increased the sensitivity issue at the cost of decreased specificity. In fact, it is challenging to drive both sensitivity and specificity and that being able to improve both would have an impact on narrowing and improving the referral population of patients for colposcopic examination. This improvement may be here in the form of a dual immunohistochemical staining for p16 and Ki67 in cervical cytology samples. And the question to be answered is, "Can dual staining effectively triage selected groups such as ASCUS, low-grade squamous intraepithelial lesions (LSIL), and high-grade squamous intraepithelial lesions (ASC-H)?" A recent study by Denton et al[1] evaluated single p16 staining alone in 810 cases of ASCUS and LSIL Pap smears and showed the high sensitivity for high-grade dysplasia and an improved specificity when compared with HPV testing. Schmidt et al expanded this study to evaluate dual staining in a similar population. The sensitivity for detecting high-grade dysplasia was 92% to 94%, and the specificity for CIN2+ increased to 80% and 68% for ASCUS and LSIL, respectively. The authors also suggested that it is the p16 and Ki67 dual positivity that is important, not the cell morphology. Some of the positive dual-stain cells morphologically look like low-grade dysplasia but had a high-grade biopsy. It is important to recognize that whether p16/Ki-67 dual staining could overrule morphology in tissue requires further exploration. Although this study benefited from having a large sample size, which, in turn, allowed the assessment of the sensitivity of p16/Ki-67 dual-stain cytology with small confidence intervals, there are a number of limitations. For instance, considering the use of liquid-based cytology, specimens that were up to 4.5 years old at the time the slide specimen preparations for the dual staining was performed may have impacted the results of the study. Further, the retrospective nature of the study, as well as a selection bias by limiting the inclusion of cases into the study where appropriate biopsy follow-up was available, may have weakened the study. Overall, the Schmidt study along with other similar studies have paved the way for large prospective studies to address the question of whether dual staining effectively triages select groups such as ASCUS, LSIL, and ASC-H.

R. Alaghehbandan, MD, MSc

Reference

1. Denton KJ, Bergeron C, Klement P, Trunk MJ, Keller T, Ridder R, European CIN-
tec Cytology Study Group. The sensitivity and specificity of p16(INK4a) cytology
vs HPV testing for detecting high-grade cervical disease in the triage of ASC-US
and LSIL pap cytology results. *Am J Clin Pathol.* 2010;134:12-21.

Usefulness of Immunohistochemical and Histochemical Studies in the Classification of Lung Adenocarcinoma and Squamous Cell Carcinoma in Cytologic Specimens

Ocque R, Tochigi N, Ohori NP, et al (Univ of Pittsburgh, PA)
Am J Clin Pathol 136:81-87, 2011

Histologic subtyping of non-small cell lung carcinoma (NSCLC) is important because the efficacy of new treatments depends on tumor histologic features. We assessed the diagnostic accuracy of classification of lung adenocarcinoma and squamous cell carcinoma (SCC) on cytologic and biopsy specimens based on cytomorphologic studies alone or in combination with ancillary studies compared with resection specimens. Compared with adenocarcinoma, the diagnosis of SCC was based more often on cytomorphologic studies alone (139/185 [75.1%] vs 107/263 [40.7%]). Significantly increased use of immunohistochemical studies in cytology was noted after introduction of targeted lung carcinoma therapies (22/156 [14.1%] for adenocarcinoma and 5/46 [11%] for SCC from 2000-2004 vs 134/156 [85.9%] for adenocarcinoma and 41/46 [89%] for SCC from 2005-2010). Use of immunohistochemical studies resulted in increased diagnostic accuracy for adenocarcinoma (56% [44/78] from 2000-2004 vs 83.2% [154/185] after 2005) but not for SCC (77% [57/74] before 2004 vs 73.9% [82/111] from 2005-2010). Adenocarcinoma showed high expression of cytokeratin (CK)7 (146/146 [100%]), thyroid transcription factor-1 (131/152 [86.2%]), surfactant A (29/36 [81%]), and periodic acid-Schiff with diastase (69/86 [80%]). All SCCs were positive for CK5/6 and p63. Use of immunohistochemical studies on cytologic cell blocks may improve classification of NSCLC.

▶ With the increasing use of cytopathology as the primary tool for the initial diagnosis of lung cancer, more information must be provided with less tissue. The article by Ocque et al shows how cytopathology is now being used to diagnose lung cancer and that immunohistochemistry is being applied to cell block sections to establish the proper classification of lung cancers. The ability to obtain sufficient material for cell block preparations is critical for services that primarily use fine-needle aspiration instead of biopsy. A number of factors affect the quality of cell block sections, and these factors include number of passes, size of needle, clinician experience, fixative, and preparation techniques. A focus on these factors is necessary to ensure that appropriate diagnoses are rendered.

S. S. Raab, MD

Cytology Workforce Study: A Report of Current Practices and Trends in New York State

Balachandran I, Friedlander M (Albany College of Pharmacy and Health Sciences, NY; Memorial Sloan-Kettering Cancer Ctr, NY)
Am J Clin Pathol 136:108-118, 2011

A survey was conducted among 130 New York State (NYS) registered cytology laboratories to better understand current and future changes in the practice of cytology, changes in the cytotechnologist (CT) scope of practice, and the future need for CTs. A 51.5% (67/130) response rate was obtained. Trends for gynecologic case volume varied across facility types. Nongynecologic volume is growing primarily in hospitals and large medical center laboratories and private laboratories; the fine-needle aspiration volume is growing in hospital and large medical center laboratories. One third of responding laboratories anticipate a continued demand for CTs within the next 3 years owing to impending retirements. Few laboratories also report the gradual adoption of molecular testing with CTs directly involved. Because 60% (3/5) of NYS CT training programs have closed since 2008, the 2 remaining programs are a valuable key staffing resource for CTs. Continued viability of these programs is essential to provide the necessary training and staffing of NYS laboratories for cytopathology practice.

▶ Cytopathology is a rapidly changing field, and the article by Balachandran and Friedlander documents interesting aspects of cytopathology practice in New York State. On average, laboratories report an increase in nongynecologic cytopathology specimen and fine-needle aspiration specimen volumes. Surprisingly, although some laboratories report a decline in the number of Pap tests, other laboratories report stability or even growth in Pap tests. These volume data indicate the cytopathology laboratories will need to maintain current levels of service and increasingly focus on the challenges of fine-needle aspiration interpretation—such as interpreting poor-quality specimens. Another interesting finding was that laboratories using the TP Imaging System for Pap tests generally did not show high levels of productivity; half of the laboratories using this system reported screening productivity levels of fewer than 50 slides per day. These results indicate that the implementation of a technology thought to improve productivity may have consequences that do not always align with predictions. For additional reading, please see the reference section.[1,2]

S. S. Raab, MD

References

1. Goulart RA. Cytotechnologists today: much more than "pap-ologists" with schools in need of our support. *Am J Clin Pathol.* 2008;129:523-524.
2. Roberson J, Eltoum IA. Cytotechnology labor market: an update. *Am J Clin Pathol.* 2010;134:820-825.

A Systematic Review and Meta-Analysis of the Diagnostic Accuracy of Fine-Needle Aspiration Cytology for Parotid Gland Lesions

Schmidt RL, Hall BJ, Wilson AR, et al (Univ of Utah School of Medicine, Salt Lake City; ARUP Laboratories, Salt Lake City, UT)
Am J Clin Pathol 136:45-59, 2011

The clinical usefulness of fine-needle aspiration cytology (FNAC) for the diagnosis of parotid gland lesions is controversial. Many accuracy studies have been published, but the literature has not been adequately summarized.

We identified 64 studies on the diagnosis of malignancy (6,169 cases) and 7 studies on the diagnosis of neoplasia (795 cases). The diagnosis of neoplasia (area under the summary receiver operating characteristic [AUSROC] curve, 0.99; 95% confidence interval [CI], 0.97-1.00) had higher accuracy than the diagnosis of malignancy (AUSROC, 0.96; 95% CI, 0.94-0.97). Several sources of bias were identified that could affect study estimates. Studies on the diagnosis of malignancy showed significant heterogeneity ($P < .001$). The subgroups of American, French, and Turkish studies showed greater homogeneity, but the accuracy of these subgroups was not significantly different from that of the remaining subgroup.

It is not possible to provide a general guideline on the clinical usefulness of FNAC for parotid gland lesions owing to the variability in study results. There is a need to improve the quality of reporting and to improve study designs to remove or assess the impact of bias (Fig 6).

▶ This study by Schmidt et al is highly informative as to the quality of our current pathology literature evaluating the diagnostic accuracy of tests and, in this case, the accuracy of fine-needle aspiration cytology of parotid gland lesions. I think their conclusion is that it is poor. I recommend this article as basic reading for any investigator who would like to evaluate the diagnostic accuracy of any pathology test. The fact that the authors could not determine the clinical usefulness of parotid gland fine-needle aspiration reflects poor study design and quality of reporting. The discussion of threshold differences (ie, study differences resulting from differences in criteria used to assign cases to categories, such as benign or neoplastic) and bias (verification [Fig 6], review, misclassification, consideration of nondefinitive diagnoses, and timing) is important to the understanding of test performance. These are sources of variation that contribute to study heterogeneity. The authors suggest more complete reporting, such as using the guidelines of the standards for reporting of diagnostic accuracy initiative. Although cytopathologists often advocate that fine-needle aspiration is sensitive and specific, evaluating their data without bias would help prove the point. For additional reading, please see reference section.[1,2]

S. S. Raab, MD

References

1. Harbord RM, Deeks JJ, Egger M, Whiting P, Sterne JA. A unification of models for meta-analysis of diagnostic accuracy studies. *Biostatistics*. 2007;8:239-251.

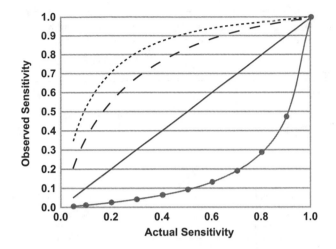

Sampling fraction, r

————— r = 0.1
————— r = 1
— — r = 5
- - - - - r = 10

FIGURE 6.—The effect of verification bias on the observed vs actual sensitivity for diagnosis of malignancy. The sampling fraction, r, is the relative proportion of malignant to benign cases that receive histologic verification. (Reprinted from Schmidt RL, Hall BJ, Wilson AR, et al. A systematic review and meta-analysis of the diagnostic accuracy of fine-needle aspiration cytology for parotid gland lesions. *Am J Clin Pathol.* 2011;136:45-59, with permission from American Society for Clinical Pathology.)

2. Bossuyt PM, Reitsma JB, Bruns DE, et al. Standards for Reporting of Diagnostic Accuracy. Towards complete and accurate reporting of studies of diagnostic accuracy: the STARD initiative. *Clin Biochem.* 2003;36:2-7.

Evaluation of HPV-16 and HPV-18 Genotyping for the Triage of Women With High-Risk HPV+ Cytology-Negative Results
Wright TC Jr, the ATHENA (Addressing THE Need for Advanced HPV Diagnostics) Study Group (Columbia Univ School of Medicine, NY; et al)
Am J Clin Pathol 136:578-586, 2011

The ATHENA (Addressing THE Need for Advanced HPV Diagnostics) HPV study evaluated the clinical usefulness of the cobas HPV Test (Roche Molecular Systems, Pleasanton, CA) for high-risk human papillomavirus (HR-HPV) testing (14 HR types) and individual HPV-16/HPV-18 genotyping in women undergoing routine cervical cytology screening in the United States. For the study, 47,208 women were recruited, including 32,260 women 30 years or older with negative cytology. All women with positive results for HR-HPV (n = 4,219) plus a subset of HR-HPV—women (n = 886) were referred for colposcopy and biopsy. The overall prevalence of HR-HPV was 6.7% and of HPV-16/HPV-18 was 1.5%. Cervical

TABLE 4.—Estimated Relative Risk of High-Grade Disease According to the HPV Test Result in Women 30 Years or Older With NILM Cytology*

HPV Test Result	Estimated Relative Risk	
	CIN 2 or Worse	CIN 3 or Worse
HPV-16+ vs HPV−	16.3 (8.2-51.3)	42.0 (15.5-695.3)
HPV-16+/HPV-18+ vs HPV−	13.7 (7.3-41.7)	35.0 (13.0-552.8)
HR-HPV+ vs HPV−	7.3 (3.9-22.0)	14.4 (5.7-227.9)
12 other HPV+ vs HPV−	5.5 (2.8-16.4)	8.7 (3.2-148.0)
HPV-18+ vs HPV−	8.4 (2.9-26.6)	20.5 (4.3-372.4)
HPV-16+ vs 12 other HPV+	3.0 (2.0-4.4)	4.8 (3.0-8.0)

CI, confidence interval; CIN, cervical intraepithelial neoplasia; HPV, human papillomavirus; HR, high-risk; NILM, negative for intraepithelial lesion or malignancy.

*Relative risk was calculated using absolute risk values to 3 decimal places. HR-HPV was detected using the cobas HPV Test. Data are given as the estimated relative risk (95% CI). HR-HPV+ includes HPV-16+ and/or HPV-18+ and/or 12 other HR-HPV+ types; HPV-16+ includes HPV-16+, with or without HPV-18+, and with or without 12 other HR-HPV+ types; HPV-18+ includes HPV-16−, HPV-18+, with or without 12 other HR-HPV+ types; 12 other HR-HPV+ types include HPV-16−, HPV-18−, 12 other HR-HPV+ types.

intraepithelial neoplasia grade 2 (CIN 2) or worse was found in 1.2% of women examined. The estimated absolute risk of CIN 2 or worse in HPV-16+ and/or HPV-18+ women was 11.4% (95% confidence interval [CI], 8.4%−14.8%) compared with 6.1% (95% CI, 4.9%−7.2%) in HR-HPV+ and 0.8% (95% CI, 0.3%−1.5%) in HR-HPV−women. These analyses validate the 2006 American Society of Colposcopy and Cervical Pathology guidelines for HPV-16/HPV-18 genotyping, which recommend referral to colposcopy of HPV-16/HPV-18+ women with negative cytology (Table 4).

▶ I find 2 important points related to the findings in this article. First, laboratories may have to be able to classify subtypes of human papilloma virus (HPV) to triage patients according to risk management strategies (Table 4). And second, laboratories need to participate in the testing process at a decision-making level. For the first point, laboratories would need to perform additional HPV testing for subtypes and increase their testing menu to accommodate these additional tests. For the second point, laboratories would need to be knowledgeable on cervical cancer Pap test and HPV test triage algorithms so that they would perform the appropriate test. As triage scenarios become more layered and complex, there is less adherence to the standardized protocols. Thus, the benefit of the additional triage must be weighed by the ability for the additional tests to be widely implemented. The assessment of laboratory capability and knowledge is generally not assessed in these studies. For additional reading, please see the reference section.[1,2]

S. S. Raab, MD

References

1. de Sanjosé S, Diaz M, Castellsagué X, et al. Worldwide prevalence and genotype distribution of cervical human papillomavirus DNA in women with normal cytology: a meta-analysis. *Lancet Infect Dis.* 2007;7:453-459.

2. Saraiya M, Berkowitz Z, Yabroff KR, Wideroff L, Kobrin S, Benard V. Cervical cancer screening with both human papillomavirus and Papanicolaou testing vs Papanicolaou testing alone: what screening intervals are physicians recommending? *Arch Intern Med.* 2010;170:977-985.

Cytologic Diagnosis and Differential Diagnosis of Lung Carcinoid Tumors: A Retrospective Study of 63 Cases With Histologic Correlation

Stoll LM, Johnson MW, Burroughs F, et al (The Johns Hopkins Hosp, Baltimore, MD)
Cancer Cytopathol 118:457-467, 2010

Background.—Neuroendocrine (NE) neoplasms of the lung are a spectrum of tumors including typical carcinoid (TC), atypical carcinoid tumor (ACT), small cell lung carcinoma (SCLC), and large cell NE carcinoma (LCNEC). Given the overlapping features within these tumors, misclassification is a known risk, with significant treatment consequences.

Methods.—A search of the pathology archives from The Johns Hopkins Hospital yielded 390 cases of TC diagnosed over 20 years. Sixty-three cytology cases with corresponding surgical material were identified. The cytology specimens were comprised of 49 cases of lung fine-needle aspiration specimens and 14 cases of lung brushings/washings.

Results.—Among 63 paired cases, 32 cases (51%) demonstrated concordant and 31 cases (49%) demonstrated discordant diagnoses. Among discordant cases, the most notable findings included overdiagnosis of TC as SCLC (4 cases; 6%), ACT (4 cases; 6%), and poorly differentiated carcinoma with NE features (5 cases; 8%) as well as misdiagnosis of other lesions as TC (4 cases; 6%) on cytology.

Conclusions.—The significant morphologic factors for distinguishing low-grade TC from ACT, SCLC, or carcinoma remain the critical evaluation of nuclear features, chromatin patterns, and assessment of nucleoli. Nuclear molding and crowding are not discernible features because they may be found on smears with increased cellularity. Crush artifact can occur in both low-grade and high-grade NE neoplasms and may cause a misinterpretation of SCLC. Other artifacts resulting from delayed fixation or poor processing and sampling error are potential causes of incorrect interpretations. Ki-67 staining may be useful in difficult cases.

▶ Stoll et al reported that the diagnosis of typical carcinoids is a challenge on cytologic specimens, and 49% of their cases were misdiagnosed (interestingly as higher-grade malignancies). Only 6 cases were of good quality and called benign. A portion of the misdiagnosed cases had poor specimen quality. Perhaps the challenge arises as these tumors are rare, although other investigators have not reported such a low correlation frequency. For additional reading, please see the reference section.[1,2]

S. S. Raab, MD

References

1. Sturgis CD, Nassar DL, D'Antonio JA, Raab SS. Cytologic features useful for distinguishing small cell from non-small cell carcinoma in bronchial brush and wash specimens. *Am J Clin Pathol.* 2000;114:197-202.
2. Crapanzano JP, Zakowski MF. Diagnostic dilemmas in pulmonary cytology. *Cancer.* 2001;93:364-375.

Current State and Future Perspective of Molecular Diagnosis of Fine-Needle Aspiration Biopsy of Thyroid Nodules

Ferraz C, Eszlinger M, Paschke R (Univ of Leipzig, Germany)
J Clin Endocrinol Metab 96:2016-2026, 2011

Context.—Fine-needle aspiration biopsy (FNAB) is the most sensitive and specific tool for the differential diagnosis of thyroid malignancy. Some limitations of FNAB can be overcome by the molecular analysis of FNAB. This review analyzes the current state and problems of the molecular analysis of FNAB as well as possible goals for increasing the diagnostic rate, especially in the indeterminate/follicular lesion cytological group.

Evidence Acquisition.—Twenty publications were evaluated for the diagnostic material and assay systems used, the type, and the number of mutations screened. Sensitivity, specificity, and false-negative and false-positive rates were calculated for all publications.

Evidence Synthesis.—Testing for a panel of somatic mutations is most promising to reduce the number of indeterminate FNAB. A mean sensitivity of 63.7% was achieved for indeterminate lesions. However, there is a broad sensitivity range for the investigation of mutations in the indeterminate lesions. Therefore, additional molecular markers should be defined by mRNA and microRNA expression studies and evaluated in FNAB samples of thyroid carcinomas without known somatic mutations, and especially for the many benign nodules in the indeterminate/follicular lesion fine-needle aspiration cytology category. This approach should improve the differential diagnosis of indeterminate/follicular lesion FNAB samples.

Conclusion.—Testing for a panel of somatic mutations has led to an improvement of sensitivity/specificity for indeterminate/follicular proliferation FNAB samples. Further methodological improvements, standardizations, and further molecular markers should soon lead to a broader application of molecular FNAB cytology for the differential diagnosis of thyroid nodules and to a substantial reduction of diagnostic surgeries (Fig 2, Table 3).

▶ The application of molecular ancillary testing to thyroid gland fine-needle aspiration (FNA) is being performed sporadically in the United States, but widespread use for specific FNA diagnoses (eg, the indeterminate nodule) is on the horizon. A contributing factor for the current use of some indeterminate diagnoses is poor specimen quality, secondary to individuals—clinicians and

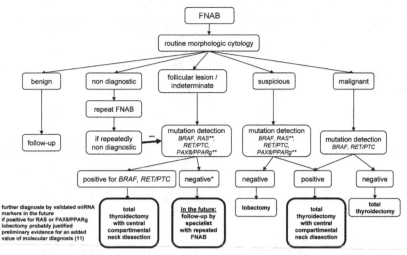

FIGURE 2.—Current and future possibilities to improve the current morphological cytological diagnosis of thyroid nodules by integrated (morphological and molecular) multilevel diagnostics of routine air-dried thyroid FNAB cytology specimens to reduce the rate of "diagnostic" surgeries and to increase the rate of primary thyroidectomies with primary central compartment neck dissection. The improvements by molecular diagnostics in comparison to conventional cytology are highlighted in *bold*. *, miRNA markers validated in future studies should allow further differentiation of *BRAF, RAS, RET/PTC,* and *PAX8/PPARG*-negative follicular lesion/indeterminate or suspicious cytologies into benign and malignant nodules and thus to further reduce the probability of having cancer without detected mutation and without miRNA malignancy markers, especially in the case of potential miRNA markers for benign nodules. **, *RAS* or *PAX8/PPARg*-positive follicular lesion/indeterminate or suspicious cytologies probably justify lobectomy even in the case of a benign histology because *RAS* mutations very likely identify a premalignant lesion (see text). ***, Preliminary evidence for an added value of molecular diagnostics according to Cantara *et al.* (39). *Editor's Note*: Please refer to original journal article for full references. (Reprinted from Ferraz C, Eszlinger M, Paschke R. Current state and future perspective of molecular diagnosis of fine-needle aspiration biopsy of thyroid nodules. *J Clin Endocrinol Metab.* 2011;96:2016-2026, Copyright 2011, with permission from The Endocrine Society.)

pathologists—who lack the skill sets in technical performance. The atypia of undetermined significance diagnostic category is 1 example. It is important to note that preanalytic failures resulting in an atypical FNA diagnosis may be targeted and improved in a number of ways, and molecular testing to differentiate benign from malignant is only 1 way. Other means to improve the poor specimen quality issue include education, skills assessment, pathologist-clinician feedback (eg, through immediate interpretation services), alternative specimen processing protocols, and clinician proficiency testing. The follicular neoplasm diagnosis represents a different type of indeterminate category, that at least for the current time, includes entities (follicular adenomas and carcinomas) that cannot be separated on the basis of cytologic light microscopic appearance alone. The utility for molecular testing in this category has not been fully evaluated (Table 3); would clinicians not perform surgery for a large follicular neoplasm that has a nonmalignant molecular profile? The application of molecular methods to thyroid gland FNA specimens will change the paradigm of diagnosis and management of patients with thyroid gland nodules (Fig 2). For additional reading, please see reference list.[1,2]

S. S. Raab, MD

TABLE 3.—Means from Studies Classified According to the Type and Number of Mutations Investigated and FNAB Category

	Several Mutations Analysis[a]	Indeterminate RET/PTC Rearrangements Analysis[b]
FP	1.25 (0–4)	0
FN	9 (1–21)	3.5 (1–6)
Sensitivity	63.7% (38–85.7%)	55% (50–60%)
Specificity	98% (95–100%)	100%

Data are expressed as means (range). The means for suspicious samples were not calculated because only data from Cantara *et al.* (39) were available. The suspicious samples from Moses *et al.* (20) were not calculated because data for a correlation of histology with mutation status were not given.

Editor's Note: Please refer to original journal article for full references.

[a]Means from four studies (20, 39–41) that analyzed a panel of mutations of indeterminate samples.
[b]RET/PTC rearrangements analysis (23, 34) of indeterminate samples.

References

1. Cantara S, Capezzone M, Marchisotta S, et al. Impact of proto-oncogene mutation detection in cytological specimens from thyroid nodules improves the diagnostic accuracy of cytology. *J Clin Endocrinol Metab.* 2010;95:1365-1369.
2. Moses W, Weng J, Sansano I, et al. Molecular testing for somatic mutations improves the accuracy of thyroid fine-needle aspiration biopsy. *World J Surg.* 2010;34:2589-2594.

The Interobserver Reproducibility of Thyroid Fine-Needle Aspiration Using the UK Royal College of Pathologists' Classification System

Kocjan G, Chandra A, Cross PA, et al (Univ College Hosp, London; St Thomas' Hosp, London; Queen Elizabeth Hosp, Tyne and Wear, UK; et al)
Am J Clin Pathol 135:852-859, 2011

The overall interobserver reproducibility of thyroid fine-needle aspiration (FNA) has not been comprehensively assessed. A blinded 6-rater interobserver reproducibility study was conducted of 200 thyroid FNA cases using the UK System, which is similar to The Bethesda System for Reporting Thyroid Cytology: Thy1, nondiagnostic; Thy2, nonneoplastic; Thy3a, atypia, probably benign; Thy3f, follicular lesion; Thy4, suspicious of malignancy; and Thy5, malignant. There was good interobserver agreement for the Thy1 ($\kappa = 0.69$) and Thy5 ($\kappa = 0.61$), moderate agreement for Thy2 ($\kappa = 0.55$) and Thy3f ($\kappa = 0.51$), and poor agreement for Thy3a ($\kappa = 0.11$) and Thy4 ($\kappa = 0.17$) categories. Combining categories implying surgical management (Thy3f, Thy4, and Thy5) achieved good agreement ($\kappa = 0.72$), as did combining categories implying medical management (Thy1, Thy2, and Thy3a; $\kappa = 0.72$). The UK thyroid FNA terminology is a reproducible and clinically relevant system for thyroid FNA reporting. This study demonstrates that international efforts to

TABLE 2.—Comparison Table of the UK Royal College of Pathologists' Thyroid FNA Classification and The Bethesda System for Reporting Thyroid Cytopathology*

RCPath	Bethesda
Nondiagnostic for cytologic diagnosis (Thy1)	I. Nondiagnostic or unsatisfactory Virtually acellular specimen Other (obscuring blood, clotting artifact, etc.)
Nondiagnostic for cytologic diagnosis—Cystic lesion (Thy1c)	Cyst fluid only
Nonneoplastic (Thy2)	II. Benign Consistent with a benign follicular nodule (includes adenomatoid nodule, colloid nodule, etc) Consistent with lymphocytic (Hashimoto) thyroiditis in the proper clinical context Consistent with granulomatous (subacute) thyroiditis Other
Nonneoplastic, cystic lesion (Thy2c)	
Neoplasm possible—atypia/nondiagnostic (Thy3a)	III. Atypia of undetermined significance or follicular lesion of undetermined significance
Neoplasm possible, suggesting follicular neoplasm (Thy3f)	IV. Follicular neoplasm or suspicious for a follicular neoplasm Specify if Hürthle cell (oncocytic) type
Suspicious for malignancy (Thy4)	V. Suspicious for malignancy Suspicious for papillary carcinoma Suspicious for medullary carcinoma Suspicious for metastatic carcinoma Suspicious for lymphoma Other
Malignant (Thy5)	VI. Malignant Papillary thyroid carcinoma Poorly differentiated carcinoma Medullary thyroid carcinoma Undifferentiated (anaplastic) carcinoma Squamous cell carcinoma Carcinoma with mixed features (specify) Metastatic carcinoma Non-Hodgkin lymphoma Other

RCPath, Royal College of Pathologists.
Editor's Note: Please refer to original journal article for full references.
*From Cross et al.[9]

harmonize and refine thyroid cytology classification systems can improve consistency in the clinical management of thyroid nodules (Table 2).

▶ Kocjan et al reported the diagnostic precision of 6 cytopathologists using the UK Royal College of Pathologists' Thyroid Fine Needle Aspiration Classification System. A comparison scorecard of the UK and the Bethesda System is shown in Table 2— they are really quite similar. It is not surprising that poor reproducibility is seen with the nondefinitive categories of atypia and suspicious. Fig 2 in the original article displays clinical management implications of the different thyroid gland fine-needle aspiration diagnoses, which also is important for pathologists to have in mind when making a diagnosis. The atypical category is the most confusing to manage, as the management in actual practice ranges from no follow-up to surgery. Cytopathologists often use the atypical category when examining poor-quality specimens; reporting the specimen quality in a comment could assist in further patient triage. For additional reading, please see reference list.[1,2]

S. S. Raab, MD

References

1. Layfield LJ, Cibas ES, Gharib H, Mandel SJ. Thyroid aspiration cytology: current status. *CA Cancer J Clin.* 2009;59:99-110.
2. Layfield LJ, Cibas ES, Baloch Z. Thyroid fine needle aspiration cytology: a review of the National Cancer Institute state of the science symposium. *Cytopathology.* 2010;21:75-85.

Implementation of Evidence-Based Guidelines for Thyroid Nodule Biopsy: A Model for Establishment of Practice Standards
Hambly NM, Gonen M, Gerst SR, et al (Memorial Sloan-Kettering Cancer Center, NY)
AJR Am J Roentgenol 196:655-660, 2011

Objective.—Multiple studies have defined criteria for the selection of thyroid nodules for biopsy. No set of criteria is sufficiently sensitive and specific. The aim of this study is to develop a method for assessing consistency of practice in an ultrasound group and to determine whether a 5-point malignancy rating scale can be used to select patients for biopsy.

Materials and Methods.—One hundred one nodules (50 benign and 51 malignant) were selected from a thyroid biopsy database. Seven radiologists were educated on evidence-based criteria used to select nodules for biopsy. Using this information, readers graded the likelihood of malignancy using a 5-point malignancy rating scale, where 1 equals the lowest probability of malignancy and 5 equals the highest probability of malignancy, on the basis of overall impression of sonographic findings. Interobserver agreement on biopsy recommendation, reader sensitivity, specificity, and accuracy were determined.

Results.—The sensitivity and specificity of biopsy recommendation were 96.1% and 52%, respectively. The misclassification rate was 25.7%, and accuracy was 74.3%. Interobserver agreement on biopsy recommendation was fair to substantial (κ, 0.38—0.69). The proportion of agreement was excellent for malignant nodules (0.88—1.0). The risk of malignancy increased with increasing malignancy rating: 4.3% of nodules with a malignancy rating of 1 were malignant versus 93.4% of those assigned a rating of 5.

Conclusion.—Our study illustrates a method to evaluate the standard of practice for thyroid nodule assessment among radiologists within an ultrasound group. Application of a 5-point malignancy rating scale to select nodules for biopsy is feasible and shows good diagnostic accuracy (Table 1).

▶ Some pathologists perform thyroid gland fine needle aspiration under ultrasound guidance. This article will be important for them, because it attempts to

TABLE 1.—Sonographic Criteria Used in This Study

Sonographic Feature	Categories
Internal content	Solid[a] [4, 5]
	Solid with cystic elements
	Predominantly cystic (> 50%)
	Cystic
	Spongiform[b] [1]
	Presence of colloid[b]
Margin	Circumscribed
	Spiculated[a] [1, 5]
	Indistinct or blurred[a] [4, 6]
Calcification	Microcalcification[a] [1—6]
	Macrocalcification[a] [1]
	Rim[a] [7]
	Absent
Hypoechoic halo	Present
	Absent
Shape	Ovoid
	Irregular[a] [3, 5]
	Taller than wide[a] [1, 4, 6]
Echo pattern	Markedly hypoechoic[a] [1, 5]
	Hypoechoic[a] [4, 6]
	Isoechoic[b] [1]
	Hyperechoic
Vascularity	Intrinsic flow
	Marked intrinsic flow
	Perinodular flow
	Avascular
Other	Innumerable tiny nodules or thyroiditis
	Other

Editor's Note: Please refer to original journal article for full references.
[a]Criteria that are most predictive of malignancy.
[b]Criteria that are most predictive of benignity.

develop a malignancy scale for thyroid gland lesions based on sonographic features (Table 1). This scale is similar in nature to the risk scale used in breast ultrasonography. If adopted, all pathologists who interpret thyroid gland cyto-pathology specimens may also want to become familiar with this risk scale, because our diagnoses will be used as the gold standard (at least initially), and we will want to correlate what we see cytologically with the risk assessed by clinicians on ultrasonographic findings. For additional reading, please see reference list.[1,2]

S. S. Raab, MD

References

1. Iannuccilli JD, Cronan JJ, Monchik JM. Risk for malignancy of thyroid nodules as assessed by sonographic criteria: the need for biopsy. *J Ultrasound Med.* 2004;23: 1455-1464.
2. American College of Radiology. *Breast Imaging and Reporting Data System: BI-RADS Atlas.* 4th ed. Retson, VA: American College of Radiology; 2003.

15 Hematolymphoid

Combined Core Needle Biopsy and Fine-Needle Aspiration With Ancillary Studies Correlate Highly With Traditional Techniques in the Diagnosis of Nodal-Based Lymphoma
Amador-Ortiz C, Chen L, Hassan A, et al (Washington Univ Med Ctr, St Louis, MO; Washington Univ School of Medicine, St Louis, MO; et al)
Am J Clin Pathol 135:516-524, 2011

Core needle biopsy (CNB) and fine needle aspiration (FNA) are increasingly replacing excisional lymph node biopsy in the diagnosis of lymphomas. However, evaluation of CNB and FNA remains challenging owing to limited architectural information and the more detailed subclassification of lymphomas required by the WHO *Classification of Tumours of Haematopoietic and Lymphoid Tissues*. Our study is the largest study to assess diagnostic accuracy of CNB and FNA in conjunction with ancillary studies. We analyzed 263 cases and a diagnosis was established in 237, of which 193 were completely subclassified. In cases in which excisional biopsy was available as a reference for comparison, CNB and FNA had a sensitivity of 96.5%, a specificity of 100%, a positive predictive value of 100%, and a negative predictive value of 90%. CNB and FNA with ancillary studies represent a viable alternative in the diagnosis of lymphoma, as long as the number and size of cores for morphologic studies are not compromised (Table 2).

▶ The best method to sample material to establish a definitive hematolymphoid diagnosis is controversial, with advocates (pathologists and clinicians) adamantly favoring some methods over others. I think a challenge in our current practice is that different institutions use different sampling methods and, therefore, publish articles reflecting the strengths and weaknesses of these sampling methods. We never get to evaluate a study in which the different services (eg, fine-needle aspiration, surgical pathology, flow cytometry) are fully discussed so we know why some aspects of the sampling may be excellent or poor. For example, large case series variably include patients who do not have lymphoid lesions; as in many scenarios, patients originally present with a mass lesion in which the differential diagnosis includes many lesions besides lymphoma or reactive hyperplasia. Or the scenario may be a patient who has a known history of lymphoma and presents with a mass that is highly suspicious for lymphoma. In an era in which medicine is moving to a paradigm of individualized care, do we even want to work up patients in these different scenarios in the same manner? I also note that even hematopathologists on the same institutional

TABLE 2.—Decisive Diagnoses of 193 Core-Needle Biopsies

Conclusive Diagnosis	No. (%)	No. (%) of New Cases*
Non-Hodgkin B-cell	111 (57.5)	76 (68.5)
DLBCL	53 (27.5)	42 (79)
Follicular	36 (18.7)	19 (53)
SLL/CLL	10 (5.2)	5 (50)
Burkitt	6 (3.1)	5 (83)
Marginal	3 (1.6)	2 (67)
Mantle	3 (1.6)	3 (100)
Benign	62 (32.1)	62 (100)
Hodgkin	16 (8.3)	9 (56)
T-cell lymphoma	4 (2.1)	1 (25)

DLBCL, diffuse large B-cell lymphoma; SLL/CLL, small lymphocytic lymphoma/chronic lymphocytic leukemia.
*Percentages are based on the number of cases in the preceding column. Of the 131 decisive lymphoma diagnoses, 86 represented a new diagnosis and 45 demonstrated a recurrence.

service work up cases differently and use different flow charts in disease exclusion and inclusion. Thus, as institutional hematopathology and cytopathology services have variable strengths, conclusions of study findings tend to apply to a limited range of institutions. The findings of Amador-Ortiz and associates indicate that combined core needle biopsy and fine-needle aspiration were highly accurate at Washington University (Table 2). However, as we do not know if both techniques needed to be performed in all cases or how these patients even fit into the larger spectrum of case presentation, we may not be able to apply their sampling methods to ours, if our institutions are different. For additional reading, please see the reference section.[1,2]

S. S. Raab, MD

References

1. Wotherspoon AC, Norton AJ, Lees WR, Shaw P, Isaacson PG. Diagnostic fine needle core biopsy of deep lymph nodes for the diagnosis of lymphoma in patients unfit for surgery. *J Pathol.* 1989;158:115-121.
2. Quinn SF, Sheley RC, Nelson HA, Demlow TA, Wienstein RE, Dunkley BL. The role of percutaneous needle biopsies in the original diagnosis of lymphoma: a prospective evaluation. *J Vasc Interv Radiol.* 1995;6:947-952.

Independent Diagnostic Accuracy of Flow Cytometry Obtained From Fine-Needle Aspirates: A 10-Year Experience With 451 Cases

Savage EC, Vanderheyden AD, Bell AM, et al (Univ of Iowa Carver College of Medicine; Pathology Associates/United Clinical Labs, Dubuque, IA)
Am J Clin Pathol 135:304-309, 2011

Although the topic is somewhat contentious, fine-needle aspiration (FNA) is frequently used in conjunction with flow cytometry (FC) to evaluate lymphoid proliferations. Despite the fact that the FNA and FC are often analyzed independently, no previous large-scale study has independently analyzed FC of FNA specimens. FC reports of 511 FNAs were retrospectively reviewed and FC diagnoses categorized as monoclonal, atypical, normal/reactive, or insufficient cellularity (3.9%). Abnormal immunophenotype was considered a positive test result. "Gold standard" diagnoses were established by histologic examination, treatment based on FNA, or clinical features. In 92.2% (451/489), there was adequate follow-up. The diagnostic accuracy of FC was 88.4%, sensitivity was 85.8%, and specificity was 92.9%. In addition, FC accuracy for classes of non-Hodgkin lymphoma was assessed. We conclude that FC is an independently accurate ancillary test in the evaluation of FNA. However, the presence of false-negative and false-positive cases supports the common practice of correlating FC with cytomorphologic findings even if performed independently.

▶ Savage et al investigated whether flow cytometry study results obtained from fine-needle aspiration biopsy specimens were accurate independently in establishing a diagnosis of hematolymphoid lesions. Several biases limit interpretation of these data. First, because different pathologists were present at the time of the fine-needle aspiration, standardized methods of immediate interpretation and specimen handling varied. The amount and quality of material obtained for flow cytometric analysis would depend on the initial diagnostic interpretation. Second, because both specimens for flow cytometric analysis and light microscopy were obtained simultaneously, in most cases, a true independent diagnosis would not have been established (ie, some form correlation occurred), and this bias leads to overestimation of test performance. I think that fine-needle aspiration flow cytometric studies would be able to establish a diagnosis independently in a subset of cases, such as recurrent lymphomas or specific types of malignant lymphoma in the appropriate clinical context (eg, plasmacytic neoplasm). However, in the bulk of cases, a pathologist would want some amount of tissue for light microscopic interpretation as well. This article illustrates that fine-needle aspiration samples generally are adequate for flow cytometric analysis, although a more detailed evaluation of the collection techniques (eg, number of passes, clinical technique) is unfortunately absent. For additional reading, please see the reference section.[1,2]

S. S. Raab, MD

References

1. Dong HY, Harris NL, Preffer FI, Pitman MB. Fine-needle aspiration biopsy in the diagnosis and classification of primary and recurrent lymphoma: a retrospective analysis of the utility of cytomorphology and flow cytometry. *Mod Pathol.* 2001;14:472-481.
2. Florentine BD, Staymates B, Rabadi M, Barstis J, Black A, Cancer Committee of the Henry Mayo Newhall Memorial Hospital. The reliability of fine-needle aspiration biopsy as the initial diagnostic procedure for palpable masses: a 4-year experience of 730 patients from a community hospital-based outpatient aspiration biopsy clinic. *Cancer.* 2006;107:406-416.

Primary Follicular Lymphoma of the Gastrointestinal Tract

Misdraji J, Harris NL, Hasserjian RP, et al (Massachusetts General Hosp, Boston)
Am J Surg Pathol 35:1255-1263, 2011

Background.—Follicular lymphoma (FL), a common nodal lymphoma, is rare in the gastrointestinal (GI) tract. We report our experience with primary FL of the GI tract.

Methods.—The surgical pathology computer files at the Massachusetts General Hospital were searched for cases of FL involving the GI tract. Patients were included if on staging, the major site of disease was the GI tract. Thirty-nine cases were identified. Clinical data were collected from electronic medical records.

Results.—The 27 women and 12 men ranged in age from 29 to 79 years (median, 59 y). Thirty tumors involved the small bowel (19 the duodenum); 8 involved the colon; and 1 involved the stomach. Eight of 10 tumors that

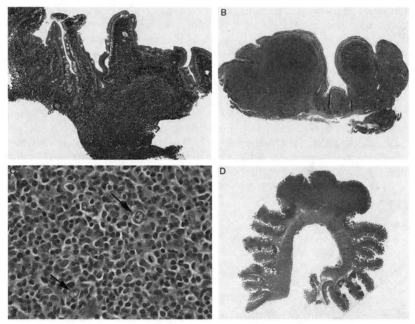

FIGURE 1.—Histologic features of primary FL of the GI tract. A, A biopsy of duodenal FL shows a large follicle composed of small lymphoid cells in the lower portion of the image. Note the dense lymphoid infiltrate of the lamina propria consistent with infiltration by neoplastic lymphoid cells. B, A biopsy of ileal FL shows polypoid nodules composed of large follicles with attenuated mantles. C, High-power magnification of a follicle in grade 1 colonic FL shows a monotonous population of centrocytes with occasional larger transformed lymphoid cells (arrows). D, A resection specimen of an ileal FL shows mucosal and submucosal involvement by the tumor, which is composed of crowded indistinct follicles. Note the involvement of MALT on either side of the tumor, in the form of expansile follicles in the mucosa. (Reprinted from Misdraji J, Harris NL, Hasserjian RP, et al. Primary follicular lymphoma of the gastrointestinal tract. *Am J Surg Pathol.* 2011;35:1255-1263, with permission from Lippincott Williams & Wilkins.)

were resected involved the small bowel (jejunum and/or ileum without duodenum) of which 5 presented with intestinal obstruction. All tumors were grade 1 or 2. Immunostains showed consistent expression of CD20 (100%), CD10 (97%), and Bcl-2 (97%). Among the 34 cases with Ann Arbor staging information, 22 were stage I, 10 were stage II, and 2 were (6%) stage IV. Of 36 cases with follow-up (median, 4.5 y), 27 patients are alive without disease, 7 are alive with disease, and 2 died of other causes. No lymphoma-related deaths were recorded.

Conclusions.—Primary FL of the GI tract occurs most often in middle-aged adults with a 2:1 female preponderance. The most frequent site of involvement is the duodenum, followed by the ileum and colon. Distal small bowel involvement is more likely to present as bowel obstruction requiring resection. The disease is localized in the bowel and regional lymph nodes in the vast majority of cases. The prognosis is favorable even when the disease is disseminated (Fig 1).

▶ The article by Misdraji et al is a good summary of 39 cases of a rare entity—primary follicular lymphoma of the gastrointestinal tract. The data show that primary follicular lymphomas comprise only 1% to 3% of all primary gastrointestinal tract lymphomas. Fig 1 shows low and small power views. The authors do not describe specific difficulties in biopsy tissue diagnosis, although they mention that some tissue fragments show patchy involvement and some tissue fragments show dense lymphocytic involvement. Knowing the clinical findings would be critical for these cases, and most cases present as solitary or multiple polyps, white patches or plaques, and mucosal nodularity. In some colonic biopsies, the lymphoma involved only the submucosa, and in other cases, the lymphoma filled the mucosa. For additional reading, please see the reference section.[1,2]

S. S. Raab, MD

References

1. LeBrun DP, Kamel OW, Cleary ML, Dorfman RF, Warnke RA. Follicular lymphomas of the gastrointestinal tract. Pathologic features in 31 cases and bcl-2 oncogenic protein expression. *Am J Pathol.* 1992;140:1327-1335.
2. Kodama M, Kitadai Y, Shishido T, et al. Primary follicular lymphoma of the gastrointestinal tract: a retrospective case series. *Endoscopy.* 2008;40:343-346.

The use of CellaVision competency software for external quality assessment and continuing professional development
Horiuchi Y, Tabe Y, Idei M, et al (Juntendo Univ School of Medicine, Bunkyo-ku, Tokyo, Japan; et al)
J Clin Pathol 64:610-617, 2011

Aims.—Quality assessment of blood cell morphological testing, such as white blood cell (WBC) differential and its interpretation, is one of the most important and difficult assignments in haematology laboratories. A monthly survey was performed to assess the possible role of the proficiency testing program produced by CellaVision competency software (CCS) in external quality assessment (EQA) of the clinical laboratories of affiliated university hospitals and the effective utilisation of this program in continuing professional development (CPD).

Methods.—Four monthly proficiency surveys were conducted in collaboration with four clinical laboratories affiliated with the teaching hospitals of Juntendo University of Medicine in Japan.

Results.—EQA results by the CCS proficiency testing program revealed a difference of performance levels of WBC differential and morphological interpretation and a discrepancy in the WBC differential criteria among laboratories. With regard to the utilisation of this proficiency program as a tool for CPD, this program successfully improved the performance of the low-scoring laboratories and less experienced individuals.

Conclusions.—The CCS proficiency testing program was useful for the quality assessment of laboratory performance, for education, and for the storage and distribution of cell images to be utilised for further standardisation and education.

▶ Horiuchi and colleagues present an interesting manuscript on an external quality assessment tool for blood smear morphologic testing that has a feedback component for improvement. The data show that the performance of laboratories and individuals improved with participation, and I believe that this is the most important point that should be emphasized. For additional reading, please see the reference section.[1,2]

S. S. Raab, MD

References

1. Saxena R, Katoch SC, Srinivas U, Rao S, Anand H. Impact of external haematology proficiency testing programme on quality of laboratories. *Indian J Med Res.* 2007;126:428-432.
2. Hilborne LH, Wenger NS, Oye RK. Physician performance of laboratory tests in self-service facilities. Residents' perceptions and performance. *JAMA.* 1990;264: 382-386.

Diagnosis and Immunophenotype of 188 Pediatric Lymphoblastic Lymphomas Treated Within a Randomized Prospective Trial: Experiences and Preliminary Recommendations From the European Childhood Lymphoma Pathology Panel

Oschlies I, Burkhardt B, Chassagne-Clement C, et al (Christian-Albrecht Univ, Kiel, Germany; Justus-Liebig-Univ, Giessen, Germany; Centre Léon Bérard, Lyon, France; et al)
Am J Surg Pathol 35:836-844, 2011

The majority of lymphoblastic (precursor cell) neoplasms presents as leukemias. Consequently, the guidelines for lineage determination and subtyping of precursor cell neoplasms were primarily established for flow cytometry methods. Large-scale studies of nonleukemic lymphoblastic

> **Myeloid lineage**
> Myeloperoxidase (flow cytometry, immunohistochemsitry or cytochemistry
> or
> monocytic differentiation (at least 2 of the following: (N)SE, CD11c, CD14,
> CD64, lysozyme)

> **T-cell lineage**
> Cytoplasmic CD3*
> or
> surface CD3

> **B-cell lineage**
> Strong CD19 with at least 1 of the following strongly expressed: CD79a,
> cytoplasmic CD22, CD10
> or
> weak CD19 with at least 2 of the following strongly expressed: CD79a,
> cytoplasmic CD22, CD10

* flow cytometry with antibodies against CD3 epsilon chain, immunhistochemistry using polyclonal anti-CD3 may detect CD3 zeta chain, which is not T-cell specific

FIGURE 4.—Requirements for assigning a lineage differentiation according to the WHO classification, which was designed primarily for FC.[26] *Editor's Note*: Please refer to original journal article for full references. (Reprinted from Oschlies I, Burkhardt B, Chassagne-Clement C, et al. Diagnosis and immunophenotype of 188 pediatric lymphoblastic lymphomas treated within a randomized prospective trial: experiences and preliminary recommendations from the European childhood lymphoma pathology panel. *Am J Surg Pathol.* 2011;35:836-844, Copyright 2011, with permission from Elsevier.)

lymphomas are lacking so far. We analyzed a large series of pediatric patients with lymphoblastic lymphoma treated within a prospective randomized trial (the Euro-LB 02 study). Among 193 lymphomas, in which a detailed immunohistochemical analysis was carried out, there were several unusual and diagnostically challenging morphologic and immunophenotypical variants. These included 11 lymphomas with mixed phenotypes expressing markers of at least 2 hematopoietic lineages, 7 terminal deoxynucleotide transferase-negative lymphoblastic lymphomas, and 3 undifferentiated hematopoietic neoplasms that could not be assigned to any lineage with certainty. Our data indicate that World Health Organization guidelines for lineage determination and subtyping of precursor cell leukemia need to be adapted before they can be applied to immunohistochemical diagnosis of lymphoma. Using the experience from this cohort we suggest a resource-saving diagnostic staining panel for the immunohistochemical analysis of precursor cell neoplasms in formalin-fixed paraffin-embedded tissue (Figs 4 and 5).

▶ Lymphoblastic (precursor) lymphoma (LBL) is the second most common type of non-Hodgkin lymphoma in western Europe. This study by Oschlies et al is the largest published series of LBL cases that were characterized by immunohistochemical study. A highly valuable resource in the article by Oschlies et al is their recommended immunohistochemical staining panel for precursor cell neoplasms (Fig 5). Fig 4 shows the requirements for assigning lineage differentiation, according to the World Health Organization classification. Panels such as these serve as a starting point for clinical practice workup and, of course, debate and refinement. The authors listed a number of challenging morphologic and immunophenotypical variants, and their recommended panel incorporates some of these challenges. It should be noted that genetic analysis was not

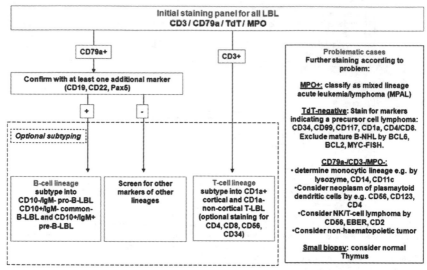

FIGURE 5.—Recommended staining algorithm for pediatric LBL for IHC on FFPE specimens. (Reprinted from Oschlies I, Burkhardt B, Chassagne-Clement C, et al. Diagnosis and immunophenotype of 188 pediatric lymphoblastic lymphomas treated within a randomized prospective trial: experiences and preliminary recommendations from the European childhood lymphoma pathology panel. *Am J Surg Pathol.* 2011;35:836-844, Copyright 2011, with permission from Elsevier.)

conducted, and specific recurrent aberrations to delineate subtypes of B-ALL and MPAL will need to be included in future studies. In addition, clinical correlations were not made and are also an important component of future research. For additional reading, please see reference list.[1,2]

S. S. Raab, MD

References

1. Reiter A. Diagnosis and treatment of childhood non-hodgkin lymphoma. *Hematology Am Soc Hematol Educ Program.* 2007:285-296.
2. Burkhardt B. Paediatric lymphoblastic T-cell leukaemia and lymphoma: one or two diseases? *Br J Haematol.* 2010;149:653-668.

Timeliness and Quality of Diagnostic Care for Medicare Recipients With Chronic Lymphocytic Leukemia

Friese CR, Earle CC, Magazu LS, et al (Univ of Michigan School of Nursing, Ann Arbor; Inst for Clinical Evaluative Sciences and Univ of Toronto, Ontario, Canada; Children's Hosp, Boston, MA; et al)
Cancer 117:1470-1477, 2011

Background.—Little is known about the patterns of care relating to the diagnosis of chronic lymphocytic leukemia (CLL), including the use of modern diagnostic techniques such as flow cytometry.

Methods.—The authors used the SEER-Medicare database to identify subjects diagnosed with CLL from 1992 to 2002 and defined diagnostic delay as present when the number of days between the first claim for a CLL-associated sign or symptom and SEER diagnosis date met or exceeded the median for the sample. The authors then used logistic regression to estimate the likelihood of delay and Cox regression to examine survival.

Results.—For the 5086 patients analyzed, the median time between sign or symptom and CLL diagnosis was 63 days (interquartile range [IQR] = 0-251). Predictors of delay included age ≥75 (OR 1.45 [1.27-1.65]), female gender (OR 1.22 [1.07-1.39]), urban residence (OR 1.46 [1.19 to 1.79]), ≥1 comorbidities (OR 2.83 [2.45-3.28]) and care in a teaching hospital (OR 1.20 [1.05-1.38]). Delayed diagnosis was not associated with survival (HR 1.11 [0.99-1.25]), but receipt of flow cytometry within thirty days before or after diagnosis was (HR 0.84 [0.76-0.91]).

Conclusions.—Sociodemographic characteristics affect diagnostic delay for CLL, although delay does not seem to impact mortality. In contrast, receipt of flow cytometry near the time of diagnosis is associated with improved survival.

▶ Friese et al present data on the timeliness and patient-centeredness of care for patients who have a chronic lymphocytic leukemia diagnosis. Most delays in cancer diagnosis are a result of failures in the pre- and/or postanalytic processes and not in the analytic phase.[1] Pathology often plays a large role in diagnostic timeliness in the reporting phase.[2] Friese et al show that the timeliness of flow cytometric results is associated with increased survival. This article is important in that it emphasizes the team nature of cancer diagnosis and that optimal care is delivered when all team members are working together.

S. S. Raab, MD

References

1. Abel GA, Friese CR, Magazu LS, et al. Delays in referral and diagnosis for chronic hematologic malignancies: a literature review. *Leuk Lymphoma.* 2008;49: 1352-1359.
2. Sekeres MA, Elson P, Kalaycio ME, et al. Time from diagnosis to treatment initiation predicts survival in younger, but not older, acute myeloid leukemia patients. *Blood.* 2009;113:28-36.

Pitfalls in bone marrow pathology: avoiding errors in bone marrow trephine biopsy diagnosis
Wilkins BS (St Thomas' Hosp and King's College, London, UK)
J Clin Pathol 64:380-386, 2011

Avoiding errors in the histological interpretation of bone marrow trephine biopsy specimens requires an unprecedented degree of collaboration between histopathologists, haematologists, specimen requesters, specimen takers, laboratory technical staff and other scientific staff. A specimen of good quality, with full, relevant clinical information is the essential

---

Box 1: Sources of Error in Interpreting BMT Histology

▶ Inadequate clinical, haematological (blood and aspirate findings), genetic and radiological information
▶ Inadequate specimen
  − Too small
  − Too crushed/distorted
  − Both
  − Poorly decalcified/processed
▶ Inadequate sections (thickness, number of levels...)
▶ Inadequate stains (poor technical quality, range too limited...)
▶ Insufficient experience to avoid common pitfalls (eg, differential diagnosis of granulomas or fibrosis)
▶ Insufficient confidence to avoid concluding 'consistent with...'
▶ 'Invisible' pathology
▶ Forgetting to look at the bone trabeculae and stroma

---

starting point. This must then be processed optimally and investigated appropriately, involving immunophenotyping and molecular testing when needed. A wide range of pathologies may involve bone marrow haemopoietic and stromal components, and a systematic approach to analysing each of the components in turn is required to avoid overlooking abnormalities; correlation with bone marrow cells aspirated in parallel is particularly important. Final interpretation should be a synthesis of the histological findings with information from such haematological and other investigations, interpreted with due regard to clinical context (Box 1).

▶ Wilkins provides a basic summary of challenges in the interpretation of bone marrow biopsy specimens. This review is for the general pathologist. Box 1 lists steps in the testing process that are error prone. Most of these steps reflect team failures or system failures rather than pitfalls in diagnostic interpretation. The team consists of the clinicians and laboratory personnel who are involved in grossing, processing, and sectioning, and clinician involvement in formulating the diagnosis is especially critical. For additional reading, please see reference list.[1,2]

S. S. Raab, MD

References

1. Bishop PW, McNally K, Harris M. Audit of bone marrow trephines. *J Clin Pathol.* 1992;45:1105-1108.
2. Charles KS, Winfield DA, Angel C, Goepel J. Audit of bone marrow aspirates and trephine biopsies in multiple myeloma—a single centre study. *Clin Lab Haematol.* 2004;26:403-406.

Pitfalls in lymphoma pathology: avoiding errors in diagnosis of lymphoid tissues
Wilkins BS (St Thomas' Hosp and King's College, London, UK)
J Clin Pathol 64:466-476, 2011

The complexity involved in the histological interpretation of lymph nodes and other lymphoid tissue specimens suspected of harbouring

---

Box 5: Errors Arising from Consideration of Insufficiently Wide Differential Diagnosis: Some Examples

Misleading range of investigations undertaken:

▶ High-grade plasmablastic tumours misinterpreted as nonhaemopoietic because of downregulation of lymphoid cellassociated antigens

▶ Extramedullary presentations of acute myeloid leukaemias mistakenly interpreted as aggressive lymphoma in the absence of screening for myeloid differentiation

▶ Neoplastic mast cell infiltrates interpreted as histiocytic, supported by CD68 expression but without concurrent staining for tryptase and/or CD117 to establish correct phenotype

Opportunity to find subtle pathology by screening missed:

▶ Missed 'in situ' follicular lymphoma in reactive-appearing germinal centres

Opportunities to maximise diagnostic/prognostic precision missed:

▶ Peripheral T-cell lymphoma, not otherwise specified, diagnosed instead of lymphomatous adult T-cell lymphoma/leukaemia, if CD25 not included in test panels

▶ DLBCL or peripheral T-cell lymphoma, not otherwise specified, diagnosed instead of distinctive B and T-cell lymphoma subtypes associated with EBV expression, if EBV−EBER in-situ hybridisation not included in test panels

---

lymphoma is underappreciated. As with other histology specimens, the quality of sections and background information are crucial but so, increasingly, is the appropriate use of immunocytochemistry and a variety of molecular analyses. Within the UK National Health Service, progressive regional centralisation is ongoing, to ensure access to specialist expertise and a full range of testing beyond traditional stains. This is to be welcomed but there remains a need to maintain skills in smaller district hospitals, to ensure lymphoma recognition in unexpected circumstances, to permit clinically useful interim diagnoses when needed urgently and to sustain training in haematopathology among junior pathologists. In this review a range of potential pitfalls in lymphoid tissue pathology is outlined, arising at all stages from specimen preparation to reporting. Knowledge of such pitfalls, some of which are common while others are rare but of vital clinical importance, should help increase confidence in lymphoma diagnosis among histopathologists (Box 5).

▶ Wilkins provides a basic and thorough overview of pitfalls in lymphoma pathology. The pearls of the article are found in the Boxes (Box 5), and the photomicrographs are excellent. Most of these data arose from audits that occurred in the United Kingdom.[1,2]

S. S. Raab, MD

References

1. National Institute for Health and Clinical Excellence. http://guidance.nice.org.uk/CSGHO. Accessed October 2011.
2. Lester JF, Dojcinov SD, Attanoos RL, et al. The clinical impact of expert pathological review on lymphoma management: a regional experience. *Br J Haematol.* 2003;123:463-468.

16 Techniques/Molecular

Gelatin foam cell blocks made from cytology fluid specimens
Mayall FG, Wood I (Musgrove Park Hosp, Taunton, Somerset, UK)
J Clin Pathol 64:818-819, 2011

This report describes a simple method of preparing cell blocks from fluids submitted for cytology, using croutons of gelatin foam surgical dressing material.

▶ Mayall and Wood describe a novel method of preparing cell blocks using surgical dressing material. The photomicrographs show well-preserved cells. No special reagents or equipment are required. This method may well be worth trying! For additional reading, please see the reference section.[1]

S. S. Raab, MD

Reference

1. Chapman CB, Whalen EJ. The examination of serous fluids by the cell-block technic. *N Eng J Med.* 1947;237:215-220.

MicroRNAs in colorectal cancer: Function, dysregulation and potential as novel biomarkers
Nugent M, Miller N, Kerin MJ (Natl Univ of Ireland, Galway)
Eur J Surg Oncol 37:649-654, 2011

Background.—MicroRNAs (miRNAs) are short non-coding segments of RNA which are involved in normal cellular development and proliferation. Recent studies have identified altered miRNA expression in both tumour tissues and circulation in the presence of colorectal cancer. These altered expression patterns may serve as novel biomarkers for colorectal cancer. This review explores recent developments in this rapidly evolving field.

Methods.—A thorough literature search was performed to identify studies describing miRNA expression in colorectal cancer. Specific areas of interest included miRNA expression patterns in relation to development, diagnosis, progression and recurrence of disease, and potential future therapeutic applications.

Results.—MiRNAs are associated with the development and progression of colorectal cancer. These may be either overexpressed or underexpressed (depending on the specific miRNA). Although there are fewer published

TABLE 1.— MiRNA Targets in Colorectal Cancer

Cyclooxygenase-2 (COX-2)	• Overexpressed in 40% of adenomas and 80% of adenocarcinomas • Strongly contributes to growth and invasiveness through inhibition of apoptosis and promotion of cell invasion via action on prostaglandin E_2 (PGE_2)[47] • Direct inhibition of COX-2 mRNA translation by *miR-101* demonstrated in vitro[47]
Adenomatous polyposis coli (APC)	• Inactivation is an initiating event in majority of colorectal carcinomas • *MiR-135a* and *miR-135b* decrease translation of APC transcript, inducing β-catenin signalling and activation of the *Wnt* pathway[11]
Kirsten retrovirusassociated sequences (KRAS) oncogene	• Direct target of *let-7a* family of miRNAs[13] • Reduced *let-7* levels shown in tumours and colon cancer cell lines • Transfection of cell lines with *let-7a-1* precursor miRNA results in growth suppression and decrease in KRAS protein levels • Also thought to be a target of *miR-143*
Epidermal growth factor receptor (EGFR)	• Phosphatidylinositol-3-kinase (PI-3-K) pathway is a central signalling pathway downstream from EGFR • p85β regulatory subunit involved in stabilising and propagating the signal is suppressed by *miR-126*
Programmed cell death 4 (PDCD4) gene	• Tumour suppressor gene (inhibits transformation and invasion) • Has conserved *miR-21* binding site within 3'UTR • Inverse correlation between *miR-21* and PDCD4 protein amounts[48]
Other possible targets[10,14]	• ERK5 (involved in the mitogen-activated protein-kinase pathway [MAPK]) • Insulin receptor substrate-1 (IRS-1) • C-Myc (oncogenic transcription factor) • DNA methyltransferase 3A • Tumour suppressor gene TP53 • Cell cycle regulator Cdc25A • Bcl-X_L oncogene

Editor's Note: Please refer to original journal article for full references.

studies regarding circulating miRNAs, these appear to be reflective of alterations in tissue expression and may have a potential role as minimally invasive biomarkers.

Conclusion.—MiRNAs have immense potential for refinement of the current processes for diagnosis, staging and prognostic prediction. They may also provide potential future therapeutic targets in the management of colorectal cancer (Table 1).

▶ Nugent et al provide a nice, to-the-point review article of microRNAs (miRNAs), which are small, single-stranded noncoding RNAs encoded in plant, invertebrate, and vertebrate genomes. miRNAs were first linked with chronic lymphocytic leukemia and then with other cancers, including colorectal cancer (Table 1). miRNAs are either overexpressed or silenced in malignancies. miRNA expression represent a means to detect or characterize specific cancers, and level of expression may have use as biomarkers of tumor presence or activity. For additional reading please see the reference section.[1,2]

S. S. Raab, MD

References

1. Mirnezami AH, Pickard K, Zhang L, Primrose JN, Packham G. MicroRNAs: key players in carcinogenesis and novel therapeutic targets. *Eur J Surg Oncol.* 2009; 35:339-347.
2. He L, He X, Lim LP, et al. A microRNA component of the p53 tumour suppressor network. *Nature.* 2007;447:1130-1134.

Evaluation of a completely automated tissue-sectioning machine for paraffin blocks
Onozato ML, Hammond S, Merren M, et al (Massachusetts General Hosp, Boston; Boston Univ, MA)
J Clin Pathol 2011 [Epub ahead of print]

Tissue-sectioning automation can be a resourceful tool in processing anatomical pathology specimens. The advantages of an automated system compared with traditional manual sectioning are the invariable thickness, uniform orientation and fewer tissue-sectioning artefacts. This short report presents the design of an automated tissue-sectioning device and compares the sectioned specimens with normal manual tissue sectioning performed by an experienced histology technician. The automated system was easy to use, safe and the sectioned material showed acceptable quality with well-preserved morphology and tissue antigenicity. It is expected that the turnaround time will be improved in the near future.

▶ As the anatomic pathology laboratory becomes more automated, a next step is automated robotic tissue sectioning. Manual sectioning still is faster, but I am impressed that the technology exists. The quality of the sections was evaluated blindly, and the robotic sectioning scored higher! The system examined in the article by Onozato is manufactured by Kurabo Industries (Osaka, Japan). For additional reading, please see reference section.[1,2]

S. S. Raab, MD

References

1. Buesa RJ. Productivity standards for histology laboratories. *Ann Diagn Pathol.* 2010;14:107-124.
2. Buesa RJ. Staffing benchmarks for histology laboratories. *Ann Diagn Pathol.* 2010;14:182-193.

Molecular Classification of Gastric Cancer: A New Paradigm
Shah MA, Khanin R, Tang L, et al (Memorial Sloan Kettering Cancer Ctr, NY)
Clin Cancer Res 17:2693-2701, 2011

Purpose.—Gastric cancer may be subdivided into 3 distinct subtypes—proximal, diffuse, and distal gastric cancer—based on histopathologic and anatomic criteria. Each subtype is associated with unique epidemiology. Our aim is to test the hypothesis that these distinct gastric cancer subtypes may also be distinguished by gene expression analysis.

Experimental Design.—Patients with localized gastric adenocarcinoma being screened for a phase II preoperative clinical trial (National Cancer Institute, NCI #5917) underwent endoscopic biopsy for fresh tumor procurement. Four to 6 targeted biopsies of the primary tumor were obtained. Macrodissection was carried out to ensure more than 80% carcinoma in the sample. HG-U133A GeneChip (Affymetrix) was used for cDNA expression analysis, and all arrays were processed and analyzed using the Bioconductor R-package.

Results.—Between November 2003 and January 2006, 57 patients were screened to identify 36 patients with localized gastric cancer who had adequate RNA for expression analysis. Using supervised analysis, we built a classifier to distinguish the 3 gastric cancer subtypes, successfully classifying each into tightly grouped clusters. Leave-one-out cross-validation error was 0.14, suggesting that more than 85% of samples were classified correctly. Gene set analysis with the false discovery rate set at 0.25 identified several pathways that were differentially regulated when comparing each gastric cancer subtype to adjacent normal stomach.

Conclusions.—Subtypes of gastric cancer that have epidemiologic and histologic distinctions are also distinguished by gene expression data. These preliminary data suggest a new classification of gastric cancer with implications for improving our understanding of disease biology and identification of unique molecular drivers for each gastric cancer subtype.

▶ Shah and colleagues histologically and anatomically defined 3 types of gastric cancer, proximal nondiffuse, diffuse, and distal nondiffuse, and then examined whether genomic signatures could significantly differentiate gastric cancer subtypes based on the histologic and anatomic subtype. A significant number of genes uniquely differentiated each subtype of gastric cancer from normal stomach. Table 2 in the original article shows the pathways and a priori—defined sets of genes that show statistically significant concordant differences between each cancer subtype and normal stomach. Why does this matter? Shah et al conclude that unique drivers may ultimately be identified among the specific genetic pathways and biomarkers, and therapeutic targets may ultimately be developed for each disease. For additional reading, please see the reference section.[1,2]

S. S. Raab, MD

References

1. Marrelli D, Roviello F, de Manzoni G, et al. Italian Research Group for Gastric Cancer. Different patterns of recurrence in gastric cancer depending on Lauren's histological type: longitudinal study. *World J Surg.* 2002;26:1160-1165.
2. Marrelli D, Pedrazzani C, Morgagni P, et al. Italian Research Group for Gastric Cancer. Changing clinical and pathological features of gastric cancer over time. *Br J Surg.* 2011;98:1273-1283.

A Comparative Analysis of Molecular Genetic and Conventional Cytogenetic Detection of Diagnostically Important Translocations in More Than 400 Cases of Acute Leukemia, Highlighting the Frequency of False-Negative Conventional Cytogenetics

King RL, Naghashpour M, Watt CD, et al (Univ of Pennsylvania, Philadelphia; H. Lee Moffitt Cancer Ctr and Res Inst, Tampa, FL)
Am J Clin Pathol 135:921-928, 2011

In this study, we correlated the results of concurrent molecular and cytogenetic detection of entity-defining translocations in adults with acute leukemia to determine the frequency of cryptic translocations missed by conventional cytogenetics (CC) and of recurrent, prognostically relevant translocations not detectable by multiplex reverse transcriptase—polymerase chain reaction (MRP). During a 5.5-year period, 442 diagnostic acute leukemia specimens were submitted for MRP-based detection of 7 common recurrent translocations: t(8;21), t(15;17), inv(16), t(9;22), t(12;21), t(4;11), and t(1;19), with a detection rate of 15.2% (67/442). CC was performed in 330 (74.7%) of 442 cases. In 7 of these 330 cases, CC missed the translocation detected by MRP. In 50 additional cases, CC revealed 1 of the MRP-detectable translocations (all were also MRP positive), yielding a false-negative rate of 12% (7/57) for the CC assay. The remaining 140 of 190 cases with clonal cytogenetic changes harbored abnormalities that were not targeted by the MRP assay, including 8 that define specific acute myeloid leukemia entities. This study revealed the frequent occurrence of false-negative, entity-defining CC analysis and highlighted the complementary nature of MRP and CC approaches in detecting genetic abnormalities in acute leukemia.

▶ King and colleagues present a large case series showing that conventional cytogenetics (CC) and multiplex reverse transcriptase polymerase chain reaction (MRP) are complementary in detecting genetic abnormalities in acute leukemia. The authors highlight the cases in which the failure to detect some specific genetic abnormalities would affect treatment protocols and prognostic parameters. However, this study did not specifically evaluate the cost and the potential patient outcomes of potentially serious safety events if these failures had been prevented by complementary running CC and MRP. From a policy or payer perspective, these data are critical in establishing this link. For additional reading, please see reference list.[1,2]

S. S. Raab, MD

References

1. Rowe D, Cotterill SJ, Ross FM, et al. Cytogenetically cryptic AML1-ETO and CBF beta-MYH11 gene rearrangements: incidence in 412 cases of acute myeloid leukaemia. *Br J Haematol.* 2000;111:1051-1056.
2. Mrózek K, Marcucci G, Paschka P, Whitman SP, Bloomfield CD. Clinical relevance of mutations and gene-expression changes in adult acute myeloid leukemia with normal cytogenetics: are we ready for a prognostically prioritized molecular classification? *Blood.* 2007;109:431-448.

Molecular Diagnostics of Lung Carcinomas

Dacic S (Univ of Pittsburgh Med Ctr, PA)
Arch Pathol Lab Med 135:622-629, 2011

Context.—The development of targeted therapies in the treatment of lung carcinoma is a rapidly growing area that requires a precise histologic classification of lung carcinomas and the implementation into clinical practice of testing for predictive biomarkers of therapy response. Molecular testing has added another layer of complexity in the routine workup of rather limited diagnostic tumor tissue.

Objective.—To review the most important lung carcinoma biomarkers predictive of response and to discuss proposed routine molecular testing in clinical practice.

Data Sources.—PubMed (US National Library of Medicine)—available review articles, peer-reviewed original articles, and experience of the author.

Conclusions.—Histologic profile, clinical characteristics, and mutational profile of lung carcinoma have all been reported as predictive factors of response to epidermal growth factor receptor—tyrosine kinase inhibitors (*EGFR*-TKIs) and other targeted therapies. Recently published results of large clinical trials indicate that mutational profiling, particularly identification of activating epidermal growth factor receptor (*EGFR*) mutations, is the best predictor for *EGFR*-TKI response. Despite all these observations, molecular profiling of lung carcinomas has not been standardized or validated in clinical practice. Rapid development of targeted therapies will probably require molecular testing for a panel of mutations to identify molecular subtypes of non—small cell lung carcinomas that will benefit from new therapeutic approaches in personalized patient care.

▶ The article by Dacic is a nice summary of the current state of molecular testing in lung cancer. Many patients who have lung cancer present with advanced-stage disease and are not candidates for surgical resection. In the past, these patients were treated with radiation therapy, platinum-based chemotherapy, or a combined regimen. More recently, oncologists have switched chemotherapeutic treatment regimens to single agent and combination therapies, such as the use of tyrosine kinase inhibitors that target the epidermal growth factor receptor. Molecular predictors of response are now important in evaluating lung adenocarcinomas. Fig 1 in the original article shows gene alterations that play a role in lung adenocarcinoma development, and developing treatment based on molecular profiles may play a role in treatment.

S. S. Raab, MD

Clinicopathologic and Molecular Profiles of Microsatellite Unstable Barrett Esophagus-associated Adenocarcinoma

Farris AB III, Demicco EG, Le LP, et al (Massachusetts General Hosp and Harvard Med School, Boston; et al)
Am J Surg Pathol 35:647-655, 2011

Microsatellite instability (MSI) has been reported in various tumors, with colon cancer as the prototype. However, little is known about MSI in Barrett esophagus (BE)-associated adenocarcinoma. Thus, the aim of this study was to compare the clinicopathologic and molecular features of BE-associated adenocarcinomas with and without MSI. The study cohort consisted of 76 patients with BE-associated adenocarcinomas (66 male, 10 female), with a mean age of 65.1 years. Immunohistochemistry (IHC) for MLH1, MSH2, MSH6, PMS2, and CD3 and in situ hybridization for Epstein-Barr virus-encoded RNA were performed. MLH1 and PMS2 expression was lost by IHC in 5 cases (6.6%); of these, 5 showed high-level MSI (MSI-H) by polymerase chain reaction assay, and 4 showed *hMLH1* promoter methylation. Histologically, tumors with MSI-H were heterogenous and included conventional adenocarcinomas with tumor-infiltrating lymphocytes (n = 1), medullary carcinoma (n = 2), signet ring cells (n = 1), and signet ring cell and mucinous components (n = 1). Compared with tumors negative for MSI by IHC, BE-associated adenocarcinomas with MSI-H were associated with older patient age ($P = 0.0060$), lymphovascular invasion ($P = 0.027$), and significantly larger numbers of tumor-infiltrating lymphocytes ($P < 0.0001$). However, there was no statistical difference in overall survival between the 2 groups ($P = 0.285$). In conclusion, MSI-H is uncommon in BE-associated adenocarcinomas, but is associated with clinicopathologic features fairly similar to sporadic microsatellite unstable colorectal cancers. Given the growing evidence that indicates lack of benefits from adjuvant therapy with fluorouracil in the colonic counterpart, it may be important to identify MSI-H in BE-associated adenocarcinomas.

▶ Ferris and coauthors evaluate microsatellite instability in Barrett esophagus (BE) adenocarcinoma. Similar to colonic adenocarcinomas, the presence or absence of this instability may affect the use of adjuvant therapy with fluorouracil in BE-associated adenocarcinomas. For additional reading, please see reference list.[1,2]

S. S. Raab, MD

References

1. Alexander J, Watanabe T, Wu T-T, Rashid A, Li S, Hamilton SR. Histopathological identification of colon cancer with microsatellite instability. *Am J Pathol.* 2001;158:527-535.
2. Muzeau F, Fléjou JF, Belghiti J, Thomas G, Hamelin R. Infrequent microsatellite instability in oesophageal cancers. *Br J Cancer.* 1997;75:1336-1339.

PART II

LABORATORY MEDICINE

17 Laboratory Management and Outcomes

Effect of Two Different FDA-approved D-dimer Assays on Resource Utilization in the Emergency Department

Sanchez LD, McGillicuddy DC, Volz KA, et al (Beth Israel Deaconess Med Ctr, Boston, MA)

Acad Emerg Med 18:317-321, 2011

Background.—The D-dimer assay has been shown to be an appropriate test to rule out pulmonary embolism (PE) in low-risk patients in the emergency department (ED). Multiple assays now are approved to measure D-dimer levels. Studies have shown a newer assay, Tina-quant, to have similar diagnostic accuracy to the VIDAS assay.

Objectives.—The objective was to determine effects of transitioning from the VIDAS assay to the Tinaquant D-dimer assay on the need for computed tomography angiogram (CTA) and ED length of stay (LOS) in patients being evaluated for PE in the ED.

Methods.—A retrospective cohort study was conducted of patients who had D-dimer levels ordered at an urban, academic, Level I trauma center with over 55,000 annual ED visits. The results of D-dimer levels in the ED were recorded over a period of 6 months prior to and 6 months after the transition to the new D-dimer assay. The numbers of positive and negative D-dimers and need for subsequent CTAs were recorded for comparison. LOS was also recorded to determine time saved. Medians were calculated and compared using Wilcoxon rank sum.

Results.—During the initial period, 875 D-dimers were ordered, with a positive rate of 41.5%. During the period after the introduction of the Tina-quant assay, 859 tests were ordered, with 25.5% having positive results. An absolute decrease of 16% in the number of necessary CTAs (p < 0.003) was seen after the transition to the Tina-quant assay. LOS data showed a mean LOS of 481 minutes in the ED for patients who underwent testing with the Tina-quant assay compared to 526 minutes with the VIDAS assay, saving an average of 45 minutes per patient (p < 0.003). The positive rate on performed imaging studies for D-dimer of >500 rose from 13 of 308 (4.2%) to 17 of 187 (9.1%).

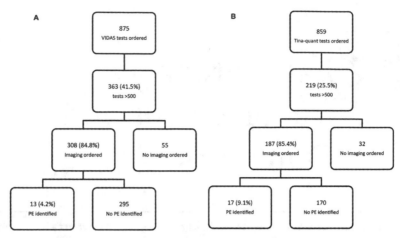

FIGURE 1.—(A) Patient flow for VIDAS D-dimer tests performed. (B) Patient flow for Tina-quant D-dimer tests performed. PE = pulmonary embolism. (Reprinted from Sanchez LD, McGillicuddy DC, Volz KA, et al. Effect of two different FDA-approved D-dimer assays on resource utilization in the emergency department. *Acad Emerg Med.* 2011;18:317-321, with permission from the Society for Academic Emergency Medicine.)

Conclusions.—Switching D-dimer assays reduced both LOS and number of imaging studies in our patient population (Fig 1).

▶ To us laboratorians, emergency departments (ED) seem universally to demand ever-faster turnaround time on any assays with which they are involved, whether based in the central lab or at the point of care. We, of course, understand these demands in terms of their impact on quality of care. Here is an example of the type of head-on comparison linked to significant ED patient care and financial outcomes that is necessary to make this case. It compares 2 assays for D-dimer to rule out pulmonary embolism (PE): the Bio-Merieux VIDAS and the Roche Tina-quant. Previous studies did not examine ED patients specifically and likely were higher in prevalence than the ED population. The Tina-quant assay has been found to be faster, with actual analysis time in the authors' laboratory of 10 to 15 minutes, compared with 30 to 35 minutes for the VIDAS assay (Fig 1). They attempted to determine the effects of transitioning from the VIDAS to the Tina-quant assay on computed tomography angiogram use and ED length of stay.

M. G. Bissell, MD, PhD, MPH

Pending Laboratory Tests and the Hospital Discharge Summary in Patients Discharged To Sub-Acute Care
Walz SE, Smith M, Cox E, et al (Univ of Wisconsin School of Medicine & Public Health, Madison)
J Gen Intern Med 26:393-398, 2011

Background.—Previous studies have noted a high (41%) prevalence and poor discharge summary communication of pending laboratory (lab) tests at the time of hospital discharge for general medical patients. However, the prevalence and communication of pending labs within a high-risk population, specifically those patients discharged to sub-acute care (i.e., skilled nursing, rehabilitation, long-term care), remains unknown.

Objective.—To determine the prevalence and nature of lab tests pending at hospital discharge and their inclusion within hospital discharge summaries, for common sub-acute care populations.

Design.—Retrospective cohort study.

Participants.—Stroke, hip fracture, and cancer patients discharged from a single large academic medical center to sub-acute care, 2003–2005 (N = 564).

Main Measures.—Pending lab tests were abstracted from the laboratory information system (LIS) and from each patient's discharge summary, then grouped into 14 categories and compared. Microbiology tests were subdivided by culture type and number of days pending prior to discharge.

Key Results.—Of sub-acute care patients, 32% (181/564) were discharged with pending lab tests per the LIS; however, only 11% (20/181) of discharge summaries documented these. Patients most often left the hospital with pending microbiology tests (83% [150/181]), particularly blood and urine cultures, and reference lab tests (17% [30/181]). However, 82% (61/74) of patients' pending urine cultures did not have 24 hour preliminary results, and 19% (13/70) of patients' pending blood cultures did not have 48 hour preliminary results available at the time of hospital discharge.

Conclusions.—Approximately one-third of the sub-acute care patients in this study had labs pending at discharge, but few were documented within hospital discharge summaries. Even after considering the availability of preliminary microbiology results, these omissions remain common. Future studies should focus on improving the communication of pending lab tests at discharge and evaluating the impact that this improved communication has on patient outcomes.

▶ As we frequently like to remind ourselves, clinical laboratory (lab) tests are an essential part of medical care, guiding approximately 70% of medical decisions. And, as we would sometimes like to forget, a lab test that was ordered during hospitalization for which the result has not returned prior to patient discharge is known as a pending lab test. General medical patients frequently (41%) leave the hospital with pending lab tests. As many as 9.4% of these pending lab test results are abnormal and would change the patient's care. Despite the high number of pending lab tests at hospital discharge for general medical patients, these tests are often omitted from the hospital discharge summary, the only document mandated by The Joint Commission to convey the patient's care plan to the next setting of care. The objectives of this study were to determine the frequency and nature of pending labs for adults discharged to subacute care, and to examine how often these pending labs were included in the hospital discharge summary. A secondary objective was to identify and determine the frequency of preliminarily available microbiology culture results for this population.

M. G. Bissell, MD, PhD, MPH

Repeated Hemoglobin A1C Ordering in the VA Health System

Laxmisan A, Vaughan-Sarrazin M, Cram P (Univ of Iowa Carver College of Medicine)
Am J Med 124:342-349, 2011

Background.—Hemoglobin A1c (HbA1c) is used to assess glycemic control in patients with diabetes. While underuse of HbA1c testing has been well studied, potential overuse is poorly characterized.

Methods.—Our objective was to examine the frequency of HbA1c testing in an integrated delivery system. We conducted a retrospective study of administrative data of 130,538 patients with newly diagnosed diabetes receiving care in the Veterans Administration Healthcare System during 2006 and 2007 (mean age 64.1 years, 97.3% male). Our main outcome measures were the proportion of patients receiving repeat HbA1c testing within 30 and 90 days and the proportion of patients receiving more than 4 repeat tests within 12 months of their initial HbA1c.

Results.—Overall 8.4% of patients (N = 11,003) received at least one repeat HbA1c within 30 days of their initial test and 30.8% (N = 40,162) within 90 days. A significantly higher proportion of patients with poor diabetes control received a repeat test within 30 days (14.7%) than patients with intermediate control (9.1%) or good control (6.8%) ($P < 0.01$). Overall, 4.2% of patients (N = 5,468) received more than 4 repeat HbA1c tests and 0.4% received more than 6 (N = 479). In logistic regression models, receipt of more than 4 repeat HbA1c tests was more common among patients age 50-70 years (compared to younger and older patients), whites (compared to blacks and Hispanics), and patients manifesting complications of diabetes ($P < 0.01$ for all).

Conclusion.—Repeat HbA1c testing appears to occur somewhat more frequently than is warranted (Fig 2).

▶ Routinely, HbAlc testing is used in clinical practice to monitor diabetes and is used as a key parameter on which to base changes in the management of patients with diabetes. Because a patient's HbAlc value reflects the blood glucose concentration over the previous 2 to 3 months, testing more frequently than this is potentially wasteful and, at worst, misleading because changes in HbAlc do not reflect short-term changes in blood sugar levels. With this background, the objective of this study was to assess the potential overuse of HbAlc testing in the entire Veterans Health Administration (VHA), an integrated health care delivery system that has focused aggressively on ambulatory quality of care. In particular, the authors sought to assess the distribution of ordering HbAlc tests among newly diagnosed patients with diabetes mellitus, examine the frequency of HbAlc test ordering among these patients, and evaluate the

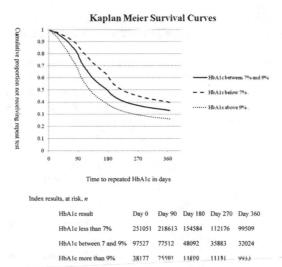

FIGURE 2.—Kaplan-Meier estimates of time to repeated testing. (Reprinted from Laxmisan A, Vaughan-Sarrazin M, Cram P. Repeated hemoglobin A1C ordering in the VA health system. *Am J Med.* 2011;124:342-349, Copyright 2011, with permission from Elsevier.)

frequency of ordering HbAlc tests in the VHA against the recommendations provided by the American Diabetes Association and the VHA Clinical Practice Guidelines (Fig 2).

M. G. Bissell, MD, PhD, MPH

Impact of Laboratory Accreditation on Patient Care and the Health System

Peter TF, Rotz PD, Blair DH, et al (Clinton Health Access Initiative, Boston, MA)

Am J Clin Pathol 134:550-555, 2010

Accreditation is emerging as a preferred framework for building quality medical laboratory systems in resource-limited settings. Despite the low numbers of laboratories accredited to date, accreditation has the potential to improve the quality of health care for patients through the reduction of testing errors and attendant decreases in inappropriate treatment. Accredited laboratories can become more accountable and less dependent on external support. Efforts made to achieve accreditation may also lead to improvements in the management of laboratory networks by focusing attention on areas of greatest need and accelerating improvement in areas such as supply chain, training, and instrument maintenance. Laboratory accreditation may also have a positive influence on performance in other areas of health care systems by allowing laboratories to demonstrate high standards of service delivery. Accreditation may, thus, provide an effective mechanism for health system improvement yielding long-term benefits in the quality, cost-effectiveness, and sustainability of public health programs. Further studies are needed to strengthen the evidence on the benefits of accreditation and to justify the resources needed to implement accreditation programs aimed at improving the performance of laboratory systems.

▶ Laboratory testing is an essential component of improved health care for patients in resource-limited settings. As we know, accurate and rapid diagnostic tests are required to diagnose illness, identify causative factors, monitor the effectiveness of treatment, perform surveillance for key diseases, and deliver high-quality patient care. However, it is not enough to invest in the expansion of diagnostic access. Simultaneous improvements in the quality of laboratory testing are needed to ensure clinician and patient confidence in test results. Accreditation is widely used in developed countries to encourage or enforce improvements in the quality and reliability of laboratories. With significant investment beginning to be channeled into recently launched laboratory accreditation initiatives in resource-limited settings, it is worthwhile evaluating the impact that accreditation can have on patient care and health systems, as the authors have attempted to do here.

M. G. Bissell, MD, PhD, MPH

The Impact of Specially Designed Digital Games-Based Learning in Undergraduate Pathology and Medical Education
Kanthan R, Senger J-L (Univ of Saskatchewan, Saskatoon, Canada)
Arch Pathol Lab Med 135:135-142, 2011

Context.—The rapid advances of computer technologies have created a new e-learner generation of "Homozappien" students that think and learn differently. Digital gaming is an effective, fun, active, and encouraging way of learning, providing immediate feedback and measurable process. Within the context of ongoing reforms in medical education, specially designed digital games, a form of active learning, are effective, complementary e-teaching/ learning resources.

Objective.—To examine the effectiveness of the use of specially designed digital games for student satisfaction and for measurable academic improvement.

Design.—One hundred fourteen students registered in first-year pathology Medicine 102 had 8 of 16 lecture sessions reviewed in specially designed content-relevant digital games. Performance scores to relevant content sessions were analyzed at midterm and final examinations. Seventy-one students who registered in second-year pathology Medicine 202 were exposed to the games only during the final examination, with the midterm examination serving as an internal matched-control group. Outcome measures included performance at midterm and final examinations. Paired 2-tailed *t* test statistics compared means. A satisfaction survey questionnaire of yes or no responses analyzed student engagement and their perceptions to digital game-based learning.

Results.—Questions relevant to the game-play sessions had the highest success rate in both examinations among 114 first-year students. In the 71

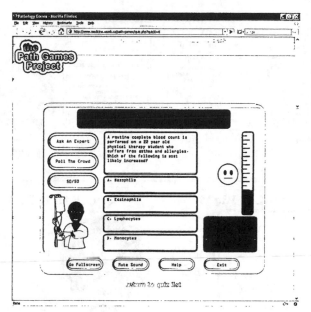

FIGURE 1.—*Path to Success* screen shot image of an interactive electronic digital game whose goal is to answer multiple choice questions to strengthen the life force of and save a dying patient. The game screen has a life force meter gauge that records the player's progress on the right and the 3 help strategies on the left: Ask An Expert, Poll The Crowd, and 50/50. (Reprinted from Kanthan R, Senger J-L. The impact of specially designed digital games-based learning in undergraduate pathology and medical education. *Arch Pathol Lab Med.* 2011;135:135-142, with permission from Archives of Pathology & Laboratory Medicine. Copyright 2011. College of American Pathologists.)

second-year students, the examination scores at the end of the final examination were significantly higher than the scores on the midterm examination. Positive satisfaction survey noted increased student engagement, enhanced personal learning, and reduced student stress.

Conclusions.—Specially constructed digital games-based learning in undergraduate pathology courses showed improved academic performance as measured by examination test scores with increased student satisfaction and engagement (Figs 1 and 2).

▶ The revolutionary change of the digital world during the last decades of the 20th century with globalization has changed the way students think and learn, thereby "prompting a need to change traditional lecture-based passive learning methodology to an active multisensory experiential learning methodology." Although digital games-based learning (DGBL) is spreading rapidly in all educational settings, the literature does not provide clear empirical evidence of its pedagogical benefits. Although theoretically, digital gaming and education fit together seamlessly, quantitative studies proving the effectiveness of this union are few in the published English literature. Although most agree that games can be engaging and instructive, it is often extremely difficult to demonstrate gains in learning that are attributable to the use of the virtual environment of video games, virtual simulations, or digital games. Learning in itself is a truly complex process to assess in

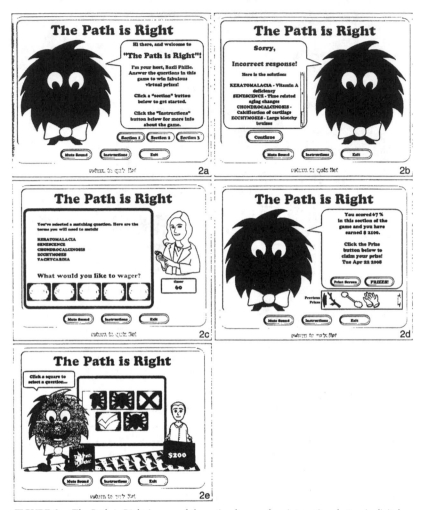

FIGURE 2.—*The Path is Right* images of the action boxes of an interactive electronic digital game with 3 sections. The host Basil Philic (a) guides the players through different challenges and offers constructive feedback with each response (b). The game is based on placing wagers with virtual money (c) with an aim to increase winnings (d) to buy virtual prizes at the end of the game. Each section has 5 options (e) leaving the players in control of their chances of winning at the game. The game design format includes multiple choice, fill in the blank, and extended matching questions. (Reprinted from Kanthan R, Senger J-L. The impact of specially designed digital games-based learning in undergraduate pathology and medical education. *Arch Pathol Lab Med.* 2011;135:135-142, with permission from Archives of Pathology & Laboratory Medicine. Copyright 2011. College of American Pathologists.)

a purely quantitative scientific paradigm. This is further compounded by the use of names other than "assessment" used in past efforts of the gaming and simulation community to demonstrate educational effectiveness of their experiential activities in the classrooms of K to 12 students. Further, although much is known about games and learning in general, little is known about game attributes that influence and contribute to learning outcomes even though simulation and gaming are used in higher education. This lack of "hard-core data" to DGBL is a further deterrent to the acceptance of the use of such active learning tools in higher education. Undergraduate medical education remains quite traditionally bound within its "evidence-based" educational paradigms, unlike engineering education with the numerous applications of simulation games. In this context, 2 specially designed content-relevant digital games were created for implementation as complementary learning tools to the first-year and second-year students registered in the undergraduate pathology courses at the College of Medicine, University of Saskatchewan, Saskatoon, Canada (Fig 1 and Fig 2). The purpose of this study was to examine the effectiveness of the implementation of such specially designed digital games in (1) improving academic performance/learning outcomes, as measured by examination test scores, and (2) examining student satisfaction and perceptions of DGBL.

M. G. Bissell, MD, PhD, MPH

Human Tissue Ownership and Use in Research: What Laboratorians and Researchers Should Know

Allen MJ, Powers MLE, Gronowski KS, et al (Washington Univ School of Medicine St Louis, MO; BJC HealthCare, St Louis, MO)
Clin Chem 56:1675-1682, 2010

Background.—The use of human blood and tissue is critical to biomedical research. A number of treaties, laws, and regulations help to guide the ethical collection of these specimens. However, there are no clearly defined regulations regarding the ownership of human tissue specimens and who can control their fate.

Content.—This review discusses the existing regulations governing human studies and the necessary components of patient consent. Legal cases that have addressed the issue of ownership of human tissue are reviewed, including recent settlements that have led to the destruction of millions of specimens of patient tissue. The unique regulations that guide the use of tissues collected postmortem are also examined. Potential changes in the future of biomedical research that uses human tissue, including genetic material, are also discussed.

Summary.—The use of human tissue is directed by numerous laws and regulations. Awareness of these rules and of how and when to obtain meaningful informed consent from patients is essential for laboratorians and researchers, who should also be familiar with situations that have led to lawsuits and in some cases the destruction of valuable human tissue specimens.

▶ Research specimens are obtained from the following 4 sources: (1) tissues collected prospectively for a research project; (2) excess tissue from samples taken specifically for clinical purposes, such as diagnosis or treatment, which are subsequently recognized as valuable for research; (3) cadaveric tissues; and (4) tissues with reproductive or "human" potential, including eggs, sperm, zygotes, embryos, and fetal tissues, which are also often collected for clinical purposes, as in (1). With the increased use of human tissue in medical research, researchers, research institutions, and human research participants have asked: Who gets to determine the fate of such specimens? In the United States, a country that prides itself on property rights, this question has prompted another: Who "owns" human tissue specimens? This question has been at the heart of several closely watched court cases. In this review, the authors explore the governing treaties, laws, and regulations that guide human studies, the necessary components of informed consent, legal cases that have examined the issue of ownership of human specimens, and the unique situation of specimens obtained postmortem. They also provide a brief look into the future of research that uses human tissue.

M. G. Bissell, MD, PhD, MPH

Intellectual Property: Turning Patent Swords into Shares
Van Overwalle G (Univ of Leuven, Belgium)
Science 330:1630-1631, 2010

Background.—Myriad Genetics was denied patent protection for genetic tests for familial breast and ovarian cancer in 2011. Product claims, describing the specific compound, were directed to isolated DNA containing human *BRCA1* and *BRCA2* gene sequences, and method claims, describing activity exercised on the compound, covered specific mutation identification. The US District Court held that both the claimed isolated DNA and the method were unpatentable. The decision has been appealed, but public policy issues associated with diagnostic gene patenting remain. The development of and access to genetic tests is a concern of the Secretary's Advisory Committee on Genetics, Health, and Society (SACGHS) of the US National Institutes of Health (NIH) and has prompted a call for focused legislative changes in this area.

Problems.—Two distinct issues arise in human genomic science and intellectual property. First, claims on genes are usually hard to circumvent, with problems stemming from licenses that are too restrictive, limiting research and development, clinical access, and the availability of high-quality tests for use with patients. The Myriad case is an example of this restrictive license policy. Second, problems arise when "patent thickets," which are webs of overlapping patents, emerge. The "stacking" of royalties to be paid in a patent thicket hinders research and development and endangers eventual clinical and patient access. Patent thickets have not yet arisen in genetics, but could emerge with changes from monogenetic to multifactorial testing and movement toward diagnostics based on genome-wide association studies driven by the high throughput of single nucleotide polymorphism platforms and next-generation sequencing efforts.

Proposed Solutions.—Patent systems are based on an implicit social contract designed to balance private and public interests. Changes to the system should acknowledge this and explore options to preserve the positive incentives while managing hindrances. Legislative measures or court decisions can be used to change policy, and the rules of contract may offer solutions. Current patent and antitrust laws allow patentees to set up licensing agreements and permit exclusive licensing. Legislation to impose compulsory licenses would force patent holders to grant use for public health purposes, an approach used in some European countries. This can avoid unduly restrictive licensing behavior by patent owners. A diagnostic-use exception would shield diagnostic testing from infringement and could apply equally to commercial and noncommercial service providers using laboratory-developed tests and to test-kit manufacturers. In addition, agencies such as the NIH could be encouraged to exercise "march-in" rights, which ignore the patent to grant licenses to others. Patent law could be altered to focus on the scope of patient rights and introduce a purpose-bound protection regimen for gene patents. The patent would be limited to the specific use described in the application and not include all possible future uses. A diagnostic method exclusion could allow patent issuance but exempt certain uses from infringement. Broadly excluding all diagnostic methods, involving the human body or not, may have more impact on patent practices.

Judicial approaches to genetic patent issues include shaping patent law to conform to the peculiarities of genetic diagnostics. Specially tailored genetic patent pools and clearinghouses could collect license fees and distribute them among those whose products are used. The sharing effect of collaborative models may safeguard the social contract and restore trust in the patent system as applied to genetic diagnostics.

Conclusions.—Gene patents and other problem areas challenge the patent system, suggesting it may be time to reconceptualize patent rights. Patents need to be viewed as a temporary permit or duty-bearing privilege that allows one to exploit monopoly rights under fair and reasonable conditions, giving technology owners the authority to invent and share.

▶ Among the United States' Founding Fathers, Benjamin Franklin and Thomas Jefferson were both distinguished inventors. Jefferson, in particular, gave serious thought to how the new Constitution should promote science and invention. He wanted a bill of rights included in the Constitution to guarantee free speech, freedom of religion, and protection against monopolies—with patents seen as temporary monopolies. In contrast, his colleague, James Madison, believed that patents represent a necessary societal trade-off of sacrifice in exchange for their benefit in stimulating practical arts, and wrote to Jefferson: "With regard to monopolies they are justly classified among the great nuisances in government. But it is clear that as encouragements to literary works and ingenious discoveries, they are too valuable to be wholly renounced." The era of the gene patent and its effects on the availability of laboratory testing has been with us long enough now to have revived the debate for a modern audience.

M. G. Bissell, MD, PhD, MPH

Determining the Optimal Approach for Government-Regulated Genetic Testing

Baudhuin LM (Mayo Clinic, Rochester, MN)
Clin Chem 57:7-8, 2011

Background.—The scope and volume of genetic tests offered, most of which are laboratory-developed tests (LDTs), have grown significantly in the past 10 years. In addition, recent tests are more complex, cover a greater scope, and focus on predicting disease rather than single-gene disorders. Spurring this growth is the arrival of direct-to-consumer (DTC) tests, which have not been under Food and Drug Administration (FDA) review. DTC genetic tests are offered over the Internet and performed in manufacturers' accredited laboratories as LDTs. The FDA has sent letters to manufacturers declaring many of these kits as medical devices and asking that the companies explain why they should not require premarket review. In addition, the FDA intends to invoke its right to oversee LDTs, although it has not specified how or when. The US Congress also held a public hearing in 2010 to focus on the Government Accountability Office (GAO) report covering DTC genetic tests' scientific validity, safety, and usefulness. Some DTC genetic-testing companies have criticized the FDA and GAO tactics, but express willingness to work with the government through the regulatory process. All are uncertain about when and how FDA regulation changes will occur.

Proposals.—In two opinion pieces published in *Nature*, authors Beaudet and Javitt agreed that some level of FDA regulation of genetic tests is needed, but disagreed about where and how this should be administered. Beaudet believes the complex nature of genetic testing in terms of evolving technology and biology requires a highly detailed approach to regulation that would require major investments of government time and money. This could impede the state of genetic testing and adversely affect patient care. He proposed that government regulation focus more on the integrity of the analytical process and data storage rather than results interpretation. DTC genetic-test results are not mediated by a healthcare practitioner and must be scrutinized further for clinical usefulness and implications, so results interpretation is not be particularly applicable.

Javitt believes that distinguishing between DTC genetic tests and those offered through healthcare professionals will be complicated and misleading. A federal shutdown of DTC testing would be difficult to justify. In her model, Javitt suggests that each test, regardless of who offers it, be regulated according to its level of risk. She sees oversight of newer, more complex tests as justified. However, the first step to take is to enforce laws that already exist concerning false advertising.

Validation Concerns.—Whether it is appropriate for genetic tests to meet certain requirements for clinical sensitivity, specificity, and utility as proposed by the Secretary's Advisory Commitment on Genetics, Health, and Society (SACGHS) is a question. Resources would likely be wasted if all laboratories must submit clinical validation data for all tests. Proper validation is suggested for tests that use novel methods or those whose results modify clinical and therapeutic approaches. Because the knowledge regarding the clinical importance of markers is growing quickly, challenges await in determining which tests and/or markers need additional scrutiny and at what level.

Conclusions.—Governmental regulation is needed for genetic-testing kits, but regulating every aspect for all genetic tests will likely prove wasteful. A reasonable approach is needed to ensure standards are met, but governmental and manufacturing parties should work together to identify what that reasonable approach will look like.

▶ The prospect of new expanded federal regulation and oversight of so-called laboratory-developed tests (LDTs) has far-reaching implications for all clinical laboratories, particularly those using mass-spectrometry-based methods. Exactly which assays end up being included in this category will affect daily lab operations, so an understanding of the background for the concerns of the US Food and Drug Administration (FDA) and the US Government Accountability Office concerns will be useful for laboratorians facing this regulatory change. In the past 10 years, the scope and volume of genetic tests (most of which fall into the LDT category) being offered has increased dramatically. Traditionally, genetic tests have been for single-gene disorders, such as cystic fibrosis and Marfan syndrome. In recent years, the scope and complexity of genetic testing has increased, and there has been a shift in emphasis toward predicting disease, especially complex disease. This shift has been mainly due to the arrival of direct-to-consumer (DTC) testing to the genetic testing market. DTC genetic tests, which have not been under the review of the FDA, are traditionally offered via the Internet and are performed in the manufacturers' accredited laboratories as LDTs. This review article outlines this important recent history.

M. G. Bissell, MD, PhD, MPH

Meeting Regulatory Requirements by the Use of Cell Phone Text Message Notification With Autoescalation and Loop Closure for Reporting of Critical Laboratory Results

Saw S, Loh TP, Ang SBL, et al (Natl Univ Hosp, Singapore)
Am J Clin Pathol 136:30-34, 2011

Critical laboratory results require timely and accurate transmission to the appropriate caregiver to provide intervention to prevent an adverse outcome. We report the use of text messages to notify critical laboratory results in a large teaching hospital to manage the documentation and audit requirements of critical result reporting by regulatory agencies. The text messaging system (critical reportable result health care messaging system [CRR-HMS]) allows a receiver to acknowledge or reject a critical result by short message service reply. Failure to obtain a confirmatory receipt within 10 minutes produces an automated escalation to an alternative physician according to a roster. The median time required for physician

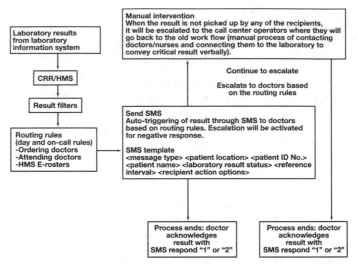

FIGURE 1.—The workflow of the CRR-HMS system. CRR, critical reportable result; HMS, health care messaging system; SMS, short message service. (Reprinted from Saw S, Loh TP, Ang SBL, et al. Meeting regulatory requirements by the use of cell phone text message notification with autoescalation and loop closure for reporting of critical laboratory results. *Am J Clin Pathol.* 2011;136:30-34, with permission from American Society for Clinical Pathology.)

response decreased from 7.3 minutes to 2 minutes after implementation of the CRR-HMS. The CRR-HMS is a clinically useful tool to rapidly communicate critical results to targeted physicians to facilitate rapid and timely intervention. This feature seems to be an important laboratory process mediator, and recent Joint Commission reviews have placed this as a requirement (Fig 1).

▶ The postanalytic phase is a vulnerable stage of laboratory testing in which between 10% and 55% of total laboratory error occurs. Failure to communicate the right laboratory result to the right person at the right time in the right context is one of the errors. A critical laboratory result is defined as a value that represents a pathophysiologic state at such variance with normal that prompt medical intervention is required to avert imminent danger for the patient concerned and for which effective action is possible. An unusually high number of critical results has been shown to be an early predictor of adverse patient events. Currently, many regulatory bodies, including the Clinical Laboratory Improvement Amendments of 1988, the Joint Commission, and the College of American Pathologists, require clinical laboratories to have in place a mechanism of disseminating critical laboratory results expediently. Information technology has been extensively explored and exploited to improve various safety aspects of clinical laboratory operations. Several studies have demonstrated the usefulness of various electronic means to improve the delivery of critical results to care providers, with a recently reported pager alert system achieving an impressive 89% first-pass communication of critical results to the appropriate care provider. The electronic modalities used in the previous studies included alphanumeric pager, electronic medical records, computer display screens, and short message service (SMS). Advantages of electronic communication include timeliness, automation, reduced waiting time for result transmission, and a captured audit trail of events. However, most clinical laboratories are likely to communicate critical results through the telephone, for which the simple practice of read-back has been suggested as a means to improve communication safety. The cellular (mobile) telephone is a communication tool prevalent in modem society. SMS is an attractive candidate for reporting of critical laboratory results for the following reasons: (1) It is a familiar software application. (2) Communication is almost instantaneous. (3) It allows an expanded word limit. (4) It provides direct 2-way communication. (5) There is an electronically captured audit trail. (6) Its hardware device, the cell phone, is in common use among health care workers, negating the cost and inconvenience of an additional portable device. This was the premise for the development and implementation of a novel, fully automated SMS (critical reportable result), which incorporates multiple reply options and autoescalation features to deliver critical laboratory results at the National University Hospital Singapore. This study reports and discusses the critical values in this hospital and the performance of the automated reporting system (Fig 1).

M. G. Bissell, MD, PhD, MPH

Maternal Serum Screening: Results Disclosure, Anxiety, and Risk Perception
Czerwinski JL, Wicklund CA, Hoskovec JM, et al (Univ of Texas Health Science Ctr at Houston; Northwestern Univ, Chicago, IL; et al)
Am J Perinatol 27:279-284, 2010

Although increased maternal anxiety following the disclosure of positive second-trimester maternal serum screen (MSS) results has been well documented, how this anxiety correlates with the method of results disclosure has not been well defined. This pilot study aimed to determine how abnormal second-trimester MSS results are disclosed, the level of anxiety experienced by women as a result of this disclosure, and the accuracy of their risk perception. Women referred for prenatal genetic counseling were asked to complete a questionnaire including demographics, standardized Spielberger State-Trait Anxiety Inventory, results disclosure information, and perceived risk. Of the 561 questionnaires distributed, 388 (69.2%) women chose to participate. Of the 136 participants referred for an abnormal MSS, 125 (91.9%) were aware of this indication and elected to complete the results disclosure portion of the questionnaire. The average anxiety level was not significantly different based on the method of results disclosure or who reported the results. We did not identify a definite cause for the anxiety experienced by women receiving abnormal MSS results; however, this study illustrates the need for further research to identify factors that contribute to the elevated anxiety experienced by these women.

▶ Women with abnormal second-trimester serum screen results are at risk for increased levels of anxiety. Additionally, these individuals may experience associated adverse outcomes, such as postpartum blues and depression. Although several studies have reported increased anxiety in women with abnormal serum screen results, no studies have determined whether the method of results disclosure correlates with anxiety levels or risk perception. Women younger than 35 years give birth to most (75%-80%) infants with Down syndrome. Less than 20% of the fetuses with Down syndrome are identified prenatally through maternal-age-indicated, second-trimester prenatal diagnosis. For this reason, identification and screening of younger women at an increased risk of having a child with a karyotypic abnormality, such as Down syndrome, is beneficial. Second-trimester maternal serum screening (MSS) is offered between 15 and 20 weeks of gestation to identify women at an increased risk of having a child with Down syndrome, trisomy 18, or an open neural tube defect from an otherwise low-risk patient population. Women who screen positive for either an open neural tube defect or a chromosomal abnormality are often referred to a genetic counselor and are given the option of additional diagnostic testing, such as genetic amniocentesis or targeted ultrasound. It has been reported that women experience an increased level of anxiety after receiving a positive MSS result. Anxiety during pregnancy has been shown to have untoward effects on the parent-infant relationship and maternal well-being and is a risk factor for postpartum depression. Anxiety resulting from an abnormal serum screen result often causes women to decline serum screening in subsequent pregnancies. The aim of this pilot study was to determine how serum screen results are typically disclosed in the population, the anxiety level of women referred for an abnormal serum screen based on how their results were disclosed, and the accuracy of the patient's perception of her risk. The results will help determine if anxiety is affected by the method of results disclosure and, if so, which method provokes the least anxiety.

M. G. Bissell, MD, PhD, MPH

18 Clinical Chemistry

Serum Bilirubin and Risk of Respiratory Disease and Death
Horsfall LJ, Rait G, Walters K, et al (Univ College London, England, UK)
JAMA 305:691-697, 2011

Context.—Serum total bilirubin levels in healthy patients reflect genetic and environmental factors that could influence the risk of developing respiratory disease.

Objective.—To examine the relationship between bilirubin levels and respiratory disease.

Design, Setting, and Participants.—Cohort study among 504 206 adults from a UK primary care research database (the Health Improvement Network) with serum bilirubin levels recorded but no evidence of hepatobiliary or hemolytic disease. Data were recorded between January 1988 and December 2008.

Main Outcome Measures.—Incidence of chronic obstructive pulmonary disease (COPD), lung cancer, and all-cause mortality.

Results.—Median bilirubin levels were 0.64 mg/dL (interquartile range, 0.47-0.88 mg/dL) in men and 0.53 mg/dL (interquartile range, 0.41-0.70 mg/dL) in women. There were 1341 cases of lung cancer, 5863 cases of COPD, and 23 103 deaths, with incidence rates of 2.5, 11.9, and 42.5 per 10 000 person-years, respectively. The incidence of lung cancer per 10 000 person-years in men was 5.0 (95% confidence interval [CI], 4.2-6.0) in the first decile category of bilirubin compared with 3.0 (95% CI, 2.3-3.8) in the fifth decile. The corresponding incidences for COPD in men were 19.5 (95% CI, 17.7-21.4) and 14.4 (95% CI, 12.7-16.2). The mortality rates per 10 000 person-years in men were 51.3 (95% CI, 48.5-54.2) in the first decile category compared with 38.1 (95% CI, 35.5-40.8) in the fifth decile. The associations were similar for women. After adjusting for other important health indicators, regression estimates for incidence rate of lung cancer per 0.1-mg/dL increase in bilirubin level were an 8% decrease (95% CI, 5%-11%) for men and an 11% decrease (95% CI, 7%-14%) for women. The regression estimate for COPD in men per 0.1-mg/dL increase in bilirubin level was a 6% decrease (95% CI, 5%-7%) and for mortality in men was a 3% decrease (95% CI, 2%-3%) after accounting for other health indicators. The results for COPD and mortality in women were very similar.

Conclusion.—Among patients with normal-range bilirubin levels in primary care practices, relatively higher levels of bilirubin were associated with a lower risk of respiratory disease and all-cause mortality.

▶ It is always interesting when a new association is discovered for an old familiar analyte. Serum total bilirubin is routinely measured in the primary care setting to identify hepatobiliary and hemolytic diseases. After excluding disease, moderately increased levels (> 1 mg/dL) generally indicate benign hereditary hyperbilirubinemia (Gilbert syndrome). This common condition is caused by a deficiency in the liver enzyme uridine diphosphate-glucuronosyltransferase 1 (UGT1A1), which converts insoluble bilirubin to a form suitable for renal and biliary excretion. Although bilirubin levels are highly heritable and genetic variation of UGT1A1 explains a large proportion of the variability, enzymes involved with bilirubin production from heme, including heme oxygenase, may also exert an influence. Elevated heme oxygenase activity, caused by genetic variation or environmental factors, appears beneficial for respiratory health. Part of this effect is purportedly because of the powerful cytoprotective properties of bilirubin, including antioxidant, anti-inflammatory, and antiproliferative effects. Experimental studies using animal models support a protective effect of increased bilirubin against respiratory injury by environmental stressors. The epidemiological relationship between bilirubin level and the risk of respiratory disease is not well characterized. The authors therefore examined the association between serum bilirubin levels and the incidence of chronic obstructive pulmonary disease (COPD), lung cancer, and all-cause mortality in a large population-based cohort of primary care patients from the United Kingdom.

M. G. Bissell, MD, PhD, MPH

Low-Dose Aspirin Use and Performance of Immunochemical Fecal Occult Blood Tests
Brenner H, Tao S, Haug U (German Cancer Res Ctr, Heidelberg, Germany)
JAMA 304:2513-2520, 2010

Context.—Immunochemical fecal occult blood tests (iFOBTs) are potentially promising tools for colorectal cancer screening. Low-dose aspirin use, which increases the likelihood of gastrointestinal bleeding, is common in the target population for colorectal cancer screening.

Objective.—To assess the association of low-dose aspirin use with the performance of 2 quantitative iFOBTs in a large sample of patients undergoing colorectal cancer screening.

Design, Setting, and Participants.—Diagnostic study conducted from 2005 through 2009 at internal medicine and gastroenterology practices in southern Germany including 1979 patients (mean age, 62.1 years): 233 regular users of low-dose aspirin (167 men, 67 women) and 1746 who never used low-dose aspirin (809 men, 937 women).

Main Outcome Measures.—Sensitivity, specificity, positive and negative predictive values, and area under receiver operating characteristic (ROC) curves in detecting advanced colorectal neoplasms (colorectal cancer or advanced adenoma) with 2 quantitative iFOBTs.

Results.—Advanced neoplasms were found in 24 users (10.3%) and 181 nonusers (10.4%) of low-dose aspirin. At the cut point recommended by the manufacturer, sensitivities of the 2 tests were 70.8% (95% confidence interval [CI], 48.9%-87.4%) for users compared with 35.9% (95% CI, 28.9%-43.4%) for nonusers and 58.3% (95% CI, 36.6%-77.9%) for users compared with 32.0% (95% CI, 25.3%-39.4%) for nonusers ($P = .001$ and $P = .01$, respectively). Specificities were 85.7% (95% CI, 80.2%-90.1%) for users compared with 89.2% (95% CI, 87.6%-90.7%) for nonusers and 85.7% (95% CI, 80.2%-90.1%) for users compared with 91.1% (95% CI, 89.5%-92.4%) for nonusers ($P = .13$ and $P = .01$, respectively). The areas under the ROC curve were 0.79 (95% CI, 0.68-0.90) for users compared with 0.67 (95% CI, 0.62-0.71) for nonusers and 0.73 (95% CI, 0.62-0.85) for users compared with 0.65 (95% CI, 0.61-0.69) for nonusers ($P = .05$ and $P = .17$, respectively). Among men, who composed the majority of low-dose aspirin users, the areas under the ROC curve were 0.87 (95% CI, 0.76-0.98) for users compared with 0.68 (95% CI, 0.63-0.74) for nonusers and 0.81 (95% CI, 0.68-0.93) for users compared with 0.67 (95% CI, 0.61-0.72) for nonusers ($P = .003$ and $P = .04$, respectively).

Conclusion.—For 2 iFOBTs, use of low-dose aspirin compared with no aspirin was associated with a markedly higher sensitivity for detecting advanced colorectal neoplasms, with only a slightly lower specificity.

▶ Screening for colorectal cancer (CRC) and its precursors by fecal occult blood tests (FOBTs), which have been shown to reduce CRC incidence and mortality in randomized trials, is widely recommended and applied in an increasing number of countries. Screening is mostly done in age groups in which use of low-dose aspirin for primary or secondary prevention of cardiovascular disease is increasingly common. Use of low-dose aspirin increases the likelihood of gastrointestinal bleeding, especially upper gastrointestinal bleeding. Because of the increased risk of bleeding from sources other than colorectal neoplasms, concerns have been raised regarding possible adverse effects on specificity of FOBT-based screening for CRC. There also have been suggestions that use of low-dose aspirin should be stopped prior to conducting FOBTs, even though results have not been consistent. Furthermore, use of low-dose aspirin might also have beneficial effects on sensitivity by increasing the likelihood of bleeding from colorectal neoplasms. The authors conducted the study because empirical evidence is sparse about the performance of FOBTs for patients who use low-dose aspirin (Fig 3 in the original article).

M. G. Bissell, MD, PhD, MPH

Effect of Screening on Ovarian Cancer Mortality: The Prostate, Lung, Colorectal and Ovarian (PLCO) Cancer Screening Randomized Controlled Trial

Buys SS, for the PLCO Project Team (Univ of Utah Health Sciences Ctr, Salt Lake City; et al)
JAMA 305:2295-2303, 2011

Context.—Screening for ovarian cancer with cancer antigen 125 (CA-125) and transvaginal ultrasound has an unknown effect on mortality.

Objective.—To evaluate the effect of screening for ovarian cancer on mortality in the Prostate, Lung, Colorectal and Ovarian (PLCO) Cancer Screening Trial.

Design, Setting, and Participants.—Randomized controlled trial of 78 216 women aged 55 to 74 years assigned to undergo either annual screening (n = 39 105) or usual care (n = 39 111) at 10 screening centers across the United States between November 1993 and July 2001.

Intervention.—The intervention group was offered annual screening with CA-125 for 6 years and transvaginal ultrasound for 4 years. Participants and their health care practitioners received the screening test results and managed evaluation of abnormal results. The usual care group was not offered annual screening with CA-125 for 6 years or transvaginal ultrasound but received their usual medical care. Participants were followed up for a maximum of 13 years (median [range], 12.4 years [10.9-13.0 years]) for cancer diagnoses and death until February 28, 2010.

Main Outcome Measures.—Mortality from ovarian cancer, including primary peritoneal and fallopian tube cancers. Secondary outcomes included ovarian cancer incidence and complications associated with screening examinations and diagnostic procedures.

Results.—Ovarian cancer was diagnosed in 212 women (5.7 per 10 000 person-years) in the intervention group and 176 (4.7 per 10 000 person-years) in the usual care group (rate ratio [RR], 1.21; 95% confidence interval [CI], 0.99-1.48). There were 118 deaths caused by ovarian cancer (3.1 per 10 000 person-years) in the intervention group and 100 deaths (2.6 per 10 000 person-years) in the usual care group (mortality RR, 1.18; 95% CI, 0.82-1.71). Of 3285 women with false-positive results, 1080 underwent surgical follow-up; of whom, 163 women experienced at least 1 serious complication (15%). There were 2924 deaths due to other causes (excluding ovarian, colorectal, and lung cancer) (76.6 per 10 000 person-years) in the intervention group and 2914 deaths (76.2 per 10 000 person-years) in the usual care group (RR, 1.01; 95% CI, 0.96-1.06).

Conclusions.—Among women in the general US population, simultaneous screening with CA-125 and transvaginal ultrasound compared with usual care did not reduce ovarian cancer mortality. Diagnostic evaluation following a false-positive screening test result was associated with complications.

Trial Registration.—clinicaltrials.gov Identifier: NCT00002540.

▶ With in vitro diagnostic tests for cancer screening, we always must ask: How well does it actually perform in terms of outcomes? In the United States, ovarian cancer is among the 5 leading causes of cancer death in women. The high case-fatality ratio of ovarian cancer may be attributed in part to its vague and nonspecific symptoms, which usually appear when the disease has reached an advanced stage. Ovarian cancer confined to the ovary has a 5-year survival of 92%; however, most women with ovarian cancer are diagnosed with advanced-stage disease, which has a 5-year survival of only 30%. The recognition that early detection of ovarian cancer may have the potential to improve prognosis prompted the development of randomized controlled trials, including the Prostate, Lung, Colorectal and Ovarian (PLCO) Cancer Screening Trial, to evaluate the efficacy of transvaginal ultrasound and serum cancer antigen 125 (CA-125) as screening tools to reduce ovarian cancer mortality. The PLCO trial's independent data and safety monitoring board, which periodically reviews the cumulative trial data, recently concluded that the predetermined end point had been reached for the ovarian cancer component of the trial and recommended that the ovarian cancer—specific mortality results be reported (Fig 2 in the original article).

M. G. Bissell, MD, PhD, MPH

A New Study of Intraosseous Blood for Laboratory Analysis

Miller LJ, Philbeck TE, Montez D, et al (Vidacare Corporation, TX; AmeriPath, Inc, San Antonio, TX)
Arch Pathol Lab Med 134:1253-1260, 2010

Context.—Intraosseous (IO) blood is frequently used to establish a blood chemistry profile in critically ill patients. Questions remain regarding the reliability of IO blood for laboratory analysis and established criteria regarding the amount of marrow/blood to waste before taking an IO sample are not available.

Objectives.—To evaluate IO-derived blood for routine laboratory blood tests needed in the care of critically ill patients and to determine the amount of marrow/blood to waste before drawing blood from the IO space for laboratory analysis.

Design.—Blood samples were drawn from peripheral veins of 10 volunteers. Within 5 minutes, 2 IO blood samples were obtained; one following 2 mL of waste and another following 6 mL of waste. Samples were analyzed for complete blood count and chemistry profile. Values were analyzed using Pearson correlation coefficients. Levels of significance were determined using the *t* distribution. Mean values for the draws were calculated and compared, with the intravenous blood sample serving as a control for the IO samples.

Results.—There was a significant correlation between intravenous and IO samples for red blood cell counts and hemoglobin and hematocrit levels but not for white blood cell counts and platelet counts. There was a significant correlation between intravenous and IO samples for glucose, blood urea nitrogen, creatinine, chloride, total protein, and albumin concentrations but not for sodium, potassium, CO_2, and calcium levels.

Conclusions.—When venous blood cannot be accessed, IO blood aspirate may serve as a reliable alternate, especially for hemoglobin and hematocrit levels and most analytes in a basic blood chemistry profile. Exceptions are CO_2 levels and platelet counts, which may be lower, and white blood cell counts, which may appear elevated.

▶ It is always of value to those of us in laboratory medicine to have updated valid information on reference ranges and preanalytical specimen requirements. This is especially true for the less frequently encountered specimen types. In this article, the authors bring us up to date on an old category of specimen that has gone out of vogue only to return once again in the modern acute/emergency care setting. This specimen type is interosseous (IO) blood, which is obtained when needles are inserted into bone marrow spaces for purposes of circulatory access in situations in which vascular access is severely limited or compromised for any number of reasons, including shock and vascular scarring with intravenous drug abuse. The IO route, popular during the 1940s, was supplanted in the postwar years by the use of disposable plastic catheters for central and peripheral venous lines. Recent studies showing the effectiveness of new devices for drug administration by the IO route to be equivalent to that via central venous catheters has led to increasing usage and, with it, increasing interest in using IO blood for clinical laboratory testing.

M. G. Bissell, MD, PhD, MPH

Inverse Log-Linear Relationship between Thyroid-Stimulating Hormone and Free Thyroxine Measured by Direct Analog Immunoassay and Tandem Mass Spectrometry
van Deventer HE, Mendu DR, Remaley AT, et al (Natl Insts of Health, Bethesda, MD; Georgetown Univ Med Ctr, Washington, DC)
Clin Chem 57:122-127, 2011

Background.—Accurate measurement of free thyroxine (FT_4) is important for diagnosing and managing thyroid disorders. Most laboratories measure FT_4 by direct analogue immunoassay methods. The validity of these methods have recently been questioned. The inverse log-linear relationship between FT_4 and thyroidstimulating hormone (TSH) is well described and provides a physiological rationale on which to base an evaluation of FT_4 assays.

Methods.—The study included 109 participants for whom FT_4 measurement was requested by their clinician. Samples were selected for inclusion to reflect a wide spectrum of TSH and albumin results. FT_4 and TSH were measured by use of the Siemens Immulite immunoassay (IA). FT_4 was also measured by liquid chromatography—tandem mass spectrometry (LC-MS/MS) (MS-FT_4).

Results.—The inverse log-linear correlation coefficient between TSH and FT$_4$ was significantly better ($P < 0.0001$) for MS-FT$_4$ (0.84, 95% CI, 0.77–0.88) than for IA-FT4 (0.45, 95% CI, 0.29–0.59). IA-FT$_4$ showed a significant correlation with albumin (Spearman correlation coefficient 0.45, 95% CI, 0.29–0.5, $P < 0.0001$) and thyroxine-binding globulin (TBG) (Spearman correlation coefficient 0.23, 95% CI, 0.05–0.41, $P < 0.02$). In contrast, FT$_4$ measurement by LC-MS/MS did not show a significant correlation with albumin or TBG.

Conclusions.—The inverse log-linear relationship between FT$_4$ and TSH was significantly better for FT$_4$ measured by LC-MS/MS than by IA. The MS-FT$_4$ method therefore provides FT$_4$ results that agree clinically with those obtained for TSH. Additionally, the significant correlation between IA-FT$_4$ with albumin and TBG suggests that this FT$_4$ method depends on binding protein concentrations and consequently does not accurately reflect FT$_4$.

▶ As witnessed by all the generations of thyroid stimulating hormone we've seen in laboratory medicine over the years, accurate measurement of both analyte and thyroxine (T4) are critical for the screening and management of thyroid disorders. In serum, the majority of thyroxine circulates bound to high-concentration, low-affinity proteins, mostly albumin and transthyretin, and to a low-concentration, high-affinity binding protein, namely thyroxine-binding globulin. Only a small percentage of total T4 circulates free. It is the free T4 (FT4) that is generally considered to be the biologically active hormone and, therefore, to be of most interest to monitor in patients with thyroid disorders. Here the authors offer us a comparison of immunoassay and mass spectrometry measurements for FT4 and derive a mathematical relationship between them.

M. G. Bissell, MD, PhD, MPH

Comparison of Urinary Albumin and Urinary Total Protein as Predictors of Patient Outcomes in CKD

Methven S, MacGregor MS, Traynor JP, et al (Crosshouse Hosp, Kilmarnock, UK; Monklands Hosp, Airdrie, UK; et al)
Am J Kidney Dis 57:21-28, 2011

Background.—Proteinuria is common and is associated with adverse patient outcomes. The optimal test of proteinuria to identify those at risk is uncertain. This study assessed albuminuria and total proteinuria as predictors of 3 patient outcomes: all-cause mortality, start of renal replacement therapy (RRT), and doubling of serum creatinine level.

Study Design.—Retrospective longitudinal cohort study.

Setting & Participants.—Nephrology clinic of a city hospital in Scotland; 5,586 patients with chronic kidney disease (CKD) and proteinuria measured in random urine samples (n = 3,378) or timed urine collections (n = 1,808).

Predictors.—Baseline measurements of albumin-creatinine ratio (ACR), total protein—creatinine ratio (PCR), 24-hour albuminuria, and total proteinuria.

Outcomes.—All-cause mortality, start of RRT, and doubling of serum creatinine level were assessed using receiver operating characteristic curves and Cox proportional hazards models.

Measurements.—Blood pressure, serum creatinine level, ACR, PCR, date of death, date of starting RRT.

Results.—Patients were followed up for a median of 3.5 (25th-75th percentile, 2.1-6.0) years. For all outcomes, adjusted HRs were similar for PCR and ACR (derived from random urine samples and timed collections): death, 1.41 (95% CI, 1.31-1.53) vs 1.38 (95% CI, 1.28-1.50); RRT, 1.96 (95% CI, 1.76-2.18) vs 2.33 (95% CI, 2.06-3.01); and doubling of serum creatinine level, 2.03 (95% CI, 1.87-2.19) vs 1.92 (95% CI, 1.78-2.08). Receiver operating characteristic curves showed almost identical performance for ACR and PCR for the 3 outcome measures. Adjusted HRs for ACR and PCR were similar when derived from random urine samples or timed collections and compared with 24-hour total protein and albumin excretion for each outcome measure.

Limitations.—This is a retrospective study.

Conclusions.—Total proteinuria and albuminuria perform equally as predictors of renal outcomes and mortality in patients with CKD. ACR and PCR were as effective as 24-hour urine samples at predicting outcomes and are more convenient for patients, clinicians, and laboratories. Both ACR and PCR stratify risk in patients with CKD.

▶ Proteinuria is always a significant clinical finding, and is both common and highly predictive of subsequent progression to frank renal disease in otherwise asymptomatic individuals; however, an outstanding question in its laboratory assessment has been which measure of proteinuria (albuminuria vs total proteinuria) is the more effective predictor of risk in this context? Specifically, albuminuria is known to best predict progressive renal disease and cardiac disease in diabetic patients, and to predict progression to end-stage renal disease in patients with lowered estimated glomerular filtration rates, but it is not known whether or not the same is true for patients who are not diabetic. Urine composition being so highly variable, typically, the measured urine protein concentration is normalized to creatinine to give the albumin-to-creatinine or total protein-to-creatinine ratio. The authors undertook to critically assess the use of these 2 measurements as predictors of mortality and morbidity in patients with chronic kidney disease.

M. G. Bissell, MD, PhD, MPH

A Combination of Serum Markers for the Early Detection of Colorectal Cancer

Wild N, Andres H, Rollinger W, et al (Roche Diagnostics GmbH, Penzberg, Germany)
Clin Cancer Res 16:6111-6121, 2010

Purpose.—Fecal occult blood testing is recommended as first-line screening to detect colorectal cancer (CRC). We evaluated markers and marker combinations in serum as an alternative to improve the detection of CRC.

Experimental Design.—Using penalized logistic regression, 6 markers were selected for evaluation in 1,027 samples (301 CRC patients, 143 patients with adenoma, 266 controls, 141 disease controls, and 176 patients with other cancer). The diagnostic performance of each marker and of marker combinations was assessed.

Results.—To detect CRC from serum samples, we tested 22 biomarkers. Six markers were selected for a marker combination, including the known tumor markers CEA (carcinoembryonic antigen) and CYFRA 21-1 as well as novel markers or markers that are less routinely used for the detection of CRC: ferritin, osteopontin (OPN), anti-p53, and seprase. CEA showed the best sensitivity at 95% specificity with 43.9%, followed by seprase (42.4%), CYFRA 21-1 (35.5%), OPN (30.2%), ferritin (23.9%), and anti-p53 (20.0%). A combination of these markers gave 69.6% sensitivity at 95% specificity and 58.7% at 98% specificity. Focusing on International Union against Cancer (UICC) stages 0—III reduced the sensitivity slightly to 68.0% and 53.3%, respectively. In a subcollective, with matched stool samples (75 CRC cases and 234 controls), the sensitivity of the marker combination was comparable with fecal immunochemical testing (FIT) with 82.4% and 68.9% versus 81.8% and 72.7% at 95% and 98% specificity, respectively.

Conclusions.—The performance of the serum marker combination is comparable with FIT. This provides a novel tool for CRC screening to trigger a follow-up colonoscopy for a final diagnosis.

▶ Colorectal cancer (CRC) screening is essential to efforts at prevention and mitigation of this devastating disease. The mainstays of CRC screening remain stool-based assays and imaging studies, ie, colonoscopy. It has always been universally recognized that a serum-based screening test would achieve wider compliance and hence more effective results, but the achievement of this has been an elusive goal. Carcinoembryonic antigen (CEA), thought at the time to be a tumor-specific antigen, was initially introduced as a universal screening test, only to be (very famously) rejected for this purpose when flaws in the design of early studies were revealed, namely that predictive values determined in high-prevalence situations do not generalize to population-based screening owing to the mathematical dependence of predictive value on the prevalence of the screened-for condition. Over the years, other markers have been advanced for this application, but to date, none has unequivocally succeeded. The current study is a new approach using a combination of biomarkers that shows some promise.

M. G. Bissell, MD, PhD, MPH

Performance Characteristics of Six Intact Parathyroid Hormone Assays
La'ulu SL, Roberts WL (Univ of Utah Health Sciences Ctr, Salt Lake City)
Am J Clin Pathol 134:930-938, 2010

The aim of this study was to evaluate the performance characteristics of 6 intact parathyroid hormone assays: Access 2 (Beckman Coulter, Fullerton, CA), ARCHITECT i2000$_{SR}$ (Abbott Diagnostics, Abbott Park, IL), ADVIA Centaur (Siemens Healthcare Diagnostics, Deerfield, IL), Modular E170 (Roche Diagnostics, Indianapolis, IN), IMMULITE 2000 (Siemens Healthcare Diagnostics), and LIAISON (DiaSorin, Stillwater, MN). Sample collection tubes and storage conditions were compared. Imprecision studies were performed using commercial quality control materials. Linearity was assessed using pools prepared from samples. For method comparison, serum and EDTA plasma samples were tested by all methods, and the ARCHITECT was used as the comparison method. Reference intervals were determined using various vitamin D cutoffs. The types of collection tubes and storage conditions are more important for some methods than others. Total coefficients of variation were 10.9% or less. The maximum deviation from the target recovery for linearity ranged from 5.0% to 82.2%. Bland-Altman plots demonstrated percentage biases ranging from −36.3% to 24.4%. The lower limit of the reference interval was not influenced by vitamin D status, whereas the upper reference limit was affected.

▶ Parathyroid hormone (PTH) measurements are a critical element in the workup of bone and mineral disorders, hypercalcemia and hypocalcemia, in assessing parathyroid function in renal failure, and in intraoperatively monitoring thyroid surgery. Reliable and specific PTH assays have made these workups considerably easier, but lack of comparability between different makes of PTH assay remain. Also, interassay variability is potentially further enhanced and complicated by the population being tested, by vitamin D status, and by a variety of preanalytic variables. PTH is a peptide of 84 amino acids in length that has a relatively short active half-life and is subject to extensive metabolism. Intact PTH assays measure not only the intact molecule (PTH 1-84) but other fragments, including PTH 7-84, that accumulate with renal insufficiency. The current study examined performance characteristics of 6 commercial intact PTH assays and included consideration of a suitable variety of preanalytic, analytic, and demographic variables to attempt to identify sources for interassay variability.

M. G. Bissell, MD, PhD, MPH

Characterization of the New Serum Protein Reference Material ERM-DA470k/IFCC: Value Assignment by Immunoassay

Zegers I, Keller T, Schreiber W, et al (Inst for Reference Materials and Measurements (IRMM), Geel, Belgium; Acomed Statistik, Leipzig, Germany; now Siemens Healthcare Diagnostics Products GmbH, Marburg, Germany; et al)
Clin Chem 56:1880-1888, 2010

Background.—The availability of a suitable matrix reference material is essential for standardization of the immunoassays used to measure serum proteins. The earlier serum protein reference material ERM-DA470 (previously called CRM470), certified in 1993, has led to a high degree of harmonization of the measurement results. A new serum protein material has now been prepared and its suitability in term of homogeneity and stability has been verified; after characterization, the material has been certified as ERM-DA470k/IFCC.

Methods.—We characterized the candidate reference material for 14 proteins by applying a protocol that is considered to be a reference measurement procedure, by use of optimized immunoassays. ERM-DA470 was used as a calibrant.

Results.—For 12 proteins [α_2 macroglobulin (A2M), α_1 acid glycoprotein (orosomucoid, AAG), α_1 antitrypsin (α_1-protease inhibitor, AAT), albumin (ALB), complement 3c (C3c), complement 4 (C4), haptoglobin (HPT), IgA, IgG, IgM, transferrin (TRF), and transthyretin (TTR)], the results allowed assignment of certified values in ERM-DA470k/IFCC. For CRP, we observed a bias between the lyophilized and liquid frozen materials, and for CER, the distribution of values was too broad. Therefore, these 2 proteins were not certified in the ERM-DA470k/IFCC. Different value transfer procedures were tested (open and closed procedures) and found to provide equivalent results.

Conclusions.—A new serum protein reference material has been produced, and values have been successfully assigned for 12 proteins.

▶ The availability of standardized reference material (SRM), such as that provided by the National Institute of Standards and Testing in the United States, is an essential component of any international effort at standardization/harmonization of clinical laboratory assays. Serum protein measurements are among the best standardized protein measurements; their quantification depends primarily on the comparison of the measurement results with those obtained with a calibrant. Here the authors used specially optimized immunoassays to characterize an SRM for serum proteins, developed by the International Federation of Clinical Chemistry (IFCC), known as ERMDA470k/IFCC, by use of protocols that can be considered as reference measurement procedures. They certified mass concentrations for the following 12 proteins: alpha-2- macroglobulin (A2M), alpha-I-acid glycoprotein (orosomucoid, AAG), alpha-I-antitrypsin (AAT), albumin (ALB), complement 3c (C3c), complement 4 (C4), haptoglobin (HPT), immunoglobulin (Ig)A, IgG, IgM, transferrin (TRF), and transthyretin (TTR). The assignment of certified values for ceruloplasmin and beta-2-microgobulin requires further investigation and is ongoing.

M. G. Bissell, MD, PhD, MPH

Initial observations regarding free cortisol quantification logistics among critically ill children
Zimmerman JJ, Barker RM, Jack R (Univ of Washington School of Medicine, Seattle)
Intensive Care Med 36:1914-1922, 2010

Purpose.—Corticosteroid insufficiency may occur among critically ill patients, but the diagnosis remains controversial. Historically assessment of free cortisol (FC) by means of equilibrium dialysis (ED) has required large blood volumes and prolonged fractionation time preceding analysis. We hypothesized that temperature-controlled centrifugal ultrafiltration with chemiluminescence immunoassay (CU/CI) would provide real-time FC data that highly correlated with ED/radioimmunoassay (ED/RI) or liquid chromatography/mass spectrometry (LC/MS) techniques.

Methods.—We quantified and correlated baseline and corticotropin-stimulated TC and FC by means of CU/CI, ED/RI, and LC/MS among healthy adults and 37 critically ill children.

Results.—Among critically ill children, FC was three- to fivefold higher than the healthy adults at baseline and increased another five- to eightfold following corticotropin administration. While TC increased approximately twofold following corticotropin administration, FC increased on average more than eightfold. Serum FC per CU/CI highly correlated with FC per ED/RI or LC/MS, but results were available in a fraction of the time. Children failing to increase TC by >9.0 µg/dL (248 nM) following corticotropin demonstrated an appropriate FC increase. Nearly 50% of critically ill children exhibited FC <2.0 µg/dL (55 nM). Neither FC nor TC concentrations correlated significantly with measures of illness severity.

Conclusions.—Quantification of FC utilizing CU/CI was fast (1—2 h) and results correlated highly with ED/RI or LC/MS methodologies. These data require validation with larger cohorts of healthy and critically ill children but indicate that real-time FC quantification is available to guide cortisol replacement therapy.

▶ The neuroendocrine response involving the adrenals represents a critical component in the overall response to stress and is a key mediator in the compensatory anti-inflammatory response. Assessing the adequacy of adrenal status and response in the context of critical illness—related stress, such as septic shock, is extremely important, yet, unfortunately, not well defined. Although total cortisol measurements have been used historically for this purpose, modern consensus favors free cortisol (FC) measurements instead, because it is this fraction, rather than the protein-bound one, that is responsible for the biochemical actions of relevance. Traditionally, a 2-step procedure is necessary for the "gold standard" measurement of FC, namely separation of the free and protein-bound fractions, classically by time-consuming equilibrium dialysis, followed by quantitation of cortisol, classically by radioimmunoassay or liquid chromatography/mass spectrometry. The current study attempts to investigate whether a combination of centrifugal ultrafiltration and a chemiluminescent immunoassay for FC measurements, a methodology requiring less time and specimen, could effectively substitute so as to have greater clinical impact with critically ill children.

M. G. Bissell, MD, PhD, MPH

An Observational Study of Early Neonatal Biochemical Parameters in Twins
Henderson P, Cordiner D, Stenson B (Royal Infirmary of Edinburgh, UK)
Am J Perinatol 28:111-116, 2011

Early neonatal biochemical values are generally considered to reflect maternal values. However, studies have been inconclusive due to the statistical methods used. We hypothesized that there would not be important differences in plasma biochemistry between newborn twins, suggesting a common mechanism of control, and that differences between unrelated infant pairs would be greater. All twins over a 5-year period who had plasma biochemistry measured within 6 hours of birth were identified retrospectively. An unrelated control infant was matched to one of each twin pair. The 95% limits of agreement for plasma urea, creatinine, and sodium were calculated for twin pairs and unrelated matched infant pairs. Fifty-three twin pairs were studied. For urea, creatinine, and sodium, 95% of differences between twins were less than or equal to 1.5 mmol/L (8.9 mg/dL), 9.2 μmol/L (0.1 mg/dL), and 5.1 mmol/L (11.7 mg/dL), respectively. In unrelated infant pairs, the corresponding values were 4.0 mmol/L (24.3 mg/dL), 33.9 μmol/L (0.4 mg/dL), and 8.2 mmol/L (18.9 mg/dL). Differences between unrelated infant pairs were significantly wider than differences between twins ($p < 0.001$). This study has demonstrated a close and significant agreement in urea, sodium, and creatinine when measured soon after birth in twin pairs compared with unrelated infants, implying a common mechanism of control (Fig 1).

▶ It is widely assumed that equilibration across the placenta ensures that serum biochemical parameters in the neonate reflect those of the mother. As a result, some may defer early biochemical assessment in sick newborn infants on this basis, even though the maternal values are not known. Data examining paired measurements of maternal and fetal/early neonatal biochemical values are surprisingly limited. These studies compared mean values in a group of mothers with the mean of the corresponding infant group. Although the studies found that the means were similar, the statistical methods did not provide a measure of the agreement between individual mother and infant pairs and could have, therefore, concealed quite large differences. The movement of individual ions and molecules across the placenta is complex and involves several mechanisms,

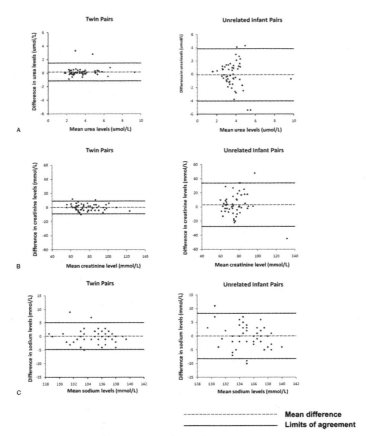

FIGURE 1.—Bland-Altman plots showing individual data points and 95% limits of agreement for twin pairs and unrelated infants for urea (A), creatinine (B), and sodium (C). (Reprinted from Henderson P, Cordiner D, Stenson B. An observational study of early neonatal biochemical parameters in twins. *Am J Perinatol.* 2011;28:111-116, with permission from Thieme Medical Publishers.)

including passive diffusion and active transport. Urea, creatinine, and sodium all cross the placenta by passive diffusion. During normal labor, it is often not necessary to measure maternal serum biochemistry and, therefore, maternal values are commonly not available when infants are admitted to the neonatal unit. Within twin pairs, the maternal serum biochemical profile is common to both twins. If neonatal plasma urea, creatinine, and sodium values are largely determined by equilibration with the mother, then they should be very similar within twin pairs. Because there is variation in these biochemical values between mothers, the differences in urea, creatinine, and sodium values between unrelated infant pairs would be expected to be larger than that seen within twin pairs. The authors hypothesized that there would not be clinically important differences in plasma urea, creatinine, and sodium between twins when measured shortly after birth and that differences between unrelated infant pairs would be greater (Fig 1).

M. G. Bissell, MD, PhD, MPH

19 Clinical Microbiology

Airborne bacteria concentrations and related factors at university laboratories, hospital diagnostic laboratories and a biowaste site
Hwang SH, Park DU, Ha KC, et al (Seoul Natl Univ, South Korea; Korea Natl Open Univ, Seoul, South Korea; Changwon Natl Univ, Gyeongnam, South Korea)
J Clin Pathol 64:261-264, 2011

Aims.—To evaluate concentrations of airborne bacteria in university laboratories, hospital diagnostic laboratories, and a biowaste site in Seoul, Korea. To measure total airborne bacteria (TAB), the authors assessed sampling site, type of ventilation system, weather and detection of Gram-negative bacteria (GNB), indoors and outdoors.

Method.—An Andersen one-stage sampler (Quick Take 30; SKC Inc) was used to sample air at a flow rate of 28.3 l/min for 5 min on nutrient medium in Petri dishes located on the impactor. A total of 236 samples (TAB, 109 indoor and nine outdoor; GNB, 109 indoor and nine outdoor) were collected three times in each spot from the 11 facilities to compare airborne bacteria concentrations.

Results.—TAB concentrations ranged from undetectable to 3451 CFU/m^3 (mean 384 CFU/m^3), and GNB concentrations from undetectable to 394 CFU/m^3 (mean 17 CFU/m^3). TAB concentrations were high in window-ventilated facilities and facilities in which GNB were detected; concentrations were also high when it was rainy (all p values <0.05). TAB concentrations correlated significantly with GNB (r = 0.548, p<0.01), number of bacteria species (r = 0.351, p<0.01) and temperature (r = 0.297, p<0.01). The presence of heating, ventilating, and air conditioning (HVAC), the number of TAB species and the detection of GNB affect TAB concentrations in laboratories.

Conclusions.—It is recommended that special attention be given to regular control of indoor environments to improve the air quality of university and hospital laboratories.

▶ It is impossible to work in a clinical laboratory and not wonder about what one is being exposed to there. Indoor environments contain a complex mixture of live (viable) and dead (nonviable) microorganisms, fragments thereof, toxins, allergens, volatile microbial organic compounds, and other chemicals. Of the microorganisms, bacteria growing actively or accumulating in indoor environments may affect health. High concentrations of airborne bacteria are indisputably harmful to public health. Previous studies have reported that airborne bacteria

297

cause respiratory conditions, such as rhinitis, asthma, and pneumonia, as well as other diseases, and these conditions can be fatal for people with other underlying health problems. Concentrations of airborne bacteria in homes, offices, air-conditioned classrooms, shopping malls, restaurants, high-rise apartment buildings, and underground railway systems have been reported. In recent years, studies have shown symptoms and physiological signs in university staff in relation to the indoor environment, bacterial infections among diagnostic laboratory workers, management programs for accreditation processes for medical laboratories, and bioaerosols around a municipal waste incinerator. Few studies, however, have examined airborne bacteria in university laboratories, hospital diagnostic laboratories, and biowaste sites. There has also been little discussion about concentrations of airborne bacteria as they relate to biosafety factors, such as ventilation systems in university laboratories, hospital diagnostic laboratories, and biowaste sites. In this study, the authors measured total airborne bacteria (TAB) and gram-negative bacteria (GNB) in university laboratories, hospital diagnostic laboratories, and a biowaste site. They hypothesized that differences in TAB concentrations would be related to indoor/outdoor sampling, type of ventilation system, detection of GNB, weather, temperature, relative humidity, number of TAB species, and laboratory area.

M. G. Bissell, MD, PhD, MPH

Interferon-γ release assays for the diagnosis of latent *Mycobacterium tuberculosis* infection: a systematic review and meta-analysis
Diel R, Goletti D, Ferrara G, et al (Med School Hanover, Germany; Natl Inst for Infectious Diseases L. Spallanzani, Rome, Italy; Univ of Perugia, Terni, Italy; et al)
Eur Respir J 37:88-99, 2011

We conducted a systematic review and meta-analysis to compare the accuracy of the QuantiFERON-TB® Gold In-Tube (QFT-G-IT) and the T-SPOT®. *TB* assays with the tuberculin skin test (TST) for the diagnosis of latent *Mycobacterium tuberculosis* infection (LTBI).

The Medline, Embase and Cochrane databases were explored for relevant articles in November 2009. Specificities, and negative (NPV) and positive (PPV) predictive values of interferon-γ release assays (IGRAs) and the TST, and the exposure gradient influences on test results among bacille Calmette-Guérin (BCG) vaccinees were evaluated.

Specificity of IGRAs varied 98–100%. In immunocompetent adults, NPV for progression to tuberculosis within 2 yrs were 97.8% for T-SPOT®. *TB* and 99.8% for QFT-G-IT. When test performance of an immunodiagnostic test was not restricted to prior positivity of another test, progression rates to tuberculosis among IGRA-positive individuals followed for 19–24 months varied 8–15%, exceeding those reported for the TST (2–3%). In multivariate analyses, the odd ratios for TST positivity following BCG vaccination varied 3–25, whereas IGRA results remained uninfluenced and IGRA positivity was clearly associated with exposure to contagious tuberculosis cases.

IGRAs may have a relative advantage over the TST in detecting LTBI and allow the exclusion of *M. tuberculosis* infection with higher reliability.

▶ This article provides important up-to-date information on the use of interferon-γ release assays (IGRAs) for the diagnosis of latent *Mycobacterium tuberculosis* infection (LTBI) useful in support of the development of evidence-based guidance for tuberculosis-screening programs. These data may also be helpful for conducting more reliable cost-effectiveness and cost-benefit analyses with respect to the use of IGRA or tuberculin skin test (TST), solely or in combination. Specifically, the diagnostic specificity of IGRAs relative to the TST, the IGRAs' negative (NPV) and positive (PPV) predictive values for the progression to active tuberculosis, the association between exposure to patients with tuberculosis, and IGRA and TST test results in contacts were evaluated. The authors present a systematic review and meta-analysis of the literature, according to evidence-based highest-standard criteria on the accuracy of commercially available IGRAs for the diagnosis of LTBI. They conducted this systematic review, according to the guidelines of the Preferred Reporting Items for Systematic Reviews and Meta-Analyses statement and the Quality Assessment of Diagnostic Accuracy Studies (QUADAS) checklist.

M. G. Bissell, MD, PhD, MPH

Saliva Polymerase-Chain-Reaction Assay for Cytomegalovirus Screening in Newborns

Boppana SB, for the National Institute on Deafness and Other Communication Disorders CHIMES Study (Univ of Alabama at Birmingham; et al)

N Engl J Med 364:2111-2118, 2011

Background.—Congenital cytomegalovirus (CMV) infection is an important cause of hearing loss, and most infants at risk for CMV-associated hearing loss are not identified early in life because of failure to test for the infection. The standard assay for newborn CMV screening is rapid culture performed on saliva specimens obtained at birth, but this assay cannot be automated. Two alternatives — real-time polymerase-chain-reaction (PCR)—based testing of a liquid-saliva or dried-saliva specimen obtained at birth — have been developed.

Methods.—In our prospective, multicenter screening study of newborns, we compared real-time PCR assays of liquid-saliva and dried-saliva specimens with rapid culture of saliva specimens obtained at birth.

Results.—A total of 177 of 34 989 infants (0.5%; 95% confidence interval [CI], 0.4 to 0.6) were positive for CMV, according to at least one of the three methods. Of 17 662 newborns screened with the use of the liquid-saliva PCR assay, 17 569 were negative for CMV, and the remaining 85 infants (0.5%; 95% CI, 0.4 to 0.6) had positive results on both culture and PCR assay. The sensitivity and specificity of the liquid-saliva PCR assay were 100% (95% CI,

95.8 to 100) and 99.9% (95% CI, 99.9 to 100), respectively, and the positive and negative predictive values were 91.4% (95% CI, 83.8 to 96.2) and 100% (95% CI, 99.9 to 100), respectively. Of 17 327 newborns screened by means of the dried-saliva PCR assay, 74 were positive for CMV, whereas 76 (0.4%; 95% CI, 0.3 to 0.5) were found to be CMV-positive on rapid culture. Sensitivity and specificity of the dried-saliva PCR assay were 97.4% (95% CI, 90.8 to 99.7) and 99.9% (95% CI, 99.9 to 100), respectively. The positive and negative predictive values were 90.2% (95% CI, 81.7 to 95.7) and 99.9% (95% CI, 99.9 to 100), respectively.

Conclusions.—Real-time PCR assays of both liquid- and dried-saliva specimens showed high sensitivity and specificity for detecting CMV infection and should be considered potential screening tools for CMV in newborns. (Funded by the National Institute on Deafness and Other Communication Disorders.)

▶ Newborn screening for congenital cytomegalovirus (CMV) infection is justified by the importance of CMV as a cause of hearing loss, especially given that most infants at risk for CMV-associated hearing loss are not identified early in life because of failure to test for the infection. The standard assay for newborn CMV screening is rapid culture performed on saliva specimens obtained at birth, but this assay cannot be automated. Two alternatives have been developed: real-time polymerase-chain-reaction (PCR)-based testing of a (1) liquid-saliva or (2) dried-saliva specimen obtained at birth. The authors compared real-time PCR assays of liquid-saliva and dried-saliva specimens with rapid culture of saliva specimens obtained at birth. The study was designed to determine the usefulness of a real-time PCR assay of saliva specimens obtained from newborns for CMV screening. During phase 1 of the study, saliva specimens were placed in transport medium and stored at 4°C before testing. PCR testing of dried saliva specimens (those that were not placed in transport medium and remained at ambient temperature during specimen storage and transport) was examined in phase 2 of the study, as dried specimens are easier to store and transport. Finally, all PCR assays were performed without a DNA extraction step to test an assay that would be more practical for screening all newborns.

M. G. Bissell, MD, PhD, MPH

Diagnostic value of laboratory tests in identifying serious infections in febrile children: systematic review
Van Den Bruel A, Thompson MJ, Haj-Hassan T, et al (Univ of Oxford, UK; et al)
BMJ 342:d3082, 2011

Objective.—To collate all available evidence on the diagnostic value of laboratory tests for the diagnosis of serious infections in febrile children in ambulatory settings.

Design.—Systematic review.

Data Sources.—Electronic databases, reference tracking, and consultation with experts.

Study Selection.—Studies were selected on six criteria: design (studies of diagnostic accuracy or deriving prediction rules), participants (otherwise healthy children and adolescents aged 1 month to 18 years), setting (first contact ambulatory care), outcome (serious infection), features assessed (in first contact care), and data reported (sufficient to construct a 2×2 table).

Data Extraction.—Quality assessment was based on the quality assessment tool of diagnostic accuracy studies (QUADAS) criteria. Meta-analyses were done using the bivariate random effects method and hierarchical summary receiver operating characteristic curves for studies with multiple thresholds.

Data Synthesis.—None of the 14 studies identified were of high methodological quality and all were carried out in an emergency department or paediatric assessment unit. The prevalence of serious infections ranged from 4.5% to 29.3%. Tests were carried out for C reactive protein (five studies), procalcitonin (three), erythrocyte sedimentation rate (one), interleukins (two), white blood cell count (seven), absolute neutrophil count (two), band count (three), and left shift (one). The tests providing most diagnostic value were C reactive protein and procalcitonin. Bivariate random effects meta-analysis (five studies, 1379 children) for C reactive protein yielded a pooled positive likelihood ratio of 3.15 (95% confidence interval 2.67 to 3.71) and a pooled negative likelihood ratio of 0.33 (0.22 to 0.49). To rule in serious infection, cut-off levels of 2 ng/mL for procalcitonin (two studies, positive likelihood ratio 13.7, 7.4 to 25.3 and 3.6, 1.4 to 8.9) and 80 mg/L for C reactive protein (one study, positive likelihood ratio 8.4, 5.1 to 14.1) are recommended; lower cut-off values of 0.5 ng/mL for procalcitonin or 20 mg/L for C reactive protein are necessary to rule out serious infection. White blood cell indicators are less valuable than inflammatory markers for ruling in serious infection (positive likelihood ratio 0.87-2.43), and have no value for ruling out serious infection (negative likelihood ratio 0.61-1.14). The best performing clinical decision rule (recently validated in an independent dataset) combines testing for C reactive protein, procalcitonin, and urinalysis and has a positive likelihood ratio of 4.92 (3.26 to 7.43) and a negative likelihood ratio of 0.07 (0.02 to 0.27).

Conclusion.—Measuring inflammatory markers in an emergency department setting can be diagnostically useful, but clinicians should apply different cut-off values depending on whether they are trying to rule in or rule out serious infection. Measuring white blood cell count is less useful for ruling in serious infection and not useful for ruling out serious infection. More rigorous studies are needed, including studies in primary care, to assess the value of laboratory tests alongside clinical diagnostic measurements, including vital signs (Fig 6).

▶ Systematic reviews of the diagnostic value of routine laboratory tests in specific clinical situations have a great deal of value. The authors recently published a systematic review of the diagnostic value of presenting clinical features in identifying serious infection in children. This review identified several important red flags; it also confirmed that consideration of symptoms and signs alone often result in residual diagnostic uncertainty, with the risk of serious infection

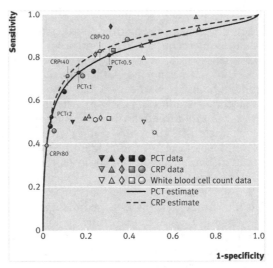

FIGURE 6.—Summary receiver operating characteristic curves for C reactive protein (CRP) and procalcitonin (PCT) levels for serious infection. Circles=Andreola 2007[16], squares=Berger 1996[39], diamonds= Galetto-Lacour 2008[21], triangles=Hsiao 2006[22], inverted triangles=Thayyil 2005[14]. *Editor's Note*: Please refer to original journal article for full references. (Reprinted from Van Den Bruel A, Thompson MJ, Haj-Hassan T, et al. Diagnostic value of laboratory tests in identifying serious infections in febrile children: systematic review. *BMJ.* 2011;342:d3082, with permission from the BMJ Publishing Group Ltd.)

being too high to ignore yet too low to justify hospital admission. The diagnostic uncertainty that clinicians are left with after clinical assessment was confirmed in a recent, large cohort study, where even a complex clinical decision rule involving 28 clinical features could not provide perfect discrimination. In situations with a significant risk of rapid progression of illness or where further refining of the risk estimate could either rule out serious infection or influence a decision to admit to the hospital or treat with antibiotics, clinicians often try to increase diagnostic certainty by measuring the white blood cell count or blood levels of inflammatory markers. Although in a hospital setting these tests are normally carried out in a laboratory, many are now available as point-of-care tests, which give an immediate result and can be used in ambulatory care settings. Earlier systematic reviews have assessed the value of 1 or 2 laboratory tests in children only or in children and adults for the diagnosis of various outcomes, such as distinguishing viral pneumonia from bacterial pneumonia or parenchymal involvement in children admitted with a urinary tract infection. Here the authors reviewed the diagnostic value of all possible blood tests for ruling in and ruling out serious infection in children in ambulatory settings and their added value after clinical signs and symptoms, using the same methods as in their previous review (Fig 6).

M. G. Bissell, MD, PhD, MPH

An Antimicrobial Stewardship Program's Impact with Rapid Polymerase Chain Reaction Methicillin-Resistant *Staphylococcus aureus/S. aureus* Blood Culture Test in Patients with *S. aureus* Bacteremia

Bauer KA, West JE, Balada-Llasat J-M, et al (The Ohio State Univ Med Ctr, Columbus; The Ohio State Univ, Columbus)
Clin Infect Dis 51:1074-1080, 2010

Rapid organism detection of *Staphylococcus aureus* bacteremia and communication to clinicians expedites antibiotic optimization. We evaluated clinical and economic outcomes of a rapid polymerase chain reaction methicillin-resistant *S. aureus/S. aureus* blood culture test (rPCR). This single-center study compared inpatients with *S. aureus* bacteremia admitted from 1 September 2008 through 31 December 2008 (pre-rPCR) and those admitted from 10 March 2009 through 30 June 2009 (post-rPCR). An infectious diseases pharmacist was contacted with results of the rPCR; effective antibiotics and an infectious diseases consult were recommended. Multivariable regression assessed clinical and economic outcomes of the 156 patients. Mean time to switch from empiric vancomycin to cefazolin or nafcillin in patients with methicillin-susceptible *S. aureus* bacteremia was 1.7 days shorter post-rPCR ($P = .002$). In the post-rPCR methicillin-susceptible and methicillin-resistant *S. aureus* groups, the mean length of stay was 6.2 days shorter ($P = .07$) and the mean hospital costs were \$21,387 less ($P = .02$). rPCR allows rapid differentiation of *S. aureus* bacteremia, enabling timely, effective therapy and is associated with decreased length of stay and health care costs.

▶ The continuing pressures for expanding careful monitoring of antibiotic utilization in so-called stewardship programs are immediately obvious: relentless proliferation of antimicrobial resistance coinciding with steadily reduced rates of development of new antibiotics. For example, because of the increased prevalence of methicillin-resistant *Staphylococcus aureus* (MRSA), vancomycin is used widely for empirical treatment. If the organism is identified as methicillin-sensitive *S aureus* (MSSA), studies have demonstrated that vancomycin is less active against MSSA than antistaphylococcal beta-lactams, including cefazolin and nafcillin. Molecular technologies for rapid multiplex detection of organisms have only recently been made available. Polymerase chain reaction (PCR) assays may improve clinical outcomes by decreasing the time to identification of coagulase-negative *Staphylococcus* species, MSSA, and MRSA and by allowing for earlier, more effective antimicrobial therapy. However, the clinical impact of a PCR assay on outcomes has not been studied. The rapid PCR MRSA/SA blood culture test (rPCR) is a novel second-generation multiplex real-time assay with results available within 1 hour. This study evaluates the clinical and economic outcomes of the rPCR with an infectious diseases pharmacist's intervention in patients with SA bacteremia.

M. G. Bissell, MD, PhD, MPH

Bacterial Vaginosis Assessed by Gram Stain and Diminished Colonization Resistance to Incident Gonococcal, Chlamydial, and Trichomonal Genital Infection

Brotman RM, Klebanoff MA, Nansel TR, et al (Univ of Maryland School of Medicine, Baltimore; Eunice Kennedy Shriver Natl Inst of Child Health and Human Bethesda, MD; et al)

J Infect Dis 202:1907-1915, 2010

Background.—We sought to assess the relationship between bacterial vaginosis (BV) assessed by Gram stain and incident trichomonal, gonococcal, and/or chlamydial genital infection.

Methods.—This longitudinal study included 3620 nonpregnant women aged 15—44 years who presented for routine care at 12 clinics in Birmingham, Alabama. Participants were assessed quarterly for 1 year. Vaginal smears were categorized by the Nugent Gram stain score (0—3, normal; 4—6, intermediate state; 7—10, BV). Pooled logistic regression was used to estimate the hazard ratios for the comparison of trichomonal, gonococcal, and chlamydial infection incidence in participants by Nugent score at the prior visit. Participants were censored at their first visit with a positive test result for trichomonal, gonococcal, and/or chlamydial infection.

Results.—Of the 10,606 eligible visits, 37.96% were classified by BV and 13.3% by positive detection of trichomonal, gonococcal, and/or chlamydial infection. An intermediate state or BV at the prior visit was associated with a 1.5—2-fold increased risk for incident trichomonal, gonococcal, and/or chlamydial infection (adjusted hazard ratio [AHR] for intermediate state, 1.41 [95% confidence interval {CI}, 1.12—1.76]; AHR for BV, 1.73 [95% CI, 1.42—2.11]; $P = .058$ for trend). Estimates were similar for trichomonal-only, gonococcal-only, and chlamydialonly infection outcomes.

Conclusions.—BV microbiota as gauged by Gram stain is associated with a significantly elevated risk for acquisition of trichomonal, gonococcal, and/or chlamydial genital infection.

▶ It is appearing increasingly likely that vaginal bacterial communities play an important role in preventing colonization by pathogenic organisms, including those responsible for sexually transmitted infections (STIs), vulvovaginal candidiasis, and urinary tract infections. Vaginal bacterial communities differ in species composition, and therefore it is also likely that they differ in how they respond to pathogens. To date, there have been relatively few studies that have prospectively assessed the association of vaginal microbiota with the incidence of *Neisseria gonorrhoeae*, *Chlamydia trachomatis*, and *Trichomonas vaginalis* infection; however, these studies were conducted among relatively high-risk women, including sex workers, women attending STI clinics, or women at risk for unplanned pregnancies. Because prior studies were conducted among high-risk populations, the authors sought to evaluate the role of the vaginal bacterial environment as a biological risk factor for trichomonal, gonococcal, and chlamydial genital infection in a large, prospective study of 3620 reproductive-age women who were recruited during routine health clinic visits.

M. G. Bissell, MD, PhD, MPH

Reducing Blood Culture Contamination by a Simple Informational Intervention
Roth A, Wiklund AE, Pålsson AS, et al (Skåne Univ Hosp, Malmö, Sweden)
J Clin Microbiol 48:4552-4558, 2010

Compared to truly negative cultures, false-positive blood cultures not only increase laboratory work but also prolong lengths of patient stay and use of broad-spectrum antibiotics, both of which are likely to increase antibiotic resistance and patient morbidity. The increased patient suffering and surplus costs caused by blood culture contamination motivate substantial measures to decrease the rate of contamination, including the use of dedicated phlebotomy teams. The present study evaluated the effect of a simple informational intervention aimed at reducing blood culture contamination at Skåne University Hospital (SUS), Malmö, Sweden, during 3.5 months, focusing on departments collecting many blood cultures. The main examined outcomes of the study were pre- and postintervention contamination rates, analyzed with a multivariate logistic regression model adjusting for relevant determinants of contamination. A total of 51,264 blood culture sets were drawn from 14,826 patients during the study period (January 2006 to December 2009). The blood culture contamination rate preintervention was 2.59% and decreased to 2.23% postintervention (odds ratio, 0.86; 95% confidence interval, 0.76 to 0.98). A similar decrease in relevant bacterial isolates was not found postintervention. Contamination rates at three auxiliary hospitals did not decrease during the same period. The effect of the intervention on phlebotomists' knowledge of blood culture routines was also evaluated, with a clear increase in level of knowledge among interviewed phlebotomists postintervention. The present study shows that a relatively simple informational intervention can have significant effects on the level of contaminated blood cultures, even in a setting with low rates of contamination where nurses and auxiliary nurses conduct phlebotomies.

▶ Blood culture contamination is an extremely common and costly occurrence, so it is reasonable to invest considerable resources in reducing blood culture contamination. Because contamination most probably is a result of personnel introducing exogenous bacteria into the blood culture, education of phlebotomists is central to prevention. Many studies advocate the effectiveness of teams of specialized phlebotomists in reducing contamination rates. Feedback, intense education in correct phlebotomy routines, and long-term monitoring programs have also been shown to be effective. In general, interventions seem less effective and contamination rates higher among nursing personnel conducting phlebotomy than those for specialized phlebotomy teams. In addition to presenting internationally comparable rates of blood culture contamination from a Swedish university hospital, the present study evaluates the effect of a simple informational intervention aimed at reducing blood culture contamination in a setting where phlebotomy for blood culture is conducted by nurses and auxiliary nurses, not by dedicated phlebotomy teams. The major examined outcome of the study was the effect of intervention on blood culture contamination rates. The effect was monitored in a novel way, by assessing the impact of the intervention on phlebotomists' knowledge of disinfection and phlebotomy routines.

M. G. Bissell, MD, PhD, MPH

Rapid Identification of 2009 H1N1 Influenza A Virus Using Fluorescent Antibody Methods
Leonardi GP (Nassau Univ Med Ctr, East Meadow, NY)
Am J Clin Pathol 134:910-914, 2010

Identification of the 2009 H1N1 influenza A virus requires emergency use authorized (EUA) molecular reverse transcriptase—polymerase chain reaction. Laboratories lacking molecular capabilities outsource testing, which is costly and may delay result reporting. A fluorescent antibody (FA; D^3 Ultra 2009 H1N1 influenza A virus ID Kit, Diagnostic Hybrids, Athens, OH) recently received Food and Drug Administration EUA status for 2009 H1N1 virus identification. The performance of this FA reagent was evaluated in this study.

Influenza A—positive nasopharyngeal specimens (seasonal H1, H3, and 2009 H1N1) were prepared for culture and FA testing and were stained using influenza A antibodies and the 2009 H1N1 reagent. Other respiratory viruses were also evaluated.

The FA reagent demonstrated 100% sensitivity and specificity. Bright, apple-green fluorescence was effortlessly identified in culture-positive cells, particularly around cell membrane perimeters. Laboratory-prepared slides were preferred over bedside-prepared specimens because background fluorescence obscured identification in the latter.

The new FA reagent provides an accurate, rapid, and inexpensive assay for identifying the 2009 H1N1 virus in nonmolecular diagnostic laboratories.

▶ Pandemic H1N1 influenza virus remains a potential worldwide threat, and work on it merits attention.

The differentiation of the 2009 H1N1 virus from seasonal H1N1 influenza A is important, but the use of molecular diagnostics is often limited in hospital laboratories. Instead, patient diagnosis relies on traditional cell culture, antigen detection, and serologic techniques. A fluorescent antibody reagent, D3 Ultra 2009 H1N1 influenza A (Diagnostic Hybrids, Athens, OH), recently became approved by the Food and Drug Administration on an emergency use authorization basis. A blend of 2009 H1N1 virus antigen-specific murine monoclonal antibodies and a fluorescein-labeled conjugate is used to identify 2009 H1N1 viral antigen in culture and in direct respiratory specimens. Thus, laboratories lacking molecular diagnostic capabilities may use this new antibody reagent to rapidly and inexpensively identify 2009 H1N1 influenza A virus in house. This study evaluated the sensitivity and specificity of this novel reagent to identify 2009 H1N1 influenza A virus in shell-vial culture and directly from patient nasopharyngeal specimens.

M. G. Bissell, MD, PhD, MPH

Diagnosis of Bacteriuria and Leukocyturia by Automated Flow Cytometry Compared with Urine Culture

Pieretti B, Brunati P, Pini B, et al (Ospedale Valduce, Como, Italy; et al)
J Clin Microbiol 48:3990-3996, 2010

Urinary tract infection (UTI) is a widespread disease, and thus, the most common samples tested in diagnostic microbiology laboratories are urine samples. The "gold standard" for diagnosis is still bacterial culture, but a large proportion of samples are negative. Unnecessary culture can be reduced by an effective screening test. We evaluated the performance of a new urine cytometer, the Sysmex UF-1000i (Dasit), on 703 urine samples submitted to our laboratory for culture. We compared bacteria and leukocyte (WBC) counts performed with the Sysmex UF-1000i to CFU-per-milliliter quantification on CPS agar to assess the best cutoff values. Different cutoff values of bacteria/ml and WBC/ml were compared to give the best discrimination. On the basis of the results obtained in this study, we suggest that when the Sysmex UF-1000i analyzer is used as a screening test for UTI the cutoff values should be 65 bacteria/ml and 100 WBC/ml. Diagnostic performance in terms of sensitivity (98.2%), specificity (62.1%), negative predictive value (98.7%), positive predictive value (53.7%), and diagnostic accuracy (73.3%) were satisfactory. Screening with the Sysmex UF-1000i is acceptable for routine use. In our laboratory, we have reduced the number of bacterial cultures by 43%, speeded up their reporting, and decreased the inappropriate use of antibiotics.

▶ The search for automatable, high-throughput methods for screening urine for bacterial infection continues on apace, fueled by the fact that the urinary tract is the most common site of infection, and urine specimens are, therefore, the most commonly encountered specimens in clinical laboratories. Because urine culture remains the standard diagnostic test for diagnosing urinary tract infection (UTI), there is a growing need to enhance the diagnostic performance of urine cultures. Because a large proportion of these urine samples are negative, the need is there to free up resources by developing the capability to reject these negative samples quickly. Thus, economics have drawn attention to solutions that can be used as screening tests to reduce the number of unnecessary culture tests performed. In this study, the authors sought to evaluate and optimize the performance of the Sysmex UF-1000i (Dasit) on 703 urine samples submitted at the same time to bacterial culture analysis.

M. G. Bissell, MD, PhD, MPH

Identification of Two Borderline Oxacillin-Resistant Strains of *Staphylococcus aureus* From Routine Nares Swab Specimens by One of Three Chromogenic Agars Evaluated for the Detection of MRSA
Buchan BW, Ledeboer NA (Med College of Wisconsin, Milwaukee)
Am J Clin Pathol 134:921-927, 2010

Methicillin-resistant *Staphylococcus aureus* (MRSA) is a leading cause of nosocomial infections that result in extended hospital stays and increased mortality. Therefore, rapid, cost-effective techniques for surveillance and detection of MRSA are critical to the containment and prevention of the spread of MRSA within the health care environment. We examined the ability of 3 chromogenic media (Spectra MRSA, Remel, Lenexa, KS; MRSA Select, Bio-Rad, Redmond, WA; and ChromID MRSA, bioMerieux, Marcy l'Etoile, France) to detect MRSA from routine surveillance specimens following 18, 24, and 48 hours of incubation. Our results indicate that detection of MRSA using all 3 chromogenic media is optimal following 24 hours of incubation. Early examination reduced sensitivity, while extended incubation reduced specificity. In addition, Spectra MRSA identified 2 borderline oxacillin-resistant strains of *S aureus* that were not detected by the other 2 chromogenic agars evaluated. These strains demonstrate increased basal and inducible resistance to β-lactam antibiotics.

▶ The usefulness of chromogenic media has been highlighted by studies that demonstrate this type of media to be superior to standard culture methods for the rapid isolation and identification of methicillin-resistant *Staphylococcus aureus* (MRSA) from typically polymicrobial specimens, such as superficial wounds, ulcers, sputum, and the anterior portion of the nares. The full benefits of chromogenic agar, however, can be realized only if the medium is able to consistently and reliably identify MRSA strains with a high sensitivity and specificity. These parameters can be affected by variables such as incubation time before inspection for typically colored colonies and bacterial load, specifically MRSA, in a given specimen. Here the authors compare performance of 3 different chromogenic agars, and found that different, less frequently identified strains could be picked up.

M. G. Bissell, MD, PhD, MPH

Detection of prion infection in variant Creutzfeldt-Jakob disease: a blood-based assay
Edgeworth JA, Farmer M, Sicilia A, et al (UCL Inst of Neurology, UK; et al)
Lancet 377:487-493, 2011

Background.—Variant Creutzfeldt-Jakob disease (vCJD) is a fatal neurodegenerative disorder originating from exposure to bovine-spongiform-encephalopathy-like prions. Prion infections are associated with long and clinically silent incubations. The number of asymptomatic individuals with vCJD prion infection is unknown, posing risk to others via blood transfusion, blood products, organ or tissue grafts, and contaminated medical instruments. We aimed to establish the sensitivity and specificity of a blood-based assay for detection of vCJD prion infection.

Methods.—We developed a solid-state binding matrix to capture and concentrate disease-associated prion proteins and coupled this method to direct immunodetection of surface-bound material. Quantitative assay sensitivity was assessed with a serial dilution series of 10^{-7} to 10^{-10} of vCJD prion-infected brain homogenate into whole human blood, with a baseline control of normal human brain homogenate in whole blood (10^{-6}). To establish the sensitivity and specificity of the assay for detection of endogenous vCJD, we analysed a masked panel of 190 whole blood samples from 21 patients with vCJD, 27 with sporadic CJD, 42 with other neurological diseases, and 100 normal controls. Samples were masked and numbered by individuals independent of the assay and analysis. Each sample was tested twice in independent assay runs; only samples that were reactive in both runs were scored as positive overall.

Findings.—We were able to distinguish a 10^{-10} dilution of exogenous vCJD prion-infected brain from a 10^{-6} dilution of normal brain (mean chemiluminescent signal, $1 \cdot 3 \times 10^5$ [SD $1 \cdot 1 \times 10^4$] for vCJD *vs* $9 \cdot 9 \times 10^4$ [$4 \cdot 5 \times 10^3$] for normal brain; $p < 0 \cdot 0001$)—an assay sensitivity that was orders of magnitude higher than any previously reported. 15 samples in the masked panel were scored as positive. All 15 samples were from patients with vCJD, showing an assay sensitivity for vCJD of $71 \cdot 4$ (95 CI $47 \cdot 8$-$88 \cdot 7$) and a specificity of 100 (95 CIs between $97 \cdot 8$ and 100).

Interpretation.—These initial studies provide a prototype blood test for diagnosis of vCJD in symptomatic individuals, which could allow development of large-scale screening tests for asymptomatic vCJD prion infection.

▶ To identify prion infection in variant Creutzfeldt-Jakob disease (vCJD) in blood, an assay must be able to detect abnormal prion protein (PrP) in a range that is several orders of magnitude lower than the sensitivity of conventionally used immunoassays. Furthermore, the ratio of background misfolded form of host cellular prion protein (PrpC; which is chemically identical to the aggregated, detergent insoluble isoforms designated PrPSc) is higher in blood than in any other tissue, with the high lipid and protein content of blood potentially contributing to nonspecific background signals. Conventionally, immunoassays for PrPSc have depended on protease pretreatment of tissues to degrade PrpC and other proteins, thereby reducing cross-reactivity. The finding that prions can bind avidly to some surfaces, including metals, has been used to develop quantitative assays for infectivity that approach the high sensitivity needed to detect the low concentrations of prions and abnormal PrP associated with blood. The authors have adopted a similar approach for the capture and enrichment of abnormal PrP from whole blood using an optimized solid-state capture matrix derived from investigation of an extensive range of potential binding surfaces coupled with direct immunodetection of the surface-bound material. This approach avoids use of any proteolytic processing, ensuring that all abnormal PrP isoforms are available for detection. They aimed to establish the sensitivity and specificity of this test for detection of vCJD prion infection in blood.

M. G. Bissell, MD, PhD, MPH

20 Hematology and Immunology

Performance characteristics of two commercially available IgG-specific immunoassays in the assessment of heparin-induced thrombocytopenia (HIT)
Bakchoul T, Giptner A, Bein G, et al (Justus Liebig Univ Giessen, Germany)
Thromb Res 127:345-348, 2011

Background.—The in vitro demonstration of antibodies against platelet factor-4/heparin (PF4/hep) complexes is an important contribution to the diagnosis of heparin-induced thrombocytopenia (HIT). The use of PF4/hep IgG-specific immunoassays enhances the specificity of HIT-investigations without any impairment of the sensitivity. Several IgG-specific immunoassays with different origin and structure of the target antigen-complex are commercially available.

Methods.—Using a retrospective cohort consisting of 459 patients suspected to have HIT, we compared the performance characteristics of two commercially available IgG-specific immunoassays, GTI- (Genetic Testing Institute) and HIA-IgG-ELISA (Hyphen Biomed Research).

Results.—PF4/hep antibodies were detected in 85 and 81 sera using GTI- and HIA-IgG-ELISA, respectively. OD values and clinical likelihood of patients who tested positive in one assay only were significantly lower than in those who tested positive in both immunoassays. Both IgG-specific assays showed high negative predictive values (100%) and similar but unsatisfactory positive predictive values, determined by a minimum clinical score of 5 and a positive HIPA result (41% and 43%, respectively). The implementation of a confirmatory step using excessive heparin increased the PPV of both assays, but results in a reduction of NPV in HIA-IgG-ELISA.

Conclusions.—The detection of IgG antibodies alone improves the clinical usefulness of immunoassays. However, functional assays remain indispensable to avoid the overdiagnosis of HIT caused by the detection of IgG non-platelet activating antibodies. The OD value in IgG immunoassays appears to correlate with the clinical relevance of the antibodies and might be used as a predictive parameter in the assessment of HIT (Fig 1).

▶ Heparin-induced thrombocytopenia (HIT) is usually caused by platelet-activating antibodies that recognize the platelet factor-4 (PF4)/heparin-complex, clinically characterized by a fall in platelet count beginning between

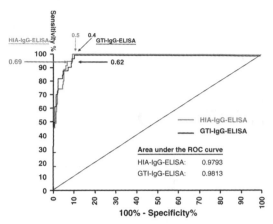

FIGURE 1.—The performance characteristics of PF4/hep immunoassays. 459 sera from patients with suspicion of HIT were re-investigated for antibodies against PF4/hep complexes to compare the operating characteristics in the diagnosis of HIT between two IgG-specific immunoassays, PF4 Enhanced (GTI Diagnostics, Waukesha, WI, USA) (GTI-IgG-ELISA, black line) and ZymutestHIA IgG (HyphenBiomed, Neuville-Sur-Oise, France) (HIA-IgG-ELISA, grey line) using the receiver-operating characteristics (ROC) curve. The diagnostic results of each immunoassay were defined to be "true positive" by a minimum clinical score of 5 and a positive result in the heparin-induced platelet activation (HIPA) test. The arrows are pointing to the sensitivity and specificity of the indicated cut-offs of each immunoassay. In this study, an optimal sensitivity but unsatisfactory specificity is obtained at standard cut-offs in both assays. Note that a cut off at OD of 0.69 and 0.62 gives the optimal compromise (trade-off) between the sensitivity and the specificity of the GTI- and HIA-IgG-ELISA, respectively. The area under the ROC curve (AUROC), which describes the ability of the each test to discriminate between individuals with/ out disease, shows that both assays have similar operating characteristics and represent informative assays in the diagnosis of HIT. (Reprinted from Bakchoul T, Giptner A, Bein G, et al. Performance characteristics of two commercially available IgG-specific immunoassays in the assessment of heparin-induced thrombocytopenia (HIT). *Thromb Res.* 2011;127:345-348, with permission from Elsevier.)

Day 5 to 10 of heparin therapy with or without thromboembolic events. The differential diagnosis of HIT is usually difficult, especially in critical care patients. HIT must be confirmed by in vitro demonstration of PF4/heparin (hep) antibodies. Currently, several immunoassays that exclusively detect immunoglobulin G (IgG) heparin-dependent antibodies are commercially available. Because various methods to immobilize different target antigens are used in these assays, the authors hypothesize that different performance characteristics may be obtained. Here they compared 2 IgG-specific immunoassays: PF4 Enhanced (GTI-IgG-enzyme-linked immunosorbent assay [ELISA]) and Zymutest HIA IgG (HIA-IgG-ELISA). Although PF4 bound to polyvinylsulfonate forms the antigen presented in GTI-IgG-ELISA, PF4 and other potential heparin-binding proteins (antigens) present in platelet lysate are added to heparin immobilized on protamine sulphate in HIA-IgG-ELISA. Both assays were evaluated using a well-characterized retrospective cohort consisting of 459 patients with suspected HIT (Fig 1).

M. G. Bissell, MD, PhD, MPH

Multiparameter Flow Cytometry in the Diagnosis and Management of Acute Leukemia

Peters JM, Ansari MQ (Univ of Texas Southwestern Med Ctr, Dallas)

Arch Pathol Lab Med 135:44-54, 2011

Context.—Timely and accurate diagnosis of hematologic malignancies is crucial to appropriate clinical management. Acute leukemias are a diverse group of malignancies with a range of clinical presentations, prognoses, and preferred treatment protocols. Historical classification systems relied predominantly on morphologic and cytochemical features, but currently, immunophenotypic, cytogenetic, and molecular data are incorporated to define clinically relevant diagnostic categories. Multiparameter flow cytometry provides rapid and detailed determination of antigen expression profiles in acute leukemias which, in conjunction with morphologic assessment, often suggests a definitive diagnosis or a narrow differential. Many recurrent molecular or cytogenetic aberrations are associated with distinct immunophenotypic features, and therefore flow cytometry is an important tool to direct further testing. In addition, detection of specific antigens may have prognostic or therapeutic implications even within a single acute leukemia subtype. After initial diagnosis, a leukemia's immunophenotypic fingerprint provides a useful reference to monitor response to therapy, minimal residual disease, and recurrence.

Objective.—To provide an overview of the application of flow cytometric immunophenotyping to the diagnosis and management of acute

---

TABLE 1.—World Health Organization (2008) Categories of Acute Leukemia[a]

Acute myeloid leukemia
    AML with recurrent cytogenetic abnormalities (see Figure 1)
    AML with myelodysplasia-related changes
    Therapy-related myeloid neoplasms
    AML NOS
        Morphologic and immunophenotypic subtypes
        Acute panmyelosis with myelofibrosis
    Myeloid sarcoma
    Myeloid leukemia associated with Down syndrome
    Blastic plasmacytoid dendritic cell neoplasm
Acute leukemia of ambiguous lineage
    Acute undifferentiated leukemia
    Mixed phenotype acute leukemia with t(9;22)(q34;q11.2); *BRC-ABL 1*
    Mixed phenotype acute leukemia with t(v;11q23); *MLL* rearranged
    Mixed phenotype acute leukemia, NOS (subclassify by phenotypes)
B-lymphoblastic leukemia/lymphoma
    B-lymphoblastic leukemia/lymphoma with recurrent genetic abnormalities
    B-lymphoblastic leukemia/lymphoma NOS
T-lymphoblastic leukemia/lymphoma

Abbreviations: AML, acute myeloid leukemia; NOS, not otherwise specified.

[a]The current World Health Organization classification includes entities defined by recurrent genetic abnormalities, cytomorphology, and clinical and immunophenotypic features. Although acute myeloid leukemias with recurrent genetic abnormalities are not strictly linked to specific morphologic or immunophenotypic characteristics, in many cases an association exists (refer to Figure 1). The unique subtypes of acute myeloid leukemia listed have a variable association with specific morphologic and immunophenotypic features. For example, the myeloid neoplasms associated with Down syndrome show a marked relative increase in apparent megakaryocytic differentiation.

leukemias, including salient features of those entities described in the 2008 World Health Organization classification.

Data Sources.—Published articles pertaining to flow cytometry, acute leukemia classification, and experiences of a reference flow cytometry laboratory.

Conclusion.—Immunophenotypic evaluation is essential to accurate diagnosis and classification of acute leukemia. Multiparameter flow cytometry provides a rapid and effective means to collect this information, as well as providing prognostic information and a modality for minimal residual disease evaluation (Table 1).

▶ As hematopathologists well know, morphologic and immunophenotypic characterization remain crucial for accurate diagnosis, as well as for monitoring response to therapy of acute leukemias, a diverse group of malignancies with a range of clinical presentations, prognoses, and preferred treatment protocols. In this area, multiparameter flow cytometry (3 or more colors) is the method of choice to determine the blast lineage and to detect aberrant antigenic profiles that may prove useful for disease monitoring. Here, the authors review some general considerations in the application of flow cytometry to the diagnosis of acute leukemias, followed by brief discussions of the characteristic immunophenotypic features of the various subtypes of acute leukemia currently recognized. A schematic summary of the current World Health Organization classification for acute leukemia is presented in Table 1.

M. G. Bissell, MD, PhD, MPH

Timeliness and Quality of Diagnostic Care for Medicare Recipients With Chronic Lymphocytic Leukemia

Friese CR, Earle CC, Magazu LS, et al (Univ of Michigan School of Nursing, Ann Arbor; Univ of Toronto, Ontario, Canada; Children's Hosp, Boston, MA; et al)
Cancer 117:1470-1477, 2011

Background.—Little is known about the patterns of care relating to the diagnosis of chronic lymphocytic leukemia (CLL), including the use of modern diagnostic techniques such as flow cytometry.

Methods.—The authors used the SEER-Medicare database to identify subjects diagnosed with CLL from 1992 to 2002 and defined diagnostic delay as present when the number of days between the first claim for a CLL-associated sign or symptom and SEER diagnosis date met or exceeded the median for the sample. The authors then used logistic regression to estimate the likelihood of delay and Cox regression to examine survival.

Results.—For the 5086 patients analyzed, the median time between sign or symptom and CLL diagnosis was 63 days (interquartile range [IQR] = 0-251). Predictors of delay included age ≥75 (OR 1.45 [1.27-1.65]), female gender (OR 1.22 [1.07-1.39]), urban residence (OR 1.46 [1.19 to 1.79]), ≥1 comorbidities (OR 2.83 [2.45-3.28]) and care in a teaching hospital (OR 1.20 [1.05-1.38]). Delayed diagnosis was not associated with survival (HR 1.11 [0.99-1.25]), but receipt of flow cytometry within thirty days before or after diagnosis was (HR 0.84 [0.76-0.91]).

Conclusions.—Sociodemographic characteristics affect diagnostic delay for CLL, although delay does not seem to impact mortality. In contrast, receipt of flow cytometry near the time of diagnosis is associated with improved survival.

▶ Delays in referral and diagnosis may negatively affect outcomes associated with many childhood malignancies and adult solid tumors. In contrast, little research has examined the relationship between diagnostic delay and outcomes for adult hematologic malignancies, despite improved techniques for pathologic diagnosis, staging, prognostication, and therapy. Such innovations may offer significant benefits for those who are referred, diagnosed, and treated in a timely manner. This has been demonstrated for younger patients with acute myelogenous leukemia and even for patients with indolent malignancies such as chronic lymphocytic leukemia (CLL). Indeed, timeliness of care was identified as 1 of 6 aims of health care quality improvement in the Institute of Medicine's Crossing the Quality Chasm report. Given that CLL is the most common type of leukemia, even small differences in outcomes driven by diagnostic delays have the potential for significant societal impact. CLL is a disease of older adults. It has a median age of diagnosis in the United States of 72 years, with 89% of patients initially diagnosed at 65 years or older. Perhaps because of its indolence and predilection for the elderly, many cases of CLL are identified incidentally or diagnosed presumptively in physicians' offices without pathologic confirmation. Moreover, even when a pathologist is involved, it is difficult to distinguish CLL from a morphologically similar disease, such as mantle cell lymphoma. Because of its utility for definitive diagnosis, confirmatory flow cytometry has been increasingly recommended as a baseline test—and a measure of quality of care—for patients with CLL. For example, the National Comprehensive Cancer Network has long recommended baseline immunophenotyping on bone marrow or peripheral blood with flow cytometry for all patients with CLL. In addition, in 2008, the National Quality Forum working with the American Society of Hematology and the American Medical Association's Physician Consortium for Performance Improvement endorsed baseline flow cytometry for all patients with CLL as a quality of care standard. It is not currently known what clinical and sociodemographic factors predict delays in CLL diagnosis and, given its mostly indolent nature, whether delays have any effect on survival. In this context, the authors sought to estimate the time between CLL-associated signs or symptoms and diagnosis and to assess several covariates of delay. They also aimed to understand the correlates of receipt of baseline flow cytometry and to evaluate the effect that delays in diagnosis and receipt of flow cytometry might have on survival after a CLL diagnosis.

M. G. Bissell, MD, PhD, MPH

Peripheral Blood Monitoring of Chronic Myeloid Leukemia During Treatment With Imatinib, Second-Line Agents, and Beyond

Lima L, Bernal-Mizrachi L, Saxe D, et al (Emory Univ School of Medicine and Winship Cancer Inst of Emory Univ, Atlanta, GA)
Cancer 117:1245-1252, 2011

Background.—The current study was conducted to compare simultaneously obtained bone marrow (BM) cytogenetics (CTG), peripheral blood (PB) and BM fluorescence in situ hybridization (FISH), and quantitative real-time polymerase chain reaction (Q-PCR) for BCR-ABL1 in monitoring response to treatment with tyrosine kinase inhibitors and homoharringtonine (HHT) in patients with chronic myeloid leukemia (CML).

Methods.—PB and BM FISH (n = 112 samples) and/or Q-PCR (n = 132 samples) for BCR-ABL1 were simultaneously obtained in 70 patients with Philadelphia chromosome-positive (Ph+) CML in chronic (68%), accelerated (16%), and blast phase (16%) before the initiation of therapy and during the course of treatment with imatinib (IM) (n = 40 patients), dasatinib (n = 20 patients), nilotinib (n = 4 patients), bosutinib (n = 18 patients), or HHT (n = 4 patients) for patients with newly diagnosed (n = 13 patients), IM-sensitive (n = 34 patients), IM-resistant (n = 30 patients), or IM-intolerant (n = 9 patients) disease. Eighteen patients were found to have Ph+ variants or karyotypic abnormalities in addition to the Ph+.

Results.—Excellent correlations (r) were observed between PB and BM FISH (r = 0.95) and PB and BM Q-PCR (r = 0.87), as well as BM CTG and PB FISH (r = 0.89) and PB Q-PCR (r = 0.82). This correlation was not affected by the presence of the Ph+ variant or additional chromosomal abnormalities, the presence of ABL1 kinase domain mutations, phase of the disease, or treatment.

Conclusions.—PB FISH and Q-PCR appear to be reliable methods with which to monitor response to modern therapy in patients with all phases of CML (Fig 4).

▶ Targeting BCR-ABL using the specific tyrosine kinase inhibitor (TKI), imatinib mesylate (IM) (Gleevec), dramatically improved outcomes in patients with chronic myeloid leukemia (CML). Similar to what was observed during treatment with interferon (IFN), the achievement of cytogenetic (CTG) remission is associated with improved disease-free and overall survivals with IM therapy. Therefore, tracking Philadelphia chromosome positivity (Ph +) yields valuable prognostic information. In addition, and with the availability of second- and third-generation TKIs, early detection, while patients are receiving IM, of suboptimal responses, loss of response, or disease progression permits treatment modifications that may favorably impact outcomes. Assessing the number of bone marrow (BM)-derived Ph+ metaphases has been the gold standard for monitoring response to therapy in CML. However, more sensitive methods, such as fluorescence in situ hybridization (FISH) and quantitative real-time polymerase chain reaction (Q-PCR), are not only more sensitive for detecting minimal residual disease but are easily measurable on peripheral blood (PB)

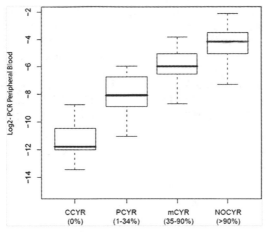

FIGURE 4.—Quantitative real-time polymerase chain reaction (Q-PCR) according to cytogenetic (CTG) responses is shown. CCYR indicates complete CTG response; PCYR, partial CTG response; mCYR, minor CTG response; NOCYR, all Philadelphia chromosome-positive metaphases. (Reprinted from Lima L, Bernal-Mizrachi L, Saxe D, et al. Peripheral blood monitoring of chronic myeloid leukemia during treatment with imatinib, second-line agents, and beyond. *Cancer.* 2011;117:1245-1252, Copyright 2011 American Cancer Society, with permission of Wiley-Liss, Inc., a subsidiary of John Wiley & Sons, Inc.)

samples. Given the need for frequent monitoring in patients with CML, interest in noninvasive methods has increased over the years. PB FISH correlated with BM CTG and BM FISH during treatment with IFN, and excellent correlations have been reported between BM and PB PCR in patients treated with IM. Correlations between PB and BM assays to detect BCR-ABL during therapy with second-line agents and beyond have not been reported; therefore, the authors herein report results in simultaneously obtained PB and BM FISH, Q-PCR, and BM CTG in this setting (Fig 4).

M. G. Bissell, MD, PhD, MPH

Prognostic Value of *FLT3* Mutations Among Different Cytogenetic Subgroups in Acute Myeloid Leukemia

Santos FPS, Jones D, Qiao W, et al (The Univ of Texas M D Anderson Cancer Ctr, Houston; et al)
Cancer 117:2145-2155, 2011

Background.—The impact of FMS-like tyrosine kinase 3 (*FLT3*) mutations and mutation burden among cytogenetic subgroups of patients with acute myeloid leukemia (AML) other than normal karyotype (NK) AML is unclear.

Methods.—Patients with newly diagnosed AML were divided among 3 cytogenetic subgroups: core binding factor (CBF) AML, NK-AML, and poor-risk AML.

Results.—In total, 481 patients were included: 13% had, CBF-AML, 57% had NK-AML, and 30% had poor risk AML, and the frequency of any *FLT3* mutations was 20%, 32%, and 7.6% in the respective cytogenetic subgroups. FLT3 mutation did not have an impact on event-free survival (EFS) in patients with CBF-AML ($P = .84$) and poor-risk AML ($P = .37$). In patients with NK-AML, EFS was worse in the *FLT3*-internal tandem duplication (ITD) group (20 weeks vs 41 weeks; $P < .00,001$) but not in the *FLT3*-tyrosine kinase domain (TKD) point mutation group (61 weeks vs 41 weeks; $P = .15$). Worse EFS and overall survival (OS) were observed among patients with NK-AML and higher *FLT3-ITD*

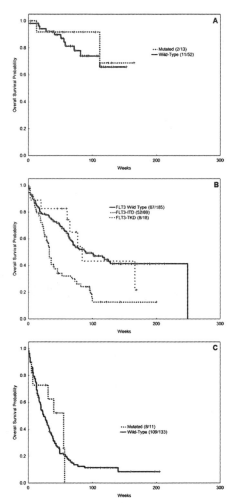

FIGURE 2.—Overall survival curves are shown for patients with (A) core binding factor-associated acute myeloid leukemia (AML); (B) normal karyotype AML (wild type FMS-like tyrosine kinase 3 [*FLT3*], *FLT3*-internal tandem duplication [*FLT3-ITD*], and *FLT3*-tyrosine kinase domain [*FLT3-TKD*] mutations); and (C) poor-risk AML. (Reprinted from Santos FPS, Jones D, Qiao W, et al. Prognostic value of FLT3 mutations among different cytogenetic subgroups in acute myeloid leukemia. *Cancer.* 2011;117:2145-2155, Copyright 2011 American Cancer Society, with permission of Wiley-Liss, Inc., a subsidary of John Wiley & Sons, Inc.)

burden but not among patients with *FLT3-TKD* mutation. In multivariate analysis, *FLT3-ITD* mutation was prognostic of EFS in patients with NK-AML (hazard ratio, 3.1; $P = .03$).

Conclusions.—FLT3 mutations did not have a prognostic impact in patients with AML who had good-risk and poor-risk karyotypes. In patients with NK-AML, *FLT3-ITD* mutations led to worse survival, which was even worse among patients who had high mutation burden (Fig 2).

▶ Acute myeloid leukemia (AML) is a heterogeneous disease, and its outcome is directed by the presence of several factors. Among the most important of these factors are age, performance status, and response to treatment. Several molecular abnormalities have been identified that have an important prognostic impact in AML, such as mutations of nucleophosmin 1, FMS-like tyrosine kinase 3 (FLT3), Wilms tumor 1, and CCAAT/enhancer binding protein alpha (CEBPA) genes. The perception that genetic and molecular abnormalities define unique subtypes of leukemias with important clinical features has led to an overall change of direction in the classification from a pure morphologic classification to a more genetic and molecular-based classification, as in the most recent World Health Organization classification. FLT3 is a receptor kinase (RTK) that belongs to the Class III RTKs (which also include KIT). FLT3 is expressed in early hematopoietic stem cells and in a subset of dendritic cell progenitors. FLT3 signaling activates intracellular pathways (eg, Ras-Raf-mitogen—activated protein kinase/extracellular signal-regulated kinase kinase [Mek], phosphatidylinositol 3-kinase) that promote proliferation and inhibition of apoptosis. In this study, the authors retrospectively evaluated the prognostic impact on survival of FLT3 mutations in well-defined cytogenetic subgroups of patients with AML (Fig 2).

M. G. Bissell, MD, PhD, MPH

Flow Cytometry Rapidly Identifies All Acute Promyelocytic Leukemias With High Specificity Independent of Underlying Cytogenetic Abnormalities
Dong HY, Kung JX, Bhardwaj V, et al (Genzyme Genetics, NY; et al)
Am J Clin Pathol 135:76-84, 2011

Acute promyelocytic leukemia (APL) is a highly aggressive disease requiring prompt diagnosis and specific early intervention. Immunophenotyping by flow cytometry (FCM) facilitates a rapid diagnosis, but commonly used criteria are neither sufficiently sensitive nor specific. With an antibody panel for diagnostic screening in routine practice, we found all 149 APL cases in this study exhibited a unique immunophenotypic profile, ie, a characteristic CD11b− myeloid population and absent CD11c expression in all myeloid populations; 96.6% of cases also lacked HLA-DR expression. These distinctive features allowed recognition of all unusual cases phenotypically resembling the regular myeloblasts (CD34+/HLA-DR+) or granulocytes (CD117−/CD34−/HLA-DR−). FCM effectively identified all 19 APL cases with variant translocations, including cases with a normal karyotype due to a cryptic submicroscopic t(15;17)(q22;q21), t(11;17)(q23;q21) that escaped the detection by fluorescence in situ hybridization for t(15;17) and der(15)ider(17)(q10) that lacked a simple reciprocal t(15;17). When APL-associated profiles were validated against 107 AML cases of non-APL subtypes, including 51 HLA-DR− cases, the diagnostic specificity and positive predictive value were 98%. FCM effectively provides independent detection of APL during diagnostic workup and harmonizes with the subsequent molecular cytogenetic diagnosis.

▶ Diagnosis of acute promyelocytic leukemia (APL) traditionally relies on the morphologic identification of the leukemic cells followed by confirmatory molecular cytogenetic detection of the t(15;17) and other rare variant translocations by karyotyping, fluorescence in situ hybridization (FISH), and reverse transcriptase-polymerase chain reaction (RT-PCR). Unfortunately, a definitive morphologic diagnosis may be difficult in many community practice settings, especially when dealing with inadequate aspirate smears and morphologic variants. Furthermore, specific FISH and RT-PCR analyses for detection of t(15;17) are typically performed only on suspected cases. Cytogenetic analysis is relatively time consuming. When there are poor culture and suboptimal resolution of chromosomes, the results will require further FISH confirmation. For cases that have a normal karyotype or a negative FISH result targeting only t(15;17), a diagnosis may be further delayed by additional studies that are done based only on a high clinical suspicion index. Here the authors report that an aberrant immunophenotypic profile of maturing myeloid cells recognizes 100% of APL cases with high specificity, including cases lacking typical flow cytometric features of APL and cases lacking straightforward cytogenetic results owing to aberrant translocations. While an accurate diagnosis always requires a multimodal approach, a flow cytometric diagnosis of APL, based on the widely used findings of CD34- and HLA-DR−blasts, is inexpedient.

M. G. Bissell, MD, PhD, MPH

Flow Cytometric Immunophenotyping of Cerebrospinal Fluid Specimens
Craig FE, Ohori NP, Gorrill TS, et al (Univ of Pittsburgh School of Medicine, PA)
Am J Clin Pathol 135:22-34, 2011

Flow cytometric immunophenotyping (FCI) is recommended in the evaluation of cerebrospinal fluid (CSF) specimens for hematologic neoplasms. This study reviewed FCI of CSF specimens collected for primary diagnosis (n = 77) and follow-up for known malignancy (n = 153). FCI was positive in 11 (4.8%) of 230 specimens: acute myeloid leukemia, 6; precursor B-acute lymphoblastic leukemia, 2; B-cell lymphoma, 2; and T-cell lymphoma, 1. Positive results were obtained in low-cellularity specimens, including 2 with fewer than 100 events in the population of interest. FCI was indeterminate in 19 (8.3%) of 230 specimens, including 3 with only sparse events, 8 with possible artifact (apparent lack of staining, nonspecific or background staining, and aspirated air), and 8 with phenotypic findings considered insufficient for diagnosis. Indeterminate specimens were often limited by low cellularity and lacked normal cell populations to evaluate for appropriate staining. FCI may be of value in low-cellularity CSF specimens, although the results should be interpreted with caution.

▶ Cerebrospinal fluid (CSF) evaluation is often used to assess patients with unexplained neurologic signs or symptoms and to stage disease in patients with neoplasms that have a predilection for central nervous system involvement. Conventional cytology has limited sensitivity in the evaluation of CSF specimens for hematologic neoplasms, and the pleocytosis seen in association with some non-neoplastic disorders may lead to false-positive results. Flow cytometric immunophenotyping (FCI) of CSF has previously been demonstrated to have high sensitivity and specificity for the detection of lymphoma and leukemia. More recent advances in multiparameter FCI, including the ability to detect more parameters in a single tube, have further enhanced the detection of phenotypic abnormalities; therefore, it has been recommended that FCI be performed routinely, in conjunction with cytology, on CSF specimens being evaluated for hematologic neoplasms. Here the authors reviewed their laboratory's experience in evaluating CSF specimens, and confirmed that FCI can be a useful diagnostic tool for the detection of hematologic malignancy in CSF specimens, even when the cellularity is low, as well as demonstrating some of the difficulties that may be encountered and recommending strategies to avoid potential misinterpretation.

M. G. Bissell, MD, PhD, MPH

Prognostic significance of the initial cerebro-spinal fluid (CSF) involvement of children with acute lymphoblastic leukaemia (ALL) treated without cranial irradiation: Results of European Organization for Research and Treatment of Cancer (EORTC) Children Leukemia Group study 58881
Sirvent N, Suciu S, Rialland X, et al (CHU Nice, France; EORTC Headquarters, Brussels, Belgium; CHU Angers, France; et al)
Eur J Cancer 47:239-247, 2011

Aim of the Study.—To evaluate the prognostic significance of the initial cerebro-spinal fluid (CSF) involvement of children with ALL enrolled from 1989 to 1996 in the EORTC 58881 trial.

Patients and Methods.—Patients (2025) were categorised according to initial central nervous system (CNS) status: CNS-1 (CNS negative, $n = 1866$), CNS-2 (<5 leucocytes/mm^3, CSF with blasts, $n = 50$), CNS-3 (CNS positive, $n = 49$), TLP+ (TLP with blasts, $n = 60$). CNS-directed therapy consisted in intravenous (i.v.) methotrexate (5 g/sqm) in 4—10 courses, and intrathecal methotrexate injections (10—20), according to CNS status. Cranial irradiation was omitted in all patients.

Results.—In the CNS1, TLP+, CNS2 and CNS3 group the 8-year EFS rate (SE%) was 69.7% (1.1%), 68.8% (6.2%), 71.3% (6.5%) and 68.3% (6.2%), respectively. The 8-year incidence of isolated CNS relapse (SE%)

was 3.4% (0.4%), 1.7% (1.7%), 6.1% (3.5%) and 9.4% (4.5%), respectively, whereas the 8-year isolated or combined CNS relapse incidence was 7.6% (0.6%), 3.5% (2.4%), 10.2% (4.4%) and 11.7% (5.0%), respectively. Patients with CSF blasts had a higher rate of initial bad risk features. Multivariate analysis indicated that presence of blasts in the CSF had no prognostic value: (i) for EFS and OS; (ii) for isolated and isolated or combined CNS relapse; WBC count <25 × 10^9/L and Medac E-coli asparaginase treatment were each related to a lower CNS relapse risk.

Conclusions.—The presence of initial CNS involvement has no prognostic significance in EORTC 58881. Intensification of CNS-directed chemotherapy, without CNS radiation, is an effective treatment of initial meningeal leukaemic involvement.

▶ Childhood acute lymphocytic leukemia (ALL) is subject to central nervous system (CNS) involvement, which is best treated presymptomatically. Cranial irradiation (XRT) in combination with intrathecal chemotherapy has been a common approach that has reduced the incidence of meningeal relapse, but the degree of radiation exposure (with resultant late CNS effects) has caused concerns and has to be based on an estimation of risk of CNS relapse. Among the initial factors that predict a higher risk, the presence of leukemic cells in a CSF containing fewer than 5 leucocytes/mm^3 has been associated with an enhanced risk of CNS relapse in some but not all clinical studies, and a poorer event-free survival (EFS) was associated with blasts in traumatic lumbar punctures at diagnosis of ALL. The European Organization for Research and Treatment of Cancer (EORTC) Children Leukemia Group (CLG) study 58881 showed that cranial XRT failed to provide any benefit to medium-risk and high-risk patients who had received high-dose methotrexate, so it was deleted from the treatment regimen of all patients with ALL, including those with overt CNS leukemia involvement. The aim of this retrospective study was to determine the prognostic significance of blasts with any number of leucocytes, with or without erythrocytes, in the CSF of patients recruited in EORTC CLG 58881. The time between the study closure and this analysis allowed the authors to identify possible late relapses, which is particularly important in a strategy that omits radiotherapy.

M. G. Bissell, MD, PhD, MPH

Transcriptomes of the B and T Lineages Compared by Multiplatform Microarray Profiling
Painter MW, The Immunological Genome Project Consortium (Harvard Med School, Boston, MA; et al)
J Immunol 186:3047-3057, 2011

T and B lymphocytes are developmentally and functionally related cells of the immune system, representing the two major branches of adaptive immunity. Although originating from a common precursor, they play very different roles: T cells contribute to and drive cell-mediated immunity, whereas B cells secrete Abs. Because of their functional importance and well-characterized differentiation pathways, T and B lymphocytes are ideal cell types with which to understand how functional differences are encoded at the transcriptional level. Although there has been a great deal of interest in defining regulatory factors that distinguish T and B cells, a truly genomewide view of the transcriptional differences between these two cells types has not yet been taken. To obtain a more global perspective of the transcriptional differences underlying T and B cells, we exploited the statistical power of combinatorial profiling on different microarray platforms, and the breadth of the Immunological Genome Project gene expression database, to generate robust differential signatures. We find that differential expression in T and B cells is pervasive, with the majority of transcripts showing statistically significant differences. These distinguishing characteristics are acquired gradually, through all stages of B and T differentiation. In contrast, very few T versus B signature genes are uniquely expressed in these lineages, but are shared throughout immune cells.

▶ As the major functional differences between B and T lymphocytes are usually assumed to be underpinned by differences in the basic cell biology of these cells, there has been some interest in determining what, beyond the Ag receptors and their ancillary factors, distinguishes B and T lymphocytes. In particular, how differently B and T lymphocytes use the blueprint of genes encoded in the genome. Although generating such data for transcripts that are strongly expressed and/or clearly differential is straightforward, there is difficulty in arriving at more general conclusions for the entire transcriptome in such comparisons. These problems lie in the confidence one can have in calls that a transcript is present or absent in a given dataset, given the difficulty in distinguishing true signals from noise owing to false negatives (nonperforming features on a microarray, subthreshold detection) or false positives (cross-hybridizing microarray features), both of which are poorly controlled on any one microarray. In addition, the use of arbitrary thresholds to define expression differentials tends to create overly simplistic distinctions. In the current study, the authors have attempted to robustly define the transcriptome differences underlying T and B lymphocytes by exploiting the unique datasets generated in the pilot phases of the Immunological Genome Project (ImmGen).

M. G. Bissell, MD, PhD, MPH

Chromosome 20q Deletion: A Recurrent Cytogenetic Abnormality in Patients With Chronic Myelogenous Leukemia in Remission
Sun J, Yin CC, Cui W, et al (The Univ of Texas M D Anderson Cancer Ctr, Houston)
Am J Clin Pathol 135:391-397, 2011

---

del(20q) can be observed in hematologic neoplasms, including chronic myelogenous leukemia (CML), and has been reported in patients undergoing blast transformation. We describe 10 patients with CML in hematologic and cytogenetic remission with del(20q) detected by conventional cytogenetics. There were 6 men and 4 women with a median age of 56 years. All patients initially had *BCR-ABL1* and t(9;22) (q34;q11.2) and achieved morphologic and cytogenetic remission after therapy. del(20q) was identified before (2/10 [20%]), at the time of (3/10 [30%]), or after (5/10 [50%]) cytogenetic remission and was not associated with morphologic evidence of dysplasia. At last follow-up, no patients had a myelodysplastic syndrome (MDS). Leukocyte and platelet counts were normal; 4 of 10 patients had mild anemia. Nine patients have remained in morphologic and cytogenetic remission with stable del(20q). *BCR-ABL1* fusion transcript levels were absent or low (median, 0.01%). Recently, in 1 patient, recurrent CML developed and del(20q) was lost. We conclude that del(20q) in the setting of CML in remission is not predictive of MDS or blast transformation (Fig 1).

▶ The natural history of chronic myelogenous leukemia (CML) is characterized by an initial indolent chronic phase (CP), followed by an accelerated phase (AP) and/or a blast phase (BP). The onset of AP or BP indicates disease progression and is often associated with additional cytogenetic abnormalities and resistance to therapy. In most patients with CML, the diagnosis is made when patients are in CP and treatment usually consists of a tyrosine kinase inhibitor and chemotherapeutic agents with or without stem cell transplantation. Complete cytogenetic

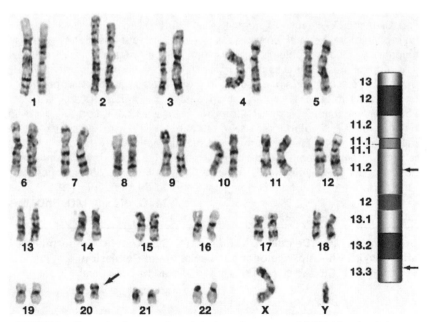

FIGURE 1.—Conventional cytogenetic analysis shows the presence of del(20q) in a female karyotype from a patient with chronic myelogenous leukemia in cytogenetic remission (left). An idiogram for normal chromosome 20 shows the location of breakpoints (arrows) that commonly occur in del(20q) (right). (Reprinted from Sun J, Yin CC, Cui W, et al. Chromosome 20q deletion: a recurrent cytogenetic abnormality in patients with chronic myelogenous leukemia in remission. *Am J Clin Pathol*. 2011;135:391-397, Copyright 2011, with permission from American Society for Clinical Pathology.)

response is achieved commonly, in up to 87% of patients in one study. The patients no longer show detectable t(9;22)(q34;ql1.2) or BCR-ABU gene rearrangement by conventional karyotyping or fluorescence in situ hybridization studies. Unbalanced chromosomal abnormalities are frequently found in hematologic neoplasms, such as myeloproliferative neoplasm, myelodysplastic syndrome (MDS), and acute myeloid leukemia, and are considered potential locations of genes responsible for pathogenesis and/or disease progression. The del(20q) (Fig 1) is one of the most common recurrent cytogenetic abnormalities in myeloid neoplasms and a known marker for MDS. In CML, del(20q) has been detected during blast transformation and is considered a potential cytogenetic marker for clonal evolution. However, rare CML cases in cytogenetic and morphologic remission in which del(20q) has been detected are reported in the literature. The clinicopathologic and follow-up data on these cases are not available. Herein the authors describe the clinical, morphologic, and molecular genetic characteristics of 10 patients with CML with del(20q) as the sole cytogenetic abnormality during morphologic and cytogenetic remission.

M. G. Bissell, MD, PhD, MPH

Automated Cerebrospinal Fluid Cell Counts Using the Sysmex XE-5000: Is It Time for New Reference Ranges?
Sandhaus LM, Ciarlini P, Kidric D, et al (Univ Hosps Case Med Ctr, Cleveland, OH)
Am J Clin Pathol 134:734-738, 2010

The main objectives of the study were to compare manual and automated WBC counts on clear cerebrospinal fluid (CSF) samples. Clear CSF samples from 200 adults and children were studied. Cell counts were performed manually using a hemocytometer and then analyzed on the Sysmex XE-5000. Descriptive statistics and Spearman correlation for nonparametric data were used for method comparison. Manual WBC counts ranged from 0 to 702 cells/µL, and Sysmex counts ranged from 0 to 629 cells/µL. The Spearman rank correlation coefficient for the entire range of data was 0.77 ($P < .001$); however, the correlation was weaker at the low end of the data spectrum. For manual WBC ranges of 0 to 5 cells/µL and 0 to 10 cells/µL, the corresponding Sysmex 0 to 95th percentile ranges were 0 to 23 cells/µL and 0 to 27 cells/µL, respectively. The results suggest that larger studies are necessary to determine new reference ranges for automated CSF WBC counts.

▶ Cerebrospinal fluid (CSF) cell counts have traditionally been performed by labor-intensive and imprecise manual methods using a hemocytometer counting chamber. Such methods are and have been obsolete for complete blood counts for more than half a century. Capabilities of some automated hematology analyzers have been extended to include automated body fluid cell counting. Implementation of such analyzers at the authors' institution presented the opportunity to evaluate their performance on clear CSF samples, many of which would be expected to have cell counts within the accepted normal ranges. It had been suggested that automated technologies might not be appropriate for such samples because a large proportion of normal samples would be misclassified as abnormal using existing reference ranges. Good laboratory practices, however, require that reference ranges be verified or new reference ranges be established when methods change. Therefore, the main objectives of this study were to compare manual hemocytometer and Sysmex XE-5000 white blood cell (WBC) counts on clear CSF samples and determine the ranges of Sysmex XE-5000 WBC counts that correspond to existing manually derived reference ranges. Secondary objectives were to evaluate the automated WBC differential count and the sensitivity and specificity of the WBC abnormal distribution flag for these samples.

M. G. Bissell, MD, PhD, MPH

Usefulness of Multiparametric Flow Cytometry in Detecting Composite Lymphoma: Study of 17 Cases in a 12-Year Period
Demurtas A, Aliberti S, Bonello L, et al (Univ of Turin, Italy)
Am J Clin Pathol 135:541-555, 2011

Composite lymphoma (CL) is a rare occurrence of 2 or more morphologically and immunophenotypically distinct lymphoma clones in a single anatomic site. A retrospective analysis of 1,722 solid tissue samples clinically suggestive of lymphoma was carried out in our institute during a 12-year period to evaluate the efficacy of flow cytometry (FC) in identifying CL. We report 17 CL cases. A strong correlation between morphologic findings and FC was observed in 13 cases (76%). In the 4 cases diagnosed as non-Hodgkin lymphoma plus Hodgkin lymphoma, although FC did not detect Reed-Sternberg cells, it accurately identified the neoplastic B- or T-cell component. In 3 cases, FC indicated the need to evaluate an additional neoplastic component that was not morphologically evident. Our data demonstrate that FC immunophenotyping of tissues may enhance the performance of the diagnostic morphologic evaluation of CL. To the best of our knowledge, this is the first report in the literature of a wide series of CL studied also by FC.

▶ Composite lymphoma (CL) was first defined as the coexistence of more than 1 type of lymphoma in the same patient. The definition was subsequently modified to include 2 or more distinct and well-demarcated types of lymphoma occurring in the same anatomic site or mass and then further expanded to include the combination of Hodgkin disease and non-Hodgkin lymphoma (NHL). Therefore, the term CL is now restricted to the rare occurrence of 2 or more morphologically and immunophenotypically distinct lymphoma clones in a single anatomic site. Besides, when 2 types of lymphomas are diagnosed at different sites, the terms simultaneous and sequential define the detection of disease at the same time or at a different time, respectively. Many combinations of CL have been reported, including multiple B-cell lymphomas, B-cell and T-cell lymphomas, NHL and Hodgkin lymphoma (HL), and complex B-cell, T-cell, and HL cases. The morphologic criteria must be confirmed by 1 or more tests, including immunohistochemical analysis, flow cytometric (FC) immuno-phenotyping, conventional cytogenetic tests, fluorescence in situ hybridization, and/or molecular biology studies. Immunophenotyping of paraffin-embedded tissue sections by immunohistochemical analysis was carried out in most cases reported in the literature, while fewer studies have reported investigation with FC. Therefore, the aim of this study was to evaluate the contribution of FC to the detection and diagnosis of CL.

M. G. Bissell, MD, PhD, MPH

21 Transfusion Medicine and Coagulation

Nucleic Acid Testing to Detect HBV Infection in Blood Donors
Stramer SL, Wend U, Candotti D, et al (American Red Cross, Gaithersburg, MD;
Univ of Giessen, Germany; the Natl Health Service Blood and Transplant,
Cambridge, UK; et al)
N Engl J Med 364:236-247, 2011

Background.—The detection of hepatitis B virus (HBV) in blood donors is achieved by screening for hepatitis B surface antigen (HBsAg) and for antibodies against hepatitis B core antigen (anti-HBc). However, donors who are positive for HBV DNA are currently not identified during the window period before seroconversion. The current use of nucleic acid testing for detection of the human immunodeficiency virus (HIV) and hepatitis C virus (HCV) RNA and HBV DNA in a single triplex assay may provide additional safety.

Methods.—We performed nucleic acid testing on 3.7 million blood donations and further evaluated those that were HBV DNA–positive but negative for HBsAg and anti-HBc. We determined the serologic, biochemical, and molecular features of samples that were found to contain only HBV DNA and performed similar analyses of follow-up samples and samples from sexual partners of infected donors. Seronegative HIV and HCV-positive donors were also studied.

Results.—We identified 9 donors who were positive for HBV DNA (1 in 410,540 donations), including 6 samples from donors who had received the HBV vaccine, in whom subclinical infection had developed and resolved. Of the HBV DNA–positive donors, 4 probably acquired HBV infection from a chronically infected sexual partner. Clinically significant liver injury developed in 2 unvaccinated donors. In 5 of the 6 vaccinated donors, a non-A genotype was identified as the dominant strain, whereas subgenotype A2 (represented in the HBV vaccine) was the dominant strain in unvaccinated donors. Of 75 reactive nucleic acid test results identified in seronegative blood donations, 26 (9 HBV, 15 HCV, and 2 HIV) were confirmed as positive.

Conclusions.—Triplex nucleic acid testing detected potentially infectious HBV, along with HIV and HCV, during the window period before seroconversion. HBV vaccination appeared to be protective, with a breakthrough subclinical infection occurring with non-A2 HBV subgenotypes and causing clinically inconsequential outcomes. (Funded by the American Red Cross and others.) (Fig 1).

▶ Although testing for hepatitis B (HBV) positivity has reduced the incidence of HBV infections among blood donors, HBV-seronegative but infected donors have been identified by means of nucleic acid testing at a rate of approximately 1 in 600 000 donations screened and have not been further studied. Although the residual risk of transmission of HBV by transfusion has decreased

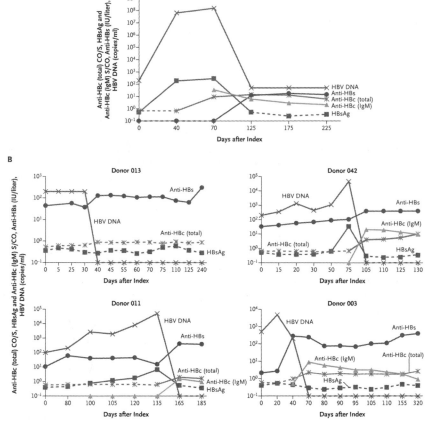

FIGURE 1.—Evolution of Serologic Markers for Hepatitis B Virus (HBV) after Index Donation from Five Donors with Acute HBV Infection. The results of follow-up analyses of virologic and serologic markers for HBV are shown for one donor who did not receive the HBV vaccine (Panel A) and for four vaccinated donors (Panel B). Included in the analyses are values for HBV DNA (in copies per milliliter). Values for hepatitis B surface antigen (HBsAg) and for IgM antibodies against hepatitis B core antigen (anti-HBc) are reported as signal-to-cutoff (S/CO) ratios, where values of 1.00 or more are considered to indicate reactivity. Values for anti-HBc (total) are reported as the reciprocal of S/CO since the assay format is based on competitive inhibition. Values of 10 or more for antibodies against hepatitis B surface antigen (anti-HBs) are considered to indicate immunity. Dashed lines indicate values below the threshold of detection. (Reprinted from Stramer SL, Wend U, Candotti D, et al. Nucleic acid testing to detect HBV infection in blood donors. *N Engl J Med.* 2011;364:236-247, Copyright 2011, with permission from Massachusetts Medical Society. All rights reserved.)

progressively, it remains higher than the estimated risks for human immunodeficiency virus (HIV) and hepatitis C virus (HCV; 1 in 1 467 000 donations and 1 in 1 149 000 donations, respectively). Here the authors conducted a study to evaluate the use of nucleic acid testing in determining the number of seronegative donors who have HBV DNA and to characterize these donors according to their risk factors and the progression of molecular, serologic, and biochemical markers (Fig 1). They used a triplex test combining the detection of HBV DNA with that of HIV and HCV RNA. They also evaluated donors who were seronegative for HIV and HCV but had positive results on nucleic acid testing.

M. G. Bissell, MD, PhD, MPH

Molecular insight into human platelet antigens: structural and evolutionary conservation analyses offer new perspective to immunogenic disorders
Landau M, Rosenberg N (Chaim Sheba Med Ctr, Tel-Hashomer, Israel; Tel-Aviv Univ, Israel)
Transfusion 51:558-569, 2011

Background.—Human platelet antigens (HPAs) are polymorphisms in platelet membrane glycoproteins (GPs) that can stimulate production of alloantibodies once exposed to foreign platelets (PLTs) with different HPAs. These antibodies can cause neonatal alloimmune thrombocytopenia, posttransfusion purpura, and PLT transfusion refractoriness. Most HPAs are localized on the main PLT receptors: 1) integrin αIIbβ3, known as the fibrinogen receptor; 2) the GPIb-IX-V complex that functions as the receptor for von Willebrand factor; and 3) integrin α2β1, which functions as the collagen receptor.

Study Design and Methods.—We analyzed the structural location and the evolutionary conservation of the residues associated with the HPAs to characterize the features that induce immunologic responses but do not cause inherited diseases.

Results.—We found that all HPAs reside in positions located on the protein surface, apart from the ligand-binding site, and are evolutionary variable.

Conclusion.—Disease-causing mutations often reside in highly conserved and buried positions. In contrast, the HPAs affect residues on the protein surface that were not conserved throughout evolution; this explains their naive effect on the protein function. Nonetheless, the HPAs involve substitutions of solvent-exposed positions that lead to altered interfaces on the surface of the protein and might present epitopes foreign to the immune system.

▶ Polymorphisms in platelet (PLT) membrane glycoproteins (GPs) are responsible for alloantibody production on exposure to PLTs with different human PLT antigens (HPA). These antibodies can cause neonatal alloimmune thrombocytopenia (NAIT), posttransfusion purpura, or PLT transfusion refractoriness after exposure to unmatched PLTs. The molecular basis of the 24 serologically defined antigens had been resolved and found to be a single-nucleotide polymorphism (SNP), resulting in an amino acid substitution in 23 of 24 antigens. The only non-SNP is HPA-14bw, an in-frame triplet deletion coding for one amino acid (beta3-Lys611). Overall, there are 17 different HPAs. In this article, the authors analyzed the structural features and evolutionary conservation of the HPAs to define the characteristics that lead to immunologic problems but not to inherited disease. They demonstrate that all HPAs studied here involve residues located on the surface of the protein far from the ligand-binding site and are not evolutionarily conserved. These criteria imply that the substitutions in these positions present a minor effect on the structure and function of the protein and, therefore, do not represent disease-causing mutations. Moreover, their location on the surface suggests that they could play a role in presenting epitopes.

M. G. Bissell, MD, PhD, MPH

The use of fresh-frozen plasma in England: high levels of inappropriate use in adults and children
Stanworth SJ, Grant-Casey J, Lowe D, et al (Univ of Oxford, UK; Royal College of Physicians, London, UK; Imperial College Academic Health Science Ctr, London, UK; et al)
Transfusion 51:62-70, 2011

Background.—Fresh-frozen plasma (FFP) is given to patients across a range of clinical settings, frequently in association with abnormalities of standard coagulation tests.

Study Design and Methods.—A UK-wide study of FFP transfusion practice was undertaken to characterize the current patterns of administration and to evaluate the contribution of pretransfusion coagulation tests.

Results.—A total of 4969 FFP transfusions given to patients in 190 hospitals were analyzed, of which 93.3% were in adults and 6.7% in children or infants. FFP transfusions to adults were given most frequently in intensive-treatment or high-dependency units (32%), in operating rooms or recovery (23%), or on medical wards (22%). In adult patients 43% of all FFP transfusions were given in the absence of documented bleeding, as prophylaxis for abnormal coagulation tests or before procedures or surgery. There was wide variation in international normalized ratio (INR) or prothrombin times before FFP administration; in 30.9% of patients where the main reason for transfusion was prophylactic in the absence of bleeding the INR was 1.5 or less. Changes in standard coagulation results after FFP administration were generally very small for adults and children.

Conclusions.—This study raises important questions about the clinical benefit of much of current FFP usage. It highlights the pressing need for better studies to inform and evaluate quantitative data for the effect of plasma on standard coagulation tests.

▶ There continues to be significant use of fresh frozen plasma (FFP) across a range of clinical specialties in hospital practice. In contrast to red blood cells, data from England and Wales for the use of FFP for transfusion show little change over the past decade, with approximately 300 000 units used annually; the latest figures for 2009 show a 4% annual increase. FFP is given primarily for 2 indications: to prevent bleeding (prophylaxis) or stop bleeding (therapeutic). National guidelines exist in many countries with broad similarities in the main recommendations for FFP use. Recommendations for transfusion of FFP include the following: active bleeding before surgery or an invasive procedure in patients with acquired deficiencies of one or more coagulation factors as demonstrated by abnormalities in the standard coagulation tests; immediate correction of vitamin K deficiency or reversal of warfarin anticoagulant effect in patients with active bleeding; disseminated intravascular coagulation or consumptive coagulopathy with active bleeding; thrombotic thrombocytopenic purpura; and patients with a congenital coagulation factor deficiency when no alternative therapies are available or appropriate. With these considerations in mind, a national study was designed to document practice for FFP transfusion, the first in England. The objectives were to understand how FFP is being used clinically, including the dose of FFP transfused, and to assess the use of standard coagulation testing before and after transfusion of FFP. A separate analysis of FFP use in infants and children was included to provide insight into current pediatric practice.

M. G. Bissell, MD, PhD, MPH

Automated mixing studies and pattern recognition for the laboratory diagnosis of a prolonged activated partial thromboplastin time using an automated coagulation analyzer
Ohsaka A, Ishii K, Yamamoto T, et al (Juntendo Univ School of Medicine, Tokyo, Japan; Juntendo Univ Hosp, Tokyo, Japan)
Thromb Res 128:86-91, 2011

Introduction.—The objective of this study was to explore whether an automated coagulation analyzer could be applied to normal plasma mixing studies for the assessment of blood samples showing a prolonged activated partial thromboplastin time (APTT).

Materials and Methods.—Ten laboratory staff members performed normal plasma mixing studies and evaluated plasma samples using 3 different methods: (1) manual dilution and analysis, (2) manual dilution and automatic analysis with STA-R®, and (3) automatic dilution and analysis with the Coapresta® 2000 (CP2000). The time from the start of the analysis to the generation of the result plots and the plasma volumes required were determined. We analyzed patient plasma samples showing a prolonged APTT using the CP2000, and the result plots were categorized into 3 curve patterns based on the area ratio values: the inhibitor type (convex pattern), deficiency type (concave pattern), and suspicious inhibitor type (approximately straight pattern).

Results.—When pooled patient plasma was used, the same patterns were obtained from normal plasma mixing studies using the 3 different methods. The time required to complete the mixing studies and the plasma volumes required were 28.2 ± 2.4 min and 350 μL for manual analysis, 23.2 ± 2.1 min and 875 μL for STA-R®, and 8.5 ± 0.1 min and 175 μL for CP2000, respectively. Of 31 patient samples, 9 were categorized into the inhibitor type, 15 were categorized into the deficiency type, and 7 were categorized into the suspicious inhibitor type.

Conclusions.—The CP2000 analyzer is applicable to the laboratory diagnosis of a prolonged APTT using pattern recognition, as it requires a shorter time to complete mixing studies and a smaller plasma volume in comparison with manual analysis (Fig 2).

▶ Antiphospholipid syndrome (APS) is an acquired thrombophilic disorder in which autoantibodies are produced in response to a variety of phospholipids and phospholipid-binding proteins. APS may be associated with venous thrombosis, arterial thrombosis, or both, and its clinical manifestations range from no symptoms to life-threatening APS. The presence of lupus anticoagulant (LA) in plasma alone or in combination with solid-phase antiphospholipid antibodies, such as anticardiolipin antibodies or antibodies to beta 2 glycoprotein I, is an important prerequisite for a diagnosis of APS. It is recommended that subjects with a prolonged activated partial thromboplastin time (APTT), patients with a history of venous and/or arterial thromboembolism (especially in cases associated with autoimmune disease), and women with a history of late pregnancy losses should be tested for LA. LA is suspected to be present when the clotting time is longer than the local cutoff value determined for the screening test. The detection of LA can be problematic in patients receiving oral anticoagulants or unfractionated heparin because the clotting times of such patients are prolonged in both screening and mixing studies, leading to false-positive results. The assessment of a prolonged APTT requires mixing studies with normal plasma, and an

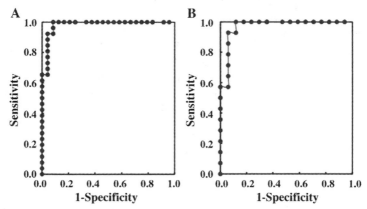

FIGURE 2.—ROC analysis of the area ratios of normal plasma mixing studies performed using the CP2000 to assess (A) commercially available plasma samples plus patient plasma samples (n = 50) and (B) patient plasma samples alone (n = 31). ROC analysis suggested that a 97% area ratio had the best sensitivity and specificity, which were 92% and 92%, respectively, in (A) and 93% and 88%, respectively, in (B). (Reprinted from Ohsaka A, Ishii K, Yamamoto T, et al. Automated mixing studies and pattern recognition for the laboratory diagnosis of a prolonged activated partial thromboplastin time using an automated coagulation analyzer. *Thromb Res.* 2011;128:86-91, with permission from Elsevier.)

additional sample may need to be collected from the patient for confirmation testing. Normal plasma mixing studies have traditionally been performed manually or mechanically, resulting in time constraints and operator-dependent variation. In this study, the authors evaluated a novel automated coagulation analyzer with a multidiluting function to explore whether it could be applied to normal plasma mixing studies for the assessment of blood samples showing a prolonged APTI. Their results indicate that the automated coagulation analyzer they used could be successfully applied to the laboratory diagnosis of a prolonged APIT by means of pattern recognition (Fig 2).

M. G. Bissell, MD, PhD, MPH

Development of a rapid emergency hemorrhage panel
Chandler WL, Ferrell C, Trimble S, et al (Univ of Washington, Seattle)
Transfusion 50:2547-2552, 2010

Background.—Evaluation of hemostasis in bleeding patients requires both accuracy and speed.

Study Design and Methods.—As an alternative to point-of-care testing, we developed an emergency hemorrhage panel (EHP: prothrombin time [PT], fibrinogen, platelet count, hematocrit) for use in making transfusion decisions on bleeding patients with a goal of less than 20-minute turnaround time (TAT) when performed in the clinical laboratory on automated instruments. Because point-of-care samples are not checked for clotting or hemolysis, we evaluated their effect on automated testing.

Results.—TAT was reduced by moving the sample immediately to testing and shortening centrifugation times. Clotting in samples was rare (1.1%) and shortened the PT by only 0.7 seconds. It lowered fibrinogen on average 18%, but resulted in only one of 2300 samples changing from normal to low fibrinogen. Hemolysis had no clinically significant effect on the PT or fibrinogen. Therefore, hemolysis checks were eliminated and clot checks minimized. Initially TAT averaged 15 ± 4 minutes (range, 8-30 min), but 9% of samples exceeded the 20-minute goal due to low fibrinogens that slowed testing. A revised fibrinogen assay with expanded calibration range resulted in a TAT of 14 ± 3 minutes (range, 6-28 min) with only 2% of samples exceeding the 20-minute goal. By limiting EHPs to patients that were actively bleeding, EHPs accounted for only 8 of 243 coagulation samples per day.

Conclusion.—Limiting EHPs to bleeding patients and modifications to the process and assays used for hemostasis testing lead to TATs of less than 20 minutes for critical testing in the clinical laboratory.

▶ Stat coagulation testing from the clinical laboratory is often felt to be too slow for use in critical situations with actively bleeding patients. This has led to the development of other approaches to improve turnaround times (TATs) for hemostasis testing, including satellite laboratories and point-of-care testing at or near critical care areas. In one study, point-of-care coagulation testing was completed in 19 ± 3 minutes, while stat coagulation testing from the clinical laboratory required 34 ± 15 minutes, with even longer TATs if sample transport times were included. Viscoelastic point-of-care coagulation assays have been reported to be useful in critical care situations by providing rapid TATs and overall assessment of the hemostatic system, including coagulation factors, platelets, and fibrinolysis. The principle drawbacks of point-of-care testing are lower accuracy, errors in predicting need for transfusion, lack of whole blood controls for these methods, and performance by non–laboratory-trained staff. The goal of this project was to evaluate critical hemostasis testing in the clinical laboratory to determine whether good accuracy and rapid TATs could be achieved using automated laboratory instruments.

M. G. Bissell, MD, PhD, MPH

Reduction of the risk of transfusion-transmitted human immunodeficiency virus (HIV) infection by using an HIV antigen/antibody combination assay in blood donation screening in Cameroon
Tagny CT, Mbanya D, Leballais L, et al (Univ Teaching Hosp, Yaoundé, Cameroon; Univ of Yaoundé I, Cameroon; Institut Natl de Transfusion Sanguine, Paris, France; et al)
Transfusion 51:184-190, 2011

Background.—Improving blood safety without introducing nucleic acid testing in blood screening may be possible using antigen/antibody (Ag/Ab) combination assays, especially in resource-poor countries.

Study Design and Methods.—To evaluate the potential reduction of human immunodeficiency virus (HIV)-transmitted infection using such an assay, a study was carried out aimed to compare the routine strategy for blood screening (S1), combining a rapid test (Determine HIV-1/-2, Inverness) and an enzyme immunoassay (human HIV-1/-2, Human Diagnostic) with an HIV Ag/Ab assay (S2, Genscreen ULTRA HIV Ag-Ab, Bio-Rad) in 2000 blood donations tested in Cameroon. Western blot and HIV RNA polymerase chain reaction were used to confirm the infection in reactive donors, and genotype was determined in HIV RNA−positive samples.

Results.—Of the 2000 donors, 3.1% were positive with S1 and 4.3% with S2. Of the 97 samples positive with S1 and/or S2 tested for confirmation, 54.7% were positive, 38.1% indeterminate, and 7.2% negative. There were significant differences between S1 and S2 in terms of sensitivity (S1, 79.2%; S2, 100%), irrespective of the genotype, and in specificity (S1, 99.0; S2, 98.3%). The most frequent genotype (49%) was CRF02_AG.

Conclusions.—A testing strategy using Genscreen ULTRA HIV Ag/Ab could prevent 55 HIV transmissions per 10,000 donations. However, this would be at a cost of discarding 170 per 10,000 negative donations that would test false positive, showing that the implementation of new techniques in blood screening need an optimization before routine use. Using confirmatory assays, HIV Ab prevalence in blood donors in Cameroon was estimated at 2.65%.

▶ Nucleic acid testing (NAT) has been effective in reducing the risk of transfusion-transmitted human immunodeficiency virus (HIV) infections, but it is too costly for application in some of the areas of the world with the greatest need for it.

Thus, most African blood banks perform HIV screening only with serologic tests. In remote areas, where difficult storage and transport conditions are frequently encountered, blood safety is based on the use of rapid tests that are affordable, easy to use and store, and do not need sophisticated equipment or electrical power. The impact of rapid test failure in blood safety is a matter of concern, particularly in areas with a high transfusion-transmitted infection prevalence rate. Improving blood safety without the use of NAT may be possible using antigen/antibody (Ag/Ab) combination assays because these methods may detect window-phase hepatitis C virus and HIV infection. Thus, the implementation of HIV Ag/Ab combination testing may be a cost-effective strategy to reduce HIV transmission risk in developing countries. To evaluate the benefit of introducing an HIV Ag/Ab combination assay in a high-HIV-prevalence African country, the authors performed a study comparing routine HIV Ab screening with a HIV Ag/Ab combination assay.

M. G. Bissell, MD, PhD, MPH

External Quality Assurance of Antithrombin, Protein C, and Protein S Assays: Results of the College of American Pathologists Proficiency Testing Program in Thrombophilia
Cunningham MT, Olson JD, Chandler WL, et al (Univ of Kansas Med Ctr; Univ of Texas Health Sciences Ctr, San Antonio; Univ of Washington, Seattle; et al)
Arch Pathol Lab Med 135:227-232, 2011

Context.—Hereditary and acquired deficiencies of antithrombin (AT), protein C (PC), and protein S (PS) are risk factors for venous thromboembolism. Proper diagnosis requires high-quality assays for these proteins.

Objective.—To determine the accuracy and interlaboratory precision of AT, PC, and PS assays used by laboratories participating in the United States College of American Pathologists proficiency testing program in thrombophilia and to grade the performance of laboratories.

Design.—Standardized normal plasma with assigned analyte values was sent in 2 separate challenges to participating laboratories. Participants measured AT, PC, and PS levels using local methods.

Results.—When compared with the assigned values for the international standard, the order of assay accuracy from highest to lowest was AT activity, PC antigen, AT antigen, total PS antigen, PC activity, PS activity, and free PS antigen (range of assay bias, 2.6%−8.8%). The order of assay precision from highest to lowest was PC activity, AT activity, AT antigen, total PS antigen, PS activity, free PS antigen, and PC antigen (range of assay coefficient of variation, 6.1%–20.0%). Most testing events (87.8%) could be graded as pass or fail using a target range of ± 3 standard deviations from the method-specific mean. The pass rate was 98.2% for all AT, PC, and PS testing events combined.

Conclusions.—Accuracy and precision were higher for AT assays and lower for PC and PS assays. It was feasible to grade individual laboratory performance.

▶ The authors' goals here were to determine the accuracy and interlaboratory precision of antithrombin, protein C, and protein S assays used by laboratories in the United States and to determine the feasibility of grading the performance of individual laboratories as pass or fail using method-specific peer group data. This was done using external quality assurance data obtained from participants of the 2008 and 2009 College of American Pathologists proficiency testing program in thrombophilia. The secondary coagulation standard Lot No.3 from the Scientific and Standardization Committee/International Society on Thrombosis and Haemostasis was used as the standardized plasma to evaluate performance. This plasma is ideal for evaluating accuracy because it has assigned concentration values for a variety of coagulation proteins and is commonly used by reagent kit manufacturers to assign calibrator values.

M. G. Bissell, MD, PhD, MPH

Development of North American Consensus Guidelines for Medical Laboratories That Perform and Interpret Platelet Function Testing Using Light Transmission Aggregometry
Hayward CPM, Moffat KA, Raby A, et al (North American Specialized Coagulation Laboratory Association, Rochester, MN; Quality Management Program—Laboratory Services, Toronto, Canada)
Am J Clin Pathol 134:955-963, 2010

Platelet function testing is important for the diagnostic evaluation of common and rare bleeding disorders. Our study goals were to promote best practices and reduce unnecessary testing variances by developing North American guidelines on platelet function testing. Guidelines were developed by consensus for expert recommendations (minimum level for approval, 70%) that included recommendations on the evaluation and interpretation of light transmission platelet aggregometry (LTA). To assess consensus, medical opinions on recommendations were gathered from diagnostic laboratories that perform LTA, in collaboration with the Quality Management Program-Laboratory Services (QMP-LS) in Ontario, Canada (10 laboratories), and the North American Specialized Coagulation Laboratory Association (NASCOLA; 47 laboratories, 5 overlapping the QMP-LS group). Adequate consensus was achieved for all and 89% of recommendations for the QMP-LS and NASCOLA groups, respectively. The recommendations adopted provide North American laboratories with additional guidance on platelet function testing, including how to interpret LTA abnormalities.

▶ Here the authors, in an effort to improve and standardize the evaluation of platelet function disorders by medical laboratories, pursued the development of consensus guidelines on platelet function testing. The guideline development was done by a process of collaboration and consultation, involving diagnostic laboratories in North America that assess platelet function and perform light transmission platelet aggregometry (LTA). Recommendations were first developed in collaboration with the Quality Management Program-Laboratory Services, a department of the Ontario Medical Association and then subsequently, the collaboration was broadened to include the medical laboratories that belong to the North American Specialized Coagulation Laboratory Association. These collaborative consultations generated consensus guidelines that cover important aspects of platelet function testing, including how to interpret and follow-up on LTA abnormalities; they are very much needed.

M. G. Bissell, MD, PhD, MPH

Reducing costs in flow-cytometric counting of residual white blood cells in blood products: utilization of a single-platform bead-free flow-rate calibration method
Fischer JC, Quenzel EM, Moog R, et al (Univ of Duesseldorf, Germany; Blood Donation Service Munich, Germany; Hosp Laboratory Network Brandenburg-Berlin, Germany; et al)
Transfusion 51:1431-1438, 2011

Background.—Commercial flow-cytometric methods for counting residual white blood cells (rWBCs) in leukoreduced blood products use calibration beads for estimation of the measured sample volume. A bead-free flow-rate calibration method is developed and validated.

Study Design and Methods.—The analyzed volume was calculated by acquisition time (ACQ). Twenty-nine spiking series of red blood cell (RBC) or platelet (PLT) products were prepared containing levels ranging from 0.08×10^6 up to 2048×10^6 WBCs/L. Nearly WBC-free triple-leukofiltered RBCs or PLT concentrates (PCs) served as background. Propidium iodide (PI) was used to identify rWBCs. Five RBC series were compared against a commercially available kit (LeukoSure, Beckman Coulter). Routine capabilities were tested on 41 RBC and 92 PC samples of two independent transfusion services.

Results.—The lower detection limit in RBC was 0.08×10^6 rWBCs/L for ACQ and 0.16 for LeukoSure. Criteria for linearity, accuracy, and precision were fulfilled within the range of 0.5×10^6 to 512×10^6 WBCs/L. For PCs, all these criteria were fulfilled between 0.5×10^6 and 32×10^6 rWBCs/L (lower detection limit of 0.25) for PI. ACQ and LeukoSure agreed sufficiently (81%) when tested on routine RBCs or PCs.

Conclusion.—A residual WBC count of fewer than 0.5×10^6 WBCs/L can be accurately counted using the ACQ approach at a total reagent cost of less than 0.5€ per sample.

▶ Before implementation of white blood cell (WBC)-reduced blood components, WBCs were one of the main reasons for adverse transfusion effects in patients. Although the benefit of universal leukoreduction could not be confirmed in all prospective studies, regulatory agencies in several countries have mandated transition to universal leukoreduced blood components. According to these regulatory requirements, at least 90% of the tested leukoreduced blood products should contain fewer than 1×10^6 WBCs per product, corresponding to 3.3×10^6 WBCs/L assuming a 300-mL blood product. Further, these guidelines require a minimum of 1% of all leukoreduced blood products to be tested for residual WBCs (rWBCs). Different manual and automated methods for assessing rWBCs are in use, including polymerase chain reaction—based, capillary volumetric, chamber counting using high-volume chambers and mostly flow cytometric methods. Because almost all common flow cytometers reveal relative concentrations rather than absolute counts, commercial kits calculate the measured neat volume by simultaneous measurement of calibration beads with known concentration. Using those calibration beads according to manufacturer recommendations will actually cost on the order of $5 per test. Based on the experience with antibody-based $CD4^+$ T-cell counting, the authors asked whether a cost-effective, bead-free, easy-to-conduct, DNA staining—based flow cytometric single-platform method could be used for the detection of rWBCs within leukoreduced blood components. They studied the limits of this method using DNA staining for detection of rWBC and assessed its suitability for routine testing of rWBCs.

M. G. Bissell, MD, PhD, MPH

Postponing or eliminating red blood cell transfusions of very low birth weight neonates by obtaining all baseline laboratory blood tests from otherwise discarded fetal blood in the placenta
Christensen RD, Lambert DK, Baer VL, et al (Intermountain Healthcare, Salt Lake City, UT; McKay-Dee Hosp Ctr, Ogden, UT; Univ of Utah School of Medicine, Salt Lake City; et al)
Transfusion 51:253-258, 2011

Background.—Safely reducing the proportion of very low birth weight neonates (<1500 g) that receive a red blood cell (RBC) transfusion would be an advance in transfusion practice.

Study Design and Methods.—We performed a prospective, single-centered, case-control, feasibility analysis, preparatory to designing a definitive trial. Specifically, we sought to determine whether we could obtain all baseline neonatal intensive care unit blood tests from the placenta, after placental delivery, thereby initially drawing no blood from the neonate.

Results.—Ten cases where all baseline blood tests were drawn from the placenta, and 10 controls where all tests were drawn from the neonate, were closely matched for birth weight, gestational age, sex, and race. Early cord clamping was used for all 20. Over the first 18 hours the hemoglobin increased in nine cases versus two controls ($p = 0.005$). During the first 72 hours one case versus five controls qualified for and received an RBC transfusion. In the first week the cases received four transfusions and the controls received 16 ($p = 0.02$). None of the cases had an intraventricular hemorrhage (IVH) but four of the controls had a Grade 1 and two had a Grade 3 ($p = 0.01$).

Conclusion.—We speculate that this method is feasible and generally postpones the first RBC transfusion until beyond the period of peak vulnerability to IVH.

▶ Very low-birth-weight (VLBW; <1500 g at birth) neonates are at risk for receiving 1 or more red blood cell (RBC) transfusions during their first week after birth. Almost every RBC transfusion administered during the first week is because a relatively large amount of blood was withdrawn for laboratory tests. Starting within minutes after birth, a battery of blood tests is generally drawn. Practice varies widely regarding which blood tests are obtained on neonatal intensive care unit (NICU) admission, but tests commonly drawn include a blood culture, complete blood cell count (CBC) with differential and platelet count, type and crossmatch, state metabolic screen, blood gas analysis, blood glucose determination, and occasionally other tests as well. Among the smallest NICU patients, the sum of this initial phlebotomy can equal 10% or more of their calculated blood volume. When these blood tests are drawn from an umbilical catheter, excess blood is withdrawn from the neonate into a flush syringe to clear the catheter of intravenous fluid. Although the blood in the flush syringe is generally returned to the neonate, this practice, in addition to the initial phlebotomy, can temporarily equate to a deficit approaching 20% of the calculated blood volume in the smallest NICU patients. The authors reasoned that phlebotomizing small ill neonates at the time of NICU admission increases their likelihood of qualifying for an RBC transfusion in the first days after birth. They hypothesized that, as an alternative, all baseline laboratory blood tests could be run on fetal blood drawn from the umbilical vein on the placenta, immediately after placental delivery. The authors suspected that doing this would be advantageous because it would leave more blood in the neonates, thereby potentially postponing the time at which they received their first RBC transfusion. As a step toward testing this hypothesis, the authors sought to determine whether it was indeed feasible to draw all baseline NICU blood tests from the placenta of 10 VLBW neonates. They also sought to determine, using a case-control approach, whether doing so would have any effect on the number of RBC transfusions administered during the first week after birth.

M. G. Bissell, MD, PhD, MPH

22 Cytogenetics and Molecular Pathology

Cancer genetics-guided discovery of serum biomarker signatures for diagnosis and prognosis of prostate cancer

Cima I, Schiess R, Wild P, et al (Eidgenössische Technische Hochschule Zurich, Switzerland; Univ Hosp Zurich, Switzerland; et al)

Proc Natl Acad Sci U S A 108:3342-3347, 2011

A key barrier to the realization of personalized medicine for cancer is the identification of biomarkers. Here we describe a two-stage strategy for the discovery of serum biomarker signatures corresponding to specific cancer-causing mutations and its application to prostate cancer (PCa) in the context of the commonly occurring phosphatase and tensin homolog (*PTEN*) tumor-suppressor gene inactivation. In the first stage of our approach, we identified 775 N-linked glycoproteins from sera and prostate tissue of wild-type and *Pten*-null mice. Using label-free quantitative proteomics, we showed that *Pten* inactivation leads to measurable perturbations in the murine prostate and serum glycoproteome. Following bioinformatic prioritization, in a second stage we applied targeted proteomics to detect and quantify 39 human ortholog candidate biomarkers in the sera of PCa patients and control individuals. The resulting proteomic profiles were analyzed by machine learning to build predictive regression models for tissue *PTEN* status and diagnosis and grading of PCa. Our approach suggests a general path to rational cancer biomarker discovery and initial validation guided by cancer genetics and based on the integration of experimental mouse models, proteomics-based technologies, and computational modeling.

▶ Molecular and genetic biomarkers play a paramount role in clinical oncology. They can help predict who will develop cancer or detect the disease at an early stage. Biomarkers also can guide treatment decisions and help identify subpopulations of patients who are most likely to respond to a specific therapy; however, the noninvasive detection and prognostic evaluation of a specific tumor by the analysis of indicators in body fluids, such as serum, remains a formidable challenge. Novel biomarkers represent today an urgent and critical medical need. Serum has long been considered a rich source for biomarkers. However, the discovery of serum biomarkers has been technically challenging and ineffectual for reasons that include the particular and variable composition

343

of the serum proteome and its enormous complexity. As the genetic alterations that cause cancer are becoming better understood, one strategy to overcome the limitations of the traditional serum proteome comparisons is to use the knowledge about specific cancer-causing mutations and the underlying disrupted signaling pathways to guide the discovery of novel cancer serum biomarkers. The tumor-suppressor gene phosphatase and tensin homolog (*PTEN*) is one of the most commonly inactivated genes in human cancer and has been identified as lost or mutated in several sporadic cancers, including endometrial carcinoma, glioblastoma, breast cancer, and prostate cancer. An established consequence of *PTEN* inactivation is the constitutive aberrant activation of the PI3 K-signaling pathway that drives uncontrolled cell growth, proliferation, and survival. It is expected that specific signaling pathway—activating mutations such as *PTEN* loss will produce changes in the surface and secreted proteomes of the affected tissue, and, in principle, these changes should be detectable as discrete biomarker signatures in the serum. Based on this conceptual consideration, the authors developed a 2-stage strategy for the discovery and initial validation of serum biomarkers in humans based on a mouse model of prostate cancer (PCa) progression caused by *PTEN* inactivation (Fig 1 in the original article).

M. G. Bissell, MD, PhD, MPH

Saliva-Derived DNA Performs Well in Large-Scale, High-Density Single-Nucleotide Polymorphism Microarray Studies
Bahlo M, Stankovich J, Danoy P, et al (The Walter and Eliza Hall Inst of Med Res, Parkville, Victoria, Australia; Univ of Tasmania, Hobart, Australia; Univ of Queensland, Brisbane, Australia; et al)
Cancer Epidemiol Biomarkers Prev 19:794-798, 2010

As of June 2009, 361 genome-wide association studies (GWAS) had been referenced by the HuGE database. GWAS require DNA from many thousands of individuals, relying on suitable DNA collections. We recently performed a multiple sclerosis (MS) GWAS where a substantial component of the cases (24%) had DNA derived from saliva. Genotyping was done on the Illumina genotyping platform using the Infinium Hap370CNV DUO microarray. Additionally, we genotyped 10 individuals in duplicate using both salivaand blood-derived DNA. The performance of blood- versus saliva-derived DNA was compared using genotyping call rate, which reflects both the quantity and quality of genotyping per sample and the "GCScore," an Illumina genotyping quality score, which is a measure of DNA quality. We also compared genotype calls and GCScores for the 10 sample pairs. Call rates were assessed for each sample individually. For the GWAS samples, we compared data according to source of DNA and center of origin. We observed high concordance in genotyping quality and quantity between the paired samples and minimal loss of quality and quantity of DNA in the saliva samples in the large GWAS sample, with the blood samples showing greater variation between centers of origin. This large data set highlights the usefulness of saliva DNA for genotyping, especially in high-density single-nucleotide polymorphism microarray studies such as GWAS.

▶ Genome-wide association studies (GWAS) require the collection of thousands of DNA samples to attain sufficient power to map loci responsible for complex diseases. DNA for such studies is usually extracted from lymphocytes, with blood collected from participants by phlebotomy. A recent study of DNA collection in a Danish nurse cohort showed a markedly greater response rate in recruitment of DNA samples from saliva versus blood (72% versus 31% of invited participants returned samples, respectively). These differences in response stemmed from a variety of issues, including the commitment required to provide blood by attending a clinic and uneasiness, or inability, to undergo phlebotomy. In comparison, saliva collection can be done at home, without professional help, and is much less invasive than phlebotomy. However, saliva-derived DNA is often contaminated with large amounts of bacterial DNA, and it is notoriously difficult to determine the relative proportion of human DNA. Moreover, different protocols are required for purification and quantitation of DNA derived from blood and saliva. It is therefore entirely plausible that DNA derived from these different sources might show systematic differences in genotyping efficiency and accuracy. The authors recently performed a multiple sclerosis (MS) GWAS with 1618 MS cases and 3413 controls under the auspices of the Australia and New Zealand MS Genetics Consortium (ANZgene). Twenty-four percent of MS cases had genotyping done on DNA derived from saliva, and the remaining samples were derived from blood. The data set used in the current study consisted of genotypes from these MS cases, some of the controls, and some samples that were not included in the published GWAS. In addition, a small data set consisting of 10 sample duplicates, where both saliva-derived and blood-derived DNAs were available, was also examined. These data were used to investigate the relative genotyping performance of blood-derived and saliva-derived genomic DNA using the Illumina single-nucleotide polymorphism (SNP) microarray platform.

M. G. Bissell, MD, PhD, MPH

Clinical Experience with the Cervista HPV HR Assay: Correlation of Cytology and HPV Status from 56,501 Specimens
Youens KE, Hosler GA, Washington PJ, et al (Duke Univ Med Ctr, Durham, NC; ProPath, Dallas, TX)
J Mol Diagn 13:160-166, 2011

Testing for high-risk (HR) human papillomavirus (HPV) is a key component of current recommendations for cervical cancer screening. Herein is described our clinical experience using Cervista HPV HR, a testing platform recently approved by the US Food and Drug Administration for clinical use. Using data from a high-volume commercial laboratory, a retrospective analysis of cytologic and Cervista HPV HR test results from 56,501 samples was performed, and an indirect comparison was made with previous experience with 53,008 samples tested using the Hybrid Capture 2 platform. Of samples analyzed using Cervista HPV HR, 1.5% were of insufficient volume for testing and 1.1% yielded an insufficient signal from the internal control to be reported. In samples with a cytological interpretation of atypical squamous cells of undetermined significance, 48.5% (95% confidence interval [CI], 47.5 to 49.5) tested positive using Cervista HPV HR, compared with 59.4% (95% CI, 58.3 to 60.5) of samples using Hybrid Capture 2. Of samples from women aged 30 years or older with a negative cytological interpretation, 5.8% (95% CI, 5.6 to 6.1) tested positive using Cervista HPV HR, compared with 5.5% (95% CI, 5.3 to 5.7) of samples using Hybrid Capture 2. When stratified by five-year age groups between 30 and 65 years, positivity rates for high-risk human papillomavirus were similar in the Cervista HPV HR and Hybrid Capture 2 populations, and were consistent with expectations established by the literature (Fig 1).

▶ The relationship of cervical cancer and cervical intraepithelial neoplasia grades 2 and 3 to persistent infection with human papillomavirus (HPV) is well established. Since the identification of HPV as the primary etiologic agent of cervical cancer, sexually transmitted oncogenic variants have been identified. These variants, referred to as the high-risk (HR) subtypes, are responsible for most cervical cancers worldwide. HR-HPV DNA testing is currently recommended by the American Society for Colposcopy and Cervical Pathology screening guidelines in 2 principal clinical settings. One setting in which HR-HPV DNA testing is beneficial is when cytologic findings are

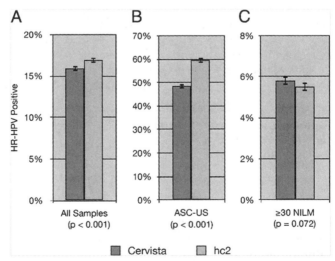

FIGURE 1.—Percent HR-HPV positive by cytologic interpretation. **A:** All samples. **B:** ASC-US. **C:** Women aged 30 years or older, NILM. All calculations are for reportable samples only. Whiskers indicate 95% confidence intervals. (Reprinted from Youens KE, Hosler GA, Washington PJ, et al. Clinical experience with the cervista HPV HR assay: correlation of cytology and HPV status from 56,501 specimens. *J Mol Diagn.* 2011;13:160-166, with permission from American Society for Investigative Pathology and the Association for Molecular Pathology.)

ambiguous or equivocal. HR-HPV DNA testing for the triage of patients with atypical squamous cells of undetermined significance (ASC-US) cytological interpretations decreases colposcopic referrals by roughly half without sacrificing screening sensitivity. A second setting in which HR-HPV testing is useful is for primary screening (co-testing, along with cytology) in patients aged 30 years or older. Women in this group with both normal cytological interpretations (ie, negative for intraepithelial lesion or malignancy [NILM]) and negative HR-HPV test results are at an extremely low risk of developing cervical cancer over the next several years. Accordingly, the current (2006) American Society for Colposcopy and Cervical Pathology screening guidelines and the 2010 American Cancer Society screening guidelines recommend that the repeat screening interval should be increased to 3 years in this double-negative population. Until 2009, clinical testing for HR-HPV was limited to a single US Food and Drug Administration (FDA)-approved method, the Hybrid Capture 2 (hc2) assay. This platform remains the most widely used clinical method for HR-HPV DNA testing. A second testing platform, the Cervista HPV HR assay, was FDA approved for clinical use in March 2009. Both tests involve hybridization of nucleic acid probes that are complementary to the viral genome, followed by a signal-amplification method for detection. Given its recent approval for clinical use, few data about Cervista clinical test performance are available. The authors present their experience using the Cervista HPV HR platform in a commercial laboratory, along with an indirect comparison with previous experience using the hc2 assay (Fig 1). In addition, estimates of the prevalence of HR-HPV infection in women with ASC-US and NILM cytologic interpretations in the present patient population are provided.

M. G. Bissell, MD, PhD, MPH

Resistance May Not Be Futile: microRNA Biomarkers for Chemoresistance and Potential Therapeutics
Allen KE, Weiss GJ (The Translational Genomics Res Inst, Phoenix, AZ)
Mol Cancer Ther 9:3126-3136, 2010

Chemoresistance to many commercially available cancer therapeutic drugs is a common occurrence and contributes to cancermortality as it often leads to disease progression. There have been a number of studies evaluating the mechanisms of resistance and the biological factors involved. microRNAs have recently been identified as playing a role in the regulation of key genes implicated as cancer therapeutic targets or in mechanisms of chemoresistance including EGFR, MDR1, PTEN, Bak1, and PDCD4 among others. This article briefly reviews chemoresistance mechanisms, discusses how microRNAs can play a role in those mechanisms, and summarizes current research involving microRNAs as both regulators of key target genes for chemoresistance and biomarkers for treatment response. It is clear from the accumulating literature that microRNAs can play an important role in chemoresistance and hold much promise for the development of targeted therapies and personalized medicine. This review brings together much of this new research as a starting point for identifying key areas of interest and potentials for future study.

▶ Using methods that tailor therapy to an individual's cancer to improve clinical benefit, so-called personalized medicine, is certainly warranted. Deciphering the mechanisms involved in chemoresistance (Fig 1 in the original article) is critical to improve the understanding of these complex pathways and to develop more effective targeted treatments. On development of chemoresistance, the alternative treatment used, which is another systemic therapy that is approved by the Food and Drug Administration for that cancer, is an investigational agent under the umbrella of a clinical trial or is an off-label use of a prescription drug. There is a burgeoning field of research to identify biomarkers that will either guide the selection of these alternate treatments by predicting the potential causes of acquired resistance or better classify the disease to improve primary treatment options and circumvent intrinsic resistance. This article seeks to review this important area of molecular testing, reviewing chemoresistance mechanisms, discussing how microRNAs (Fig 2 in the original article) can play a role in those mechanisms, and summarizing current research involving microRNAs as both regulators of key target genes for chemoresistance and biomarkers for treatment response.

M. G. Bissell, MD, PhD, MPH

Assay Design Affects the Interpretation of T-Cell Receptor Gamma Gene Rearrangements: Comparison of the Performance of a One-Tube Assay with the BIOMED-2-Based TCRG Gene Clonality Assay
Cushman-Vokoun AM, Connealy S, Greiner TC (Univ of Nebraska Med Ctr, Omaha)
J Mol Diagn 12:787-796, 2010

Interpretation of capillary electrophoresis results derived from multiplexed fluorochrome-labeled primer sets can be complicated by small peaks, which may be incorrectly interpreted as clonal T-cell receptor-γ gene rearrangements. In this report, different assay designs were used to illustrate how design may adversely affect specificity. Ten clinical cases, with subclonal peaks containing one of the two infrequently used joining genes, were identified with a tri-color, one-tube assay. The DNA was amplified with the same NED fluorochrome on all three joining primers, first combined (one-color assay) and then amplified separately using a single NED-labeled joining primer. The single primer assay design shows how insignificant peaks could easily be wrongly interpreted as clonal T-cell receptor-γ gene rearrangements. Next, the performance of the one-tube assay was compared with the two-tube BIOMED-2-based TCRG Gene Clonality Assay in a series of 44 cases. Whereas sensitivity was similar between the two methods (92.9% vs. 96.4%; $P = 0.55$), specificity was significantly less in the BIOMED-2 assay (87.5% vs. 56.3%;

$P = 0.049$) when a 2× ratio was used to define clonality. Specificity was improved to 81.3% by the use of a 5× peak height ratio ($P = 0.626$). These findings illustrate how extra caution is needed in interpreting a design with multiple, separate distributions, which is more difficult to interpret than a single distribution assay.

▶ Evaluation of clonal T-cell receptor-γ gene rearrangements (TCRγGR) using various polymerase chain reaction (PCR)-based methods is useful in the diagnosis of T-cell malignancies. Most laboratories use labeled joining region primers in capillary electrophoresis separation of PCR products. There are 3 possible approaches to evaluate TCRγGR using multiple fluorescent-labeled joining region primer sets. The first approach consists of a complete multiplex assay using multiple variables and joining region primers within a single tube. In this tricolor approach, each primer in a set of joining region primers is labeled with a different fluorochrome tag. The second complete multiplex approach is similar; however, instead of a different fluorescent label on each primer, the joining primers are labeled with the same fluorochrome tag (one color, eg, NED). The third approach involves a partial multiplex reaction using a single fluorochrome-labeled primer for each joining gene segment in separate tubes. This report is intended to show how assay design can heavily influence the likelihood of generating pseudoclonal peaks that can result in a false-positive interpretation of a TCRγGR and to compare the performance of 2 assays with divergent designs: a 1-tube assay with 1 size distribution versus the 2-tube TCRG gene clonality assay based on the BIOMED-2 design.

M. G. Bissell, MD, PhD, MPH

Effect of Direct-to-Consumer Genomewide Profiling to Assess Disease Risk

Bloss CS, Schork NJ, Topol EJ (Scripps Translational Science Inst, La Jolla, CA)
N Engl J Med 364:524-534, 2011

Background.—The use of direct-to-consumer genomewide profiling to assess disease risk is controversial, and little is known about the effect of this technology on consumers. We examined the psychological, behavioral, and clinical effects of risk scanning with the Navigenics Health Compass, a commercially available test of uncertain clinical validity and utility.

Methods.—We recruited subjects from health and technology companies who elected to purchase the Health Compass at a discounted rate. Subjects reported any changes in symptoms of anxiety, intake of dietary fat, and exercise behavior at a mean (±SD) of $5.6 ± 2.4$ months after testing, as compared with baseline, along with any testrelated distress and the use of health-screening tests.

Results.—From a cohort of 3639 enrolled subjects, 2037 completed follow-up. Primary analyses showed no significant differences between baseline and follow-up in anxiety symptoms (P=0.80), dietary fat intake (P=0.89), or exercise behavior (P=0.61). Secondary analyses revealed that test-related distress was positively correlated with the average estimated lifetime risk among all the assessed conditions ($\beta=0.117$, P<0.001). However, 90.3% of subjects who completed follow-up had scores indicating no test-related distress. There was no significant increase in the rate of use of screening tests associated with genomewide profiling, most of which are not considered appropriate for screening asymptomatic persons in any case.

Conclusions.—In a selected sample of subjects who completed follow-up after undergoing consumer genomewide testing, such testing did not result in any measurable short-term changes in psychological health, diet or exercise behavior, or use of screening tests. Potential effects of this type of genetic testing on the population at large are not known. (Funded by the National Institutes of Health and Scripps Health.)

▶ The US Food and Drug Administration's recent moves to actively intervene on the regulation of so-called "laboratory-defined tests" or LDTs is said to have originated from a concern over genomic profiling results being offered directly to the public, accompanied by interpretations of disease risk. The use of direct-to-consumer genomewide profiling to assess disease risk is controversial, and little is known about the effect of this technology on consumers. Studies of the psychological, behavioral, and clinical effects of genetic-risk disclosure for single diseases have generally been small and have yielded somewhat mixed findings. The Scripps Genomic Health Initiative was designed as a longitudinal cohort study to measure the effects of direct-to-consumer genomewide scans. Subjects purchased a commercially available genomewide risk scan at a subsidized rate and underwent Web-based standardized assessments at baseline and during follow-up, with the aim of gauging changes in anxiety level, diet, exercise, test-related distress, and use of screening tests.

M. G. Bissell, MD, PhD, MPH

A Novel and Rapid Method of Determining the Effect of Unclassified *MLH1* Genetic Variants on Differential Allelic Expression

Perera S, Li B, Tsitsikotas S, et al (Univ of Toronto, Ontario; Mt. Sinai Hosp, Toronto, Ontario, Canada)
J Mol Diagn 12:757-764, 2010

Germline mutations in mismatch repair genes predispose patients to Lynch Syndrome and the majority of these mutations have been detected in two key genes, *MLH1* and *MSH2*. In particular, about a third of the missense variants identified in *MLH1* are of unknown clinical significance. Using the Peak-Picker software program, we have conducted a proof-of-principle study to investigate whether missense variants in *MLH1* lead to allelic imbalances. Lymphocyte RNA extracted from patients harboring known *MLH1* variants was used to quantify the ratio of variant to wild-type transcript, while patient lymphocyte DNA was used to establish baseline allelic expression levels. Our analysis indicated that the missense variants c.350C>T, c.793C>T, and c.1852_1853AA>GC, as well as the truncating variant c.1528C>T were all associated with significantly unbalanced allelic expression. However, the variants c.55A>T and c.2246T>C did not demonstrate an allelic imbalance. These results illustrate a novel and efficient method to investigate the pathogenicity of unclassified genetic variants discovered in mismatch repair genes, as well as genes implicated in other inherited diseases. In addition, the PeakPicker methodology has the potential to be applied in the diagnostic setting, which, in conjunction with results from other assays, will help increase both the accuracy and efficiency of genetic testing of colorectal cancer, as well as other inherited diseases.

▶ Lynch syndrome, or hereditary nonpolyposis colorectal cancer (HNPCC; MIM 120435), which accounts for about 2% of all colorectal cancer cases, is one of the most common cancer predisposition syndromes. Those affected have about an 80% lifetime risk of developing colorectal cancer. In addition, malignancies of the endometrium, skin, bladder, ovaries, kidney, and small intestine are also associated with this syndrome. Lynch syndrome is an autosomal dominant condition that is characterized by germline mutations in mismatch repair (MMR) genes, about 90% of which are found in the 2 MMR genes, *MLH1* and *MSH2*. Determining unbalanced allelic expression offers an alternative method of investigating the pathogenic nature of a variant. Several studies in other genes have demonstrated that single-nucleotide substitutions are capable of altering the levels of messenger RNA (mRNA) transcripts. Furthermore, it has been proposed that such cis-acting functional variants can affect transcription, mRNA processing, and mRNA stability. The authors have conducted a proof-of-principle study to investigate whether missense variants in MLH1 lead to an allelic imbalance by measuring levels of transcript present in lymphocytes of individuals carrying 6 specific variants using the PeakPicker method.

M. G. Bissell, MD, PhD, MPH

Necessity of Bilateral Bone Marrow Biopsies for Ancillary Cytogenetic Studies in the Pediatric Population
Grimm KE, Chen C, Weiss LM (City of Hope Natl Med Ctr, Duarte, CA)
Am J Clin Pathol 134:982-986, 2010

The need for bilateral pediatric bone marrow biopsies for cytogenetic and fluorescent in situ hybridization (FISH) studies has not been clearly delineated. We retrospectively identified 166 pediatric bilateral bone marrow biopsy specimens obtained from patients with a variety of clinical diagnoses, including solid tumors, lymphoma, leukemia, and other hematologic conditions. The cases included all pediatric bilateral bone marrow biopsies performed at our hospital spanning the years of 1992 to 2008. Agreement of FISH and classical cytogenetic results between the 2 sides was assessed. Of a total of 166 bilateral cases, 2 cases showed disagreement (1.2%), both from patients with solid tumors. One case was a rhabdomyosarcoma, in which FISH only was performed; the second was a neuroblastoma in which FISH and cytogenetics were performed (both

FISH and classical cytogenetic results disagreed). The remainder of the cases showed complete agreement between the 2 sides (total 98.8%). We conclude that it is usually not necessary to perform bilateral bone marrow biopsies for FISH and cytogenetics in the pediatric population outside of the setting of solid tumor staging.

▶ Bone marrow biopsy, although a low-risk procedure, is not entirely without risks. In the pediatric population, the risks and benefits of an invasive procedure must be balanced with the benefit of the information provided by the study. Histologic evaluation of bilateral bone marrow biopsies is often necessary in lymphoma or solid tumor staging. Ancillary studies are important tools in monitoring minimal residual disease or assessing current disease status. Molecular studies have become more important in determining the diagnosis and prognosis of pediatric leukemia. The role of bilateral versus unilateral biopsies for ancillary studies such as fluorescence in situ hybridization (FISH) and classical cytogenetics is less well defined. Such studies are expensive and should not be performed unless they contribute to the diagnosis or prognosis in a meaningful way. This retrospective study examined the agreement of classical cytogenetics and FISH studies between the 2 sides of bilateral bone marrow specimens.

M. G. Bissell, MD, PhD, MPH

Cancer: Missing the mark
Buchen L (San Francisco, CA)
Nature 471:428-432, 2011

Background.—It has been hypothesized that early-detection biomarkers will be discovered and change the way cancer is found and treated. A review of 35 protein biomarkers, including 5 panels of proteins, was conducted by researchers coordinated by the Early Detection Research Network (EDRN), with rigorous testing of blood samples from over 1000 women. It was hoped that some would perform better than CA-125, which has several drawbacks. None of the candidates was better than CA-125, however. The poorest performance was turned in by biomarker panels identified by Gil Mor, a cancer biologist at Yale University. This 6-protein panel detected ovarian cancer in just 34% of the women diagnosed with the disease within 1 year, whereas the CA-125 found 63% of cases. The tale of Mor's work was offered as an example of what can go wrong.

Mor's Story.—Mor holds a PhD and began Discovery to Cure, a program designed to speed cancer research to the clinic. The group built a bank of blood and tissue samples that included some from a Yale clinic for women at high risk of ovarian cancer based on family history. David Ward, a geneticist, developed a "high-throughput" technique to quantify multiple proteins in blood using arrays of antibodies and wanted to use Mor's samples to search for biomarkers of early ovarian cancer. The blood samples from women newly diagnosed with ovarian cancer from Yale's high-risk clinic and from women coming for routine gynecologic examinations were screened for a panel of four proteins: leptin, prolactin, osteopontin, and insulin-like growth factor II. Mor developed an algorithm to classify women as having cancer or not based on these four proteins. The test's sensitivity was 95% and specificity was 95%, better than CA-125 tests, which have a sensitivity between 70% and 80% and a specificity of about 95%. Their findings were published and a patent application made for the panel.

Researchers from EDRN were performing a validation study and wanted to include Mor's panel. Their trial included 155,000 women and men whose blood samples had been accumulated and were being screened for ovarian or closely related cancers. Problems were detected in data analysis and statistics with Mor's material. For example the positive predictive value (PPV) was reported by Mor to be 99.3% but only 6.5% by the EDRN biostatistician, which is too low to be of much use for screening. This resulted when Mor used the PPVspecific to the study population (46%), whereas the EDRN used the accepted prevalence in postmenopausal women (0.04%). The high value was published, and LabCorp offered to begin marketing the panel as OvaSure, designed for use by women at high risk for ovarian cancer and claiming that it would help physicians detect and treat ovarian cancer in its earliest stages. With use, reasons for concern arose, such as prolactin being highly sensitive to stress and therefore elevated for reasons unrelated to cancer, uncertainties, evidence of biases, and no mention of cautions to be observed. The Food and Drug Administration (FDA) eventually became involved and LabCorp, while it disagreed with FDA assertions, pulled OvaSure from the market.

Analysis.—The biomarker field is still young and has drawn many cancer biologists who lack the expertise or resources to pursue translational or clinical work. Experts agree that potential biomarkers for early cancer detection should be validated on samples taken before diagnosis, but few groups attempt to take this step and the biomarkers tested for ovarian cancer have failed.

Conclusions.—The EDRN's study was one of the largest and most systematic validation studies of biomarkers. The findings revealed that biomarker research is falling short of expectations, perhaps because these biological molecules do not work or because rigorous scientific approaches are not being used.

▶ Simple blood tests that are practically useful for the screening and early detection of cancer have remained the "holy grail" of laboratorians for many decades. The checkered story of the introduction of carcinoembryonic antigen (CEA) into the marketplace well illustrates some of the many problems that have been involved, and indeed, this story was featured in that now-classic book *Beyond Normality* by Galen and Gambino in 1975. Similar lessons can be found in the stories behind many cancer biomarkers that have sputtered and failed on their way to the clinic. Those tests that are in clinical use—including prostate-specific antigen (PSA) for prostate cancer, mammogram-detected masses for breast cancer, and CA-125—fail to detect all cancers and sometimes "detect" ones that are not there. This story is updated and brought into the molecular diagnostics age with this *Nature* article: genomics, proteomics, and other such technologies promised to help by finding combinations of markers that are more powerful and cancer-specific than individual ones, but that promise has not been realized.

M. G. Bissell, MD, PhD, MPH

Design and Multiseries Validation of a Web-Based Gene Expression Assay for Predicting Breast Cancer Recurrence and Patient Survival
Van Laar RK (ChipDX LLC, NY)
J Mol Diagn 13:297-304, 2011

Gene expression analysis is a valuable tool for determining the risk of disease recurrence and overall survival of an individual patient with breast cancer. The purpose of this study was to create and validate a robust prognostic algorithm and implement it within an online analysis environment. Genomic and clinical data from 477 clinically diverse patients with breast cancer were analyzed with Cox regression models to identify genes associated with outcome, independent of standard prognostic factors. Percentile-ranked expression data were used to train a "metagene" algorithm to stratify patients as having a high or low risk of recurrence. The classifier was applied to 1016 patients from five independent series. The 200-gene algorithm stratifies patients into risk groups with statistically and clinically significant differences in recurrence-free and overall survival. Multivariate analysis revealed the classifier to be the strongest predictor of outcome in each validation series. In untreated node-negative patients, 88% sensitivity and 44% specificity for 10-year recurrence-free survival was observed, with positive and negative predictive values of 32% and 92%, respectively. High-risk patients appear to significantly benefit from systemic adjuvant therapy. A 200-gene prognosis signature has been developed and validated using genomic and clinical data representing a range of breast cancer clinicopathological subtypes. It is a strong independent predictor of patient outcome and is available for research use (Fig 2).

▶ Genomic profiling is increasingly being incorporated into the clinical management of patients with breast cancer, specifically the use of multigene algorithms to predict an individual patient's risk of disease recurrence, overall survival (OS), and potential benefit from adjuvant therapy. Since the advent of high-throughput genomics, multiple gene "signatures" associated with disease progression have been identified, several of which are sold as commercially available diagnostic tests. A training series of genomic data from patients with breast cancer with diverse clinicopathological variables was compiled from public data repositories. This information was analyzed using a statistical approach designed to identify individual genes associated with recurrence, independent of other prognostic factors. A predictive algorithm was formed on the gene set identified by this strategy and then applied to multiple independent breast cancer series, representing a range of clinicopathological variables. The resulting algorithm outputs an easily interpretable robust prognostic index

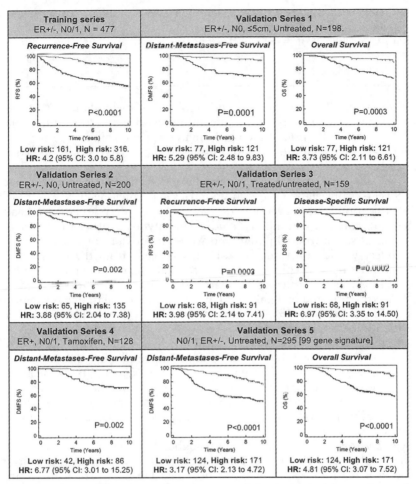

Training series ER+/-, N0/1, N = 477	Validation Series 1 ER+/-, N0, ≤5cm, Untreated, N=198.	
Recurrence-Free Survival	Distant-Metastases-Free Survival	Overall Survival
P<0.0001	P=0.0001	P=0.0003
Low risk: 161, High risk: 316. HR: 4.2 (95% CI: 3.0 to 5.8)	Low risk: 77, High risk: 121 HR: 5.29 (95% CI: 2.48 to 9.83)	Low risk: 77, High risk: 121 HR: 3.73 (95% CI: 2.11 to 6.61)

Validation Series 2 ER+/-, N0, Untreated, N=200	Validation Series 3 ER+/-, N0/1, Treated/untreated, N=159	
Distant-Metastases-Free Survival	Recurrence-Free Survival	Disease-Specific Survival
P=0.002	P=0.0003	P=0.0002
Low risk: 65, High risk: 135 HR: 3.88 (95% CI: 2.04 to 7.38)	Low risk: 68, High risk: 91 HR: 3.98 (95% CI: 2.14 to 7.41)	Low risk: 68, High risk: 91 HR: 6.97 (95% CI: 3.35 to 14.50)

Validation Series 4 ER+, N0/1, Tamoxifen, N=128	Validation Series 5 N0/1, ER+/-, Untreated, N=295 [99 gene signature]	
Distant-Metastases-Free Survival	Distant-Metastases-Free Survival	Overall Survival
P=0.002	P<0.0001	P<0.0001
Low risk: 42, High risk: 86 HR: 6.77 (95% CI: 3.01 to 15.25)	Low risk: 124, High risk: 171 HR: 3.17 (95% CI: 2.13 to 4.72)	Low risk: 124, High risk: 171 HR: 4.81 (95% CI: 3.07 to 7.52)

FIGURE 2.—Kaplan-Meier analysis of risk-group—stratified training and validation series. *P* values are from log-rank testing of the high- versus the low-risk group. Validation series 5 was analyzed using a 99-gene subset classifier, generated using 99 of 200 genes available on the NKI custom microarray used (see Supplemental Figure S1 at http://jmd.amjpathol.org). (Reprinted from Van Laar RK. Design and multiseries validation of a web-based gene expression assay for predicting breast cancer recurrence and patient survival. *J Mol Diagn.* 2011;13:297-304, with permission from American Society for Investigative Pathology and the Association for Molecular Pathology.)

and risk group assignment. Prognostic indexes and risk group assignments for all patients were evaluated in the context of the available clinical and survival data to assess clinical utility (Fig 2). The algorithm is implemented in an online diagnostic environment (ChipDX), available for evaluation.

M. G. Bissell, MD, PhD, MPH

DNA yield and quality of saliva samples and suitability for large-scale epidemiological studies in children

Koni AC, on behalf of the IDEFICS Consortium (Univ of Glasgow, Scotland, UK; et al)
Int J Obes 35:S113-S118, 2011

Objective.—To evaluate two saliva collection methods for DNA yield and quality as applied to a large, integrated, multicentre, European project involving the collection of biological material from children.

Design.—Cross-sectional multicentre comparative study in young children.

Methods.—Saliva samples were collected from 14 019 children aged 2–9 years from eight European countries participating in the IDEFICS (Identification and prevention of dietary- and lifestyle-induced health effects in children and infants) study. This involved either the collection of 2 ml of saliva from children who were able to spit, or using a sponge to collect whole saliva and buccal mucosal cells from the inside of the mouth of younger children unable to spit. Samples were assembled centrally in each participating centre and subsequently despatched for DNA extraction and biobanking to the University of Glasgow. A subgroup of 4678 samples ($\sim$33% of sampled individuals) were chosen for DNA extraction before genotyping.

Results.—The whole-saliva collection method resulted in a higher DNA yield than the sponge collection method (mean $\pm$ s.d.; saliva: 20.95 $\pm$ 2.35 µg, sponge: 9.13 $\pm$ 2.25 µg; $P < 0.001$). DNA quality as measured by A_{260}/A_{280} was similar for the two collection methods. A minimum genotype calling success rate of 95% showed that both methods provide good-quality DNA for genotyping using *TaqMan* allelic discrimination assays.

Conclusions.—Our results showed higher DNA yield from the whole-saliva collection method compared with the assisted sponge collection. However, both collection methods provided DNA of sufficient quantity and quality for large-scale genetic epidemiological studies (Table 3).

▶ Genetic epidemiological studies and clinical trials involving genetic association analysis are highly dependent on collecting, storing, and distributing DNA of good quality from a representative sample of participants to examine genetic influences on treatment response and disease risk. The success rates of genotyping depend on DNA quality and yield. The traditional method of collecting genetic material suitable for epidemiological studies and multiplex genotyping assays has been based on the use of blood samples, but this poses challenges, both financial and practical, in large studies, particularly when children are studied. Saliva is increasingly being collected in large studies because of its potential as diagnostic material and has previously been shown to be a reliable source of human genomic DNA suitable for large genetic epidemiological studies. The noninvasive nature of this collection method makes it particularly suitable for children. Buccal swabs are convenient and relatively inexpensive compared with blood sampling. Saliva

TABLE 3.—Comparison of DNA Yield and Quality by Method of Collection

Collection Method	n	DNA Yield (µg)		A_{260}/A_{280} Ratio	
		Mean (s.d.)	Median (IQ)	Mean (s.d.)	Median (IQ)
Total sample	4584	14.36 (2.83)	13.88 (7.35−27.26)	1.78 (0.27)	1.80 (1.67−1.91)
Whole saliva	1962	20.95 (2.35)	21.76 (11.93−38.21)	1.77 (0.18)	1.79 (1.67−1.89)
Sponge	2108	9.13 (2.25)	9.24 (5.23−15.90)	1.80 (0.20)	1.82 (1.69−1.93)

Abbreviation: IQ, limits of the interquartile range.

sampling has therefore become more popular as the methods for extraction of high-quality DNA have developed and costs have reduced. Saliva-based methods typically yield DNA of sufficient quantity and quality to carry out extensive genotyping. It would also appear that these convenient and noninvasive methods considerably increase the response rate in epidemiological studies. However, most previous studies using saliva-based methods have used relatively small numbers of adult subjects, and it therefore remains to be determined whether these methods are suitable for producing DNA of high quality and yield in larger studies, especially those involving young children. The IDEFICS (Identification and Prevention of Dietary- and Lifestyle-Induced Health Effects in Children and Infants) study is an integrated project funded by the Sixth Framework Program of the European Commission, and with a cohort size of 16 224 young children is one of the largest single studies to undertake saliva/DNA collection. In this study, the authors describe the design and methodological approaches used for DNA collection, extraction, biobanking, and genotyping in the IDEFICS study on the basis of the analysis of a subgroup of 4678 samples selected from the full IDEFICS cohort (Table 3).

M. G. Bissell, MD, PhD, MPH

Article Index

Chapter 1: Outcomes Analysis

Resident education and quality of gross tissue examination practices of benign
uteri   3

Pathology Review of Outside Material: When Does It Help and When Can It Hurt?   4

Certification and maintenance of certification: updates from the American Board of
Pathology   5

Biopsy Misidentification Identified by DNA Profiling in a Large Multicenter Trial   6

The College of American pathologists and National Society for Histotechnology
Workload Study   7

Are There Barriers to the Release of Paraffin Blocks for Clinical Research Trials?
A College of American Pathologists Survey of 609 Laboratories   9

Pathology subspecialty fellowship application reform 2007 to 2010   10

Mislabeling of Cases, Specimens, Blocks, and Slides: A College of American
Pathologists Study of 136 Institutions   12

Current experience and attitudes to biomedical scientist cut-up; results of an online
survey of UK consultant histopathologists   14

Inappropriate calibration and optimisation of pan-keratin (pan-CK) and low
molecular weight keratin (LMWCK) immunohistochemistry tests: Canadian
Immunohistochemistry Quality Control (CIQC) experience   15

Error rates in reporting prostatic core biopsies   17

Chapter 2: Breast

Effect of Occult Metastases on Survival in Node-Negative Breast Cancer   19

Prognostic Value of a Combined Estrogen Receptor, Progesterone Receptor, Ki-67,
and Human Epidermal Growth Factor Receptor 2 Immunohistochemical Score
and Comparison With the Genomic Health Recurrence Score in Early Breast
Cancer   20

The effect of delay in fixation, different fixatives, and duration of fixation in
estrogen and progesterone receptor results in breast carcinoma   22

Assessment of Ki67 in Breast Cancer: Recommendations from the International
Ki67 in Breast Cancer Working Group   23

Accuracy and Completeness of Pathology Reporting - Impact on Partial Breast
Irradiation Eligibility   25

ER, HER2, and TOP2A expression in primary tumor, synchronous axillary nodes,
and asynchronous metastases in breast cancer   26

All atypia diagnosed at stereotactic vacuum-assisted breast biopsy do not need
surgical excision   27

A multisite performance study comparing the reading of immunohistochemical
slides on a computer monitor with conventional manual microscopy for estrogen
and progesterone receptor analysis   29

Benign epithelial inclusions in axillary lymph nodes: report of 18 cases and review of the literature   30

Anaplastic large cell lymphoma and breast implants: results from a structured expert consultation process   31

Chapter 3: Gastrointestinal System

A quantitative assessment of the risks and cost savings of forgoing histologic examination of diminutive polyps   33

How to Classify Adenocarcinomas of the Esophagogastric Junction: As Esophageal or Gastric Cancer?   34

Gastric Hyperplastic Polyps: A Heterogeneous Clinicopathologic Group Including a Distinct Subset Best Categorized as Mucosal Prolapse Polyp   36

Virtual microscopy for histology quality assurance of screen-detected polyps   38

Adenoma detection rate increases with each decade of life after 50 years of age   39

A Prospective Study of Duodenal Bulb Biopsy in Newly Diagnosed and Established Adult Celiac Disease   40

Inter-observer variation in the histological diagnosis of polyps in colorectal cancer screening   42

Current practice patterns among pathologists in the assessment of venous invasion in colorectal cancer   43

What Impact Has the Introduction of a Synoptic Report for Rectal Cancer Had on Reporting Outcomes for Specialist Gastrointestinal and Nongastrointestinal Pathologists?   45

Chapter 4: Hepatobiliary System and Pancreas

Fibrolamellar carcinomas are positive for CD68   47

The steatohepatitic variant of hepatocellular carcinoma and its association with underlying steatohepatitis   49

Telangiectatic Variant of Hepatic Adenoma: Clinicopathologic Features and Correlation Between Liver Needle Biopsy and Resection   50

Identification of Malignant Cytologic Criteria in Pancreatobiliary Brushings With Corresponding Positive Fluorescence In Situ Hybridization Results   52

Diagnostic Utility of CD10 in Benign and Malignant Extrahepatic Bile Duct Lesions   53

Costaining for keratins 8/18 plus ubiquitin improves detection of hepatocyte injury in nonalcoholic fatty liver disease   55

The Liver in Celiac Disease: Clinical Manifestations, Histologic Features, and Response to Gluten-Free Diet in 30 Patients   57

The role of the pathologist in diagnosing and grading biliary diseases   57

Hepatic granulomas: A clinicopathologic analysis of 86 cases   59

Autoimmune Pancreatitis (AIP) Type 1 and Type 2: An International Consensus Study on Histopathologic Diagnostic Criteria   61

The Concept of Hepatic Artery-Bile Duct Parallelism in the Diagnosis of
Ductopenia in Liver Biopsy Samples   62

Histologic characteristics of pancreatic intraepithelial neoplasia associated with
different pancreatic lesions   63

Chapter 5: Dermatopathology

Assessment of Copy Number Status of Chromosomes 6 and 11 by FISH Provides
Independent Prognostic Information in Primary Melanoma   65

Fluorescence *in situ* hybridization, a diagnostic aid in ambiguous melanocytic
tumors: European study of 113 cases   66

Atypical Intradermal Smooth Muscle Neoplasms: Clinicopathologic Analysis of 84
Cases and a Reappraisal of Cutaneous "Leiomyosarcoma"   68

Sebaceous Carcinoma: An Immunohistochemical Reappraisal   69

A two-antibody mismatch repair protein immunohistochemistry screening approach
for colorectal carcinomas, skin sebaceous tumors, and gynecologic tract carcinomas   71

Mitotic Activity Within Dermal Melanocytes of Benign Melanocytic Nevi: A Study
of 100 Cases With Clinical Follow-up   72

Proliferative Nodules Arising Within Congenital Melanocytic Nevi: A Histologic,
Immunohistochemical, and Molecular Analyses of 43 Cases   74

Poikilodermatous mycosis fungoides: A study of its clinicopathological,
immunophenotypic, and prognostic features   75

Superficial Ewing's sarcoma family of tumors: a clinicopathological study with
differential diagnoses   77

Pseudomyogenic Hemangioendothelioma: A Distinctive, Often Multicentric
Tumor With Indolent Behavior   78

Melanocytes in nonlesional sun-exposed skin: A multicenter comparative study   80

p16 Expression: A marker of differentiation between childhood malignant
melanomas and Spitz nevi   82

Specificity of *IRF4* translocations for primary cutaneous anaplastic large cell
lymphoma: a multicenter study of 204 skin biopsies   83

Chapter 6: Lung and Mediastinum

Thymic Carcinoma Associated With Multilocular Thymic Cyst: A Clinicopathologic
Study of 7 Cases   85

High-grade neuroendocrine carcinomas of the lung highly express enhancer of
zeste homolog 2, but carcinoids do not   86

Pax8 Expression in Thymic Epithelial Neoplasms: An Immunohistochemical
Analysis   87

Small Neuroendocrine Lesions in Intrathoracic Lymph Nodes of Patients With
Primary Lung Adenocarcinoma: Real Metastasis?   88

Lymphomatoid Granulomatosis: Insights Gained Over 4 Decades   89

Optimal Immunohistochemical Markers for Distinguishing Lung Adenocarcinomas
From Squamous Cell Carcinomas in Small Tumor Samples   91

Chapter 7: Cardiovascular

Importance of specimen length during temporal artery biopsy 93

Endomyocardial biopsy—when and how? 94

Chapter 8: Soft Tissue and Bone

Low-Grade Fibromyxoid Sarcoma: A Clinicopathologic Study of 33 Cases With Long-Term Follow-Up 97

Percutaneous CT-guided biopsy of the musculoskeletal system: Results of 2027 cases 98

BCL-6 expression in mesenchymal tumours: an immunohistochemical and fluorescence in situ hybridisation study 100

Chapter 9: Female Genital Tract

Correlation between invasive pattern and immunophenotypic alterations in endocervical adenocarcinoma 103

Significant Variation in the Assessment of Cervical Involvement in Endometrial Carcinoma: An Interobserver Variation Study 105

Mutation and Loss of Expression of ARID1A in Uterine Low-grade Endometrioid Carcinoma 107

Immunoexpression of PAX 8 in Endometrial Cancer: Relation to High-Grade Carcinoma and p53 109

IMP2 Expression Distinguishes Endometrioid From Serous Endometrial Adenocarcinomas 110

Should grade 3 endometrioid endometrial carcinoma be considered a type 2 cancer—A clinical and pathological evaluation 112

Liposarcoma Arising in Uterine Lipoleiomyoma: A Report of 3 Cases and Review of the Literature 114

Correlation of macroscopic and microscopic pathology in risk reducing salpingo-oophorectomy: Implications for intraoperative specimen evaluation 115

FOXL2 Is a Sensitive and Specific Marker for Sex Cord-Stromal Tumors of the Ovary 117

Patterns of Low-grade Serous Carcinoma With Emphasis on the Nonepithelial-lined Spaces Pattern of Invasion and the Disorganized Orphan Papillae 119

Emergence of CA125 Immunoreactivity in Recurrent or Metastatic Primary Ovarian Mucinous Neoplasms of the Intestinal Type 121

Placenta weight percentile curves for singleton and twins deliveries 123

Placental Mesenchymal Dysplasia Presenting as a Twin Gestation With Complete Molar Pregnancy 124

Eosinophilic/T-cell Chorionic Vasculitis: A Clinicopathologic and Immunohistochemical Study of 51 Cases 126

Chapter 10: Urinary Bladder and Male Genital Tract

Epithelial Proliferations in Prostatic Stromal Tumors of Uncertain Malignant Potential (STUMP) — 129

Epithelial Proliferations in Prostatic Stromal Tumors of Uncertain Malignant Potential (STUMP) — 130

Immunohistochemical Analysis in a Morphologic Spectrum of Urachal Epithelial Neoplasms: Diagnostic Implications and Pitfalls — 135

Identification of Gleason Pattern 5 on Prostatic Needle Core Biopsy: Frequency of Underdiagnosis and Relation to Morphology — 138

Routine dual-color immunostaining with a 3-antibody cocktail improves the detection of small cancers in prostate needle biopsies — 139

Should Intervening Benign Tissue Be Included in the Measurement of Discontinuous Foci of Cancer on Prostate Needle Biopsy? Correlation With Radical Prostatectomy Findings — 141

Plasmacytoid urothelial carcinoma of the urinary bladder: clinicopathologic, immunohistochemical, ultrastructural, and molecular analysis of a case series — 143

Initial High-grade Prostatic Intraepithelial Neoplasia With Carcinoma on Subsequent Prostate Needle Biopsy: Findings at Radical Prostatectomy — 148

Initial High-grade Prostatic Intraepithelial Neoplasia With Carcinoma on Subsequent Prostate Needle Biopsy: Findings at Radical Prostatectomy — 149

PAX8 and PAX2 Immunostaining Facilitates the Diagnosis of Primary Epithelial Neoplasms of the Male Genital Tract — 151

Flat urothelial carcinoma in situ of the bladder with glandular differentiation — 153

D2-40 immunoreactivity in penile squamous cell carcinoma: a marker of aggressiveness — 157

Gleason Score 7 Prostate Cancer on Needle Biopsy: Relation of Primary Pattern 3 or 4 to Pathological Stage and Progression After Radical Prostatectomy — 159

Chapter 11: Kidney

Role of Immunohistochemistry in the Evaluation of Needle Core Biopsies in Adult Renal Cortical Tumors: An Ex Vivo Study — 161

Immunohistochemical Distinction of Primary Adrenal Cortical Lesions From Metastatic Clear Cell Renal Cell Carcinoma: A Study of 248 Cases — 163

Handling and reporting of nephrectomy specimens for adult renal tumours: a survey by the European Network of Uropathology — 165

Pure Epithelioid PEComas (So-Called Epithelioid Angiomyolipoma) of the Kidney: A Clinicopathologic Study of 41 Cases: Detailed Assessment of Morphology and Risk Stratification — 166

Immunohistochemical markers of tissue injury in biopsies with transplant glomerulitis — 168

The Nature of Biopsies with "Borderline Rejection" and Prospects for Eliminating This Category — 170

Overlapping pathways to transplant glomerulopathy: chronic humoral rejection, hepatitis C infection, and thrombotic microangiopathy — 171

Low glomerular density is a risk factor for progression in idiopathic membranous nephropathy 173

Postinfectious Glomerulonephritis in the Elderly 174

A composite urine biomarker reflects interstitial inflammation in lupus nephritis kidney biopsies 176

Immunohistochemical evaluation of podocalyxin expression in glomerulopathies associated with nephrotic syndrome 178

The Relevance of Periglomerular Fibrosis in the Evaluation of Routine Needle Core Renal Biopsies 179

Chapter 12: Head and Neck

Salivary gland carcinoma in Denmark 1990–2005: A national study of incidence, site and histology. Results of the Danish Head and Neck Cancer Group (DAHANCA) 181

Cribriform Adenocarcinoma of Minor Salivary Gland Origin Principally Affecting the Tongue: Characterization of New Entity 183

Lymphadenoma of the salivary gland: clinicopathological and immunohistochemical analysis of 33 tumors 186

Salivary Gland Anlage Tumor: A Clinicopathological Study of Two Cases 190

A Histologic and Immunohistochemical Study Describing the Diversity of Tumors Classified as Sinonasal High-grade Nonintestinal Adenocarcinomas 194

Sinonasal neuroendocrine carcinoma: impact of differentiation status on response and outcome 198

Basal cell carcinoma on the ear is more likely to be of an aggressive phenotype in both men and women 201

A Combined Molecular-Pathologic Score Improves Risk Stratification of Thyroid Papillary Microcarcinoma 204

Adenomatous tumors of the middle ear and temporal bone: clinical, morphological and tumor biological characteristics of challenging neoplastic lesions 207

The Chernobyl Thyroid Cancer Experience: Pathology 210

Molecular, Morphologic, and Outcome Analysis of Thyroid Carcinomas According to Degree of Extrathyroid Extension 215

Chapter 13: Neuropathology

TDP-43 Proteinopathy and Motor Neuron Disease in Chronic Traumatic Encephalopathy 219

Altered microRNA expression in frontotemporal lobar degeneration with TDP-43 pathology caused by progranulin mutations 220

Subtypes of medulloblastoma have distinct developmental origins 221

Amyloid Triggers Extensive Cerebral Angiogenesis Causing Blood Brain Barrier Permeability and Hypervascularity in Alzheimer's Disease 222

Toward Brain Tumor Gene Therapy Using Multipotent Mesenchymal Stromal Cell Vectors 224

Enhanced invasion *in vitro* and the distribution patterns *in vivo* of CD133⁺ glioma stem cells — 224

Inducible nitric oxide synthase is present in motor neuron mitochondria and Schwann cells and contributes to disease mechanisms in ALS mice — 226

Chapter 14: Cytopathology

Randomized healthservices study of human papillomavirus-based management of low-grade cytological abnormalities — 229

p16/Ki-67 Dual-Stain Cytology in the Triage of ASCUS and LSIL Papanicolaou Cytology: Results From the European Equivocal or Mildly Abnormal Papanicolaou Cytology Study — 230

Usefulness of Immunohistochemical and Histochemical Studies in the Classification of Lung Adenocarcinoma and Squamous Cell Carcinoma in Cytologic Specimens — 232

Cytology Workforce Study: A Report of Current Practices and Trends in New York State — 233

A Systematic Review and Meta-Analysis of the Diagnostic Accuracy of Fine-Needle Aspiration Cytology for Parotid Gland Lesions — 234

Evaluation of HPV-16 and HPV-18 Genotyping for the Triage of Women With High-Risk HPV+ Cytology-Negative Results — 235

Cytologic Diagnosis and Differential Diagnosis of Lung Carcinoid Tumors: A Retrospective Study of 63 Cases With Histologic Correlation — 237

Current State and Future Perspective of Molecular Diagnosis of Fine-Needle Aspiration Biopsy of Thyroid Nodules — 238

The Interobserver Reproducibility of Thyroid Fine-Needle Aspiration Using the UK Royal College of Pathologists' Classification System — 240

Implementation of Evidence-Based Guidelines for Thyroid Nodule Biopsy: A Model for Establishment of Practice Standards — 242

Chapter 15: Hematolymphoid

Combined Core Needle Biopsy and Fine-Needle Aspiration With Ancillary Studies Correlate Highly With Traditional Techniques in the Diagnosis of Nodal-Based Lymphoma — 245

Independent Diagnostic Accuracy of Flow Cytometry Obtained From Fine-Needle Aspirates: A 10-Year Experience With 451 Cases — 246

Primary Follicular Lymphoma of the Gastrointestinal Tract — 248

The use of CellaVision competency software for external quality assessment and continuing professional development — 249

Diagnosis and Immunophenotype of 188 Pediatric Lymphoblastic Lymphomas Treated Within a Randomized Prospective Trial: Experiences and Preliminary Recommendations From the European Childhood Lymphoma Pathology Panel — 250

Timeliness and Quality of Diagnostic Care for Medicare Recipients With Chronic Lymphocytic Leukemia — 252

Pitfalls in bone marrow pathology: avoiding errors in bone marrow trephine biopsy
diagnosis   253

Pitfalls in lymphoma pathology: avoiding errors in diagnosis of lymphoid tissues   254

Chapter 16: Techniques/Molecular

Gelatin foam cell blocks made from cytology fluid specimens   257

MicroRNAs in colorectal cancer: Function, dysregulation and potential as novel
biomarkers   257

Evaluation of a completely automated tissue-sectioning machine for paraffin
blocks   259

Molecular Classification of Gastric Cancer: A New Paradigm   260

A Comparative Analysis of Molecular Genetic and Conventional Cytogenetic
Detection of Diagnostically Important Translocations in More Than 400 Cases
of Acute Leukemia, Highlighting the Frequency of False-Negative Conventional
Cytogenetics   261

Molecular Diagnostics of Lung Carcinomas   262

Clinicopathologic and Molecular Profiles of Microsatellite Unstable Barrett
Esophagus-associated Adenocarcinoma   263

Chapter 17: Laboratory Management and Outcomes

Effect of Two Different FDA-approved D-dimer Assays on Resource Utilization
in the Emergency Department   267

Pending Laboratory Tests and the Hospital Discharge Summary in Patients
Discharged To Sub-Acute Care   268

Repeated Hemoglobin A1C Ordering in the VA Health System   270

Impact of Laboratory Accreditation on Patient Care and the Health System   271

The Impact of Specially Designed Digital Games-Based Learning in Undergraduate
Pathology and Medical Education   272

Human Tissue Ownership and Use in Research: What Laboratorians and
Researchers Should Know   275

Intellectual Property: Turning Patent Swords into Shares   276

Determining the Optimal Approach for Government-Regulated Genetic Testing   278

Meeting Regulatory Requirements by the Use of Cell Phone Text Message
Notification With Autoescalation and Loop Closure for Reporting of Critical
Laboratory Results   279

Maternal Serum Screening: Results Disclosure, Anxiety, and Risk Perception   281

Chapter 18: Clinical Chemistry

Serum Bilirubin and Risk of Respiratory Disease and Death   283

Low-Dose Aspirin Use and Performance of Immunochemical Fecal Occult Blood
Tests   284

Effect of Screening on Ovarian Cancer Mortality: The Prostate, Lung, Colorectal and Ovarian (PLCO) Cancer Screening Randomized Controlled Trial 286

A New Study of Intraosseous Blood for Laboratory Analysis 287

Inverse Log-Linear Relationship between Thyroid-Stimulating Hormone and Free Thyroxine Measured by Direct Analog Immunoassay and Tandem Mass Spectrometry 288

Comparison of Urinary Albumin and Urinary Total Protein as Predictors of Patient Outcomes in CKD 289

A Combination of Serum Markers for the Early Detection of Colorectal Cancer 291

Performance Characteristics of Six Intact Parathyroid Hormone Assays 292

Characterization of the New Serum Protein Reference Material ERM-DA470k/IFCC: Value Assignment by Immunoassay 293

Initial observations regarding free cortisol quantification logistics among critically ill children 294

An Observational Study of Early Neonatal Biochemical Parameters in Twins 295

Chapter 19: Clinical Microbiology

Airborne bacteria concentrations and related factors at university laboratories, hospital diagnostic laboratories and a biowaste site 297

Interferon-γ release assays for the diagnosis of latent *Mycobacterium tuberculosis* infection: a systematic review and meta-analysis 298

Saliva Polymerase-Chain-Reaction Assay for Cytomegalovirus Screening in Newborns 299

Diagnostic value of laboratory tests in identifying serious infections in febrile children: systematic review 300

An Antimicrobial Stewardship Program's Impact with Rapid Polymerase Chain Reaction Methicillin-Resistant *Staphylococcus aureus/S. aureus* Blood Culture Test in Patients with *S. aureus* Bacteremia 303

Bacterial Vaginosis Assessed by Gram Stain and Diminished Colonization Resistance to Incident Gonococcal, Chlamydial, and Trichomonal Genital Infection 304

Reducing Blood Culture Contamination by a Simple Informational Intervention 305

Rapid Identification of 2009 H1N1 Influenza A Virus Using Fluorescent Antibody Methods 306

Diagnosis of Bacteriuria and Leukocyturia by Automated Flow Cytometry Compared with Urine Culture 307

Identification of Two Borderline Oxacillin-Resistant Strains of *Staphylococcus aureus* From Routine Nares Swab Specimens by One of Three Chromogenic Agars Evaluated for the Detection of MRSA 308

Detection of prion infection in variant Creutzfeldt-Jakob disease: a blood-based assay 308

Chapter 20: Hematology and Immunology

Performance characteristics of two commercially available IgG-specific immunoassays in the assessment of heparin-induced thrombocytopenia (HIT)   311

Multiparameter Flow Cytometry in the Diagnosis and Management of Acute Leukemia   313

Timeliness and Quality of Diagnostic Care for Medicare Recipients With Chronic Lymphocytic Leukemia   314

Peripheral Blood Monitoring of Chronic Myeloid Leukemia During Treatment With Imatinib, Second-Line Agents, and Beyond   316

Prognostic Value of *FLT3* Mutations Among Different Cytogenetic Subgroups in Acute Myeloid Leukemia   317

Flow Cytometry Rapidly Identifies All Acute Promyelocytic Leukemias With High Specificity Independent of Underlying Cytogenetic Abnormalities   319

Flow Cytometric Immunophenotyping of Cerebrospinal Fluid Specimens   320

Prognostic significance of the initial cerebro-spinal fluid (CSF) involvement of children with acute lymphoblastic leukaemia (ALL) treated without cranial irradiation: Results of European Organization for Research and Treatment of Cancer (EORTC) Children Leukemia Group study 58881   321

Transcriptomes of the B and T Lineages Compared by Multiplatform Microarray Profiling   322

Chromosome 20q Deletion: A Recurrent Cytogenetic Abnormality in Patients With Chronic Myelogenous Leukemia in Remission   323

Automated Cerebrospinal Fluid Cell Counts Using the Sysmex XE-5000: Is It Time for New Reference Ranges?   325

Usefulness of Multiparametric Flow Cytometry in Detecting Composite Lymphoma: Study of 17 Cases in a 12-Year Period   326

Chapter 21: Transfusion Medicine and Coagulation

Nucleic Acid Testing to Detect HBV Infection in Blood Donors   329

Molecular insight into human platelet antigens: structural and evolutionary conservation analyses offer new perspective to immunogenic disorders   331

The use of fresh-frozen plasma in England: high levels of inappropriate use in adults and children   332

Automated mixing studies and pattern recognition for the laboratory diagnosis of a prolonged activated partial thromboplastin time using an automated coagulation analyzer   333

Development of a rapid emergency hemorrhage panel   335

Reduction of the risk of transfusion-transmitted human immunodeficiency virus (HIV) infection by using an HIV antigen/antibody combination assay in blood donation screening in Cameroon   336

External Quality Assurance of Antithrombin, Protein C, and Protein S Assays: Results of the College of American Pathologists Proficiency Testing Program in Thrombophilia   337

Development of North American Consensus Guidelines for Medical Laboratories That Perform and Interpret Platelet Function Testing Using Light Transmission Aggregometry   338

Reducing costs in flow-cytometric counting of residual white blood cells in blood products: utilization of a single-platform bead-free flow-rate calibration method   339

Postponing or eliminating red blood cell transfusions of very low birth weight neonates by obtaining all baseline laboratory blood tests from otherwise discarded fetal blood in the placenta   340

Chapter 22: Cytogenetics and Molecular Pathology

Cancer genetics-guided discovery of serum biomarker signatures for diagnosis and prognosis of prostate cancer   343

Saliva-Derived DNA Performs Well in Large-Scale, High-Density Single-Nucleotide Polymorphism Microarray Studies   344

Clinical Experience with the Cervista HPV HR Assay: Correlation of Cytology and HPV Status from 56,501 Specimens   345

Resistance May Not Be Futile: microRNA Biomarkers for Chemoresistance and Potential Therapeutics   347

Assay Design Affects the Interpretation of T-Cell Receptor Gamma Gene Rearrangements: Comparison of the Performance of a One-Tube Assay with the BIOMED-2-Based TCRG Gene Clonality Assay   348

Effect of Direct-to-Consumer Genomewide Profiling to Assess Disease Risk   349

A Novel and Rapid Method of Determining the Effect of Unclassified *MLH1* Genetic Variants on Differential Allelic Expression   350

Necessity of Bilateral Bone Marrow Biopsies for Ancillary Cytogenetic Studies in the Pediatric Population   351

Cancer: Missing the mark   352

Design and Multiseries Validation of a Web-Based Gene Expression Assay for Predicting Breast Cancer Recurrence and Patient Survival   354

DNA yield and quality of saliva samples and suitability for large-scale epidemiological studies in children   356

Author Index

A

Abbott RA, 75
Abrosimov AA, 210
Agersborg SS, 29
Agoumi M, 82
A'Hern R, 23
Al Dhaybi R, 82
Al-Agha OM, 117
Al-Ahmadie HA, 161
Al-Hussain TO, 148, 149
Alden D, 161
Algaba F, 165
Aliberti S, 326
Aljabri S, 123
Allen KE, 347
Allen MJ, 275
Almog B, 123
Amador-Ortiz C, 245
Amin A, 159
Andres H, 291
Ang SBL, 279
Ansai S-I, 69
Ansari MQ, 313
Antic T, 53
Apple S, 22
Arase S, 69
Asad-Syed M, 27
Ashikaga T, 19
Aziz I, 40
Azzi J, 168

B

Baer VL, 340
Bahlo M, 344
Baid-Agrawal S, 171
Bakchoul T, 311
Baker M, 220
Balachandran I, 233
Balada-Llasat J-M, 303
Barkan GA, 135
Barker RM, 294
Barr Fritcher EG, 52
Bartalena T, 98
Batal I, 168
Baudhuin LM, 278
Bauer KA, 303
Bein G, 311
Bell AM, 246
Bengzon J, 224
Bennett BD, 5
Bernal-Mizrachi L, 316
Berney DM, 165

Bexell D, 224
Bhardwaj V, 319
Biron KE, 222
Bjørndal K, 181
Black-Schaffer WS, 10
Blair DH, 271
Bloss CS, 349
Blue JE, 52
Bogdanova T, 210
Bonello L, 326
Boppana SB, 299
Brenner H, 284
Brodsky SV, 179
Brotman RM, 304
Brouste V, 27
Brunati P, 307
Brunner AH, 109
Buchan BW, 308
Buchen L, 352
Burkhardt B, 250
Burroughs F, 237
Bussolati G, 38
Buys SS, 286

C

Calabuig-Fariñas S, 77
Candotti D, 329
Carcangiu ML, 30
Carr RA, 14
Caudill JL, 52
Chandler WL, 335, 337
Chandra A, 240
Chari S, 61
Chassagne-Clement C, 250
Chen C, 351
Chen K, 226
Chen L, 245
Chopp W, 62
Chopra N, 93
Chow C, 117
Christensen RD, 340
Ciarlini P, 325
Cima I, 343
Coffinet L, 190
Cohen C, 29
Colarossi C, 151
Connealy S, 348
Copete M, 15
Cordiner D, 295
Courtney ED, 93
Cox E, 268
Craig FE, 320
Cram P, 270
Crawford JM, 10

Crook ML, 103
Cross PA, 240
Cross SS, 40
Cui W, 323
Cunningham MT, 337
Cushman-Vokoun AM, 348
Cuzick J, 20
Czerwinski JL, 281

D

Dacic S, 262
Dal Cin P, 114
Daniel HDJ, 47
Danoy P, 344
d'Anzeo G, 157
de Freitas DG, 170
de la Fouchardière A, 66
de Mascarel I, 27
Deavers MT, 119
Delahunt B, 165
Demicco EG, 263
Demurtas A, 326
Deshpande V, 36
Diamond SJ, 39
Dickstein DL, 222
Diel R, 298
Dillner L, 229
Dizon DS, 124
Dong HY, 319
Dowsett M, 20, 23
Doxtader E, 89
Driman DK, 43
Duderstadt M, 207

E

Earle CC, 252, 314
Edgeworth JA, 308
El-Haddad N, 168
Elfgren K, 229
Enestvedt BK, 39
Epstein JI, 129, 130, 148, 149, 159
Eszlinger M, 238
Evans HL, 97
Evans KE, 40
Ewertz M, 26

F

Fajardo DA, 138
Farmer M, 308

Farris AB III, 171, 263
Fellegara G, 30
Ferrara G, 298
Ferraz C, 238
Ferrell C, 335
Fidler ME, 174
Findeis-Hosey JJ, 86
Fine SW, 161
Fischer JC, 339
Fitzgibbons PL, 9
Fletcher CD, 166
Fletcher CDM, 68, 78
Ford JM, 71
Förster C, 207
Fowler I, 6
Friedlander M, 233
Friese CR, 252, 314
Fujita H, 36
Fujiwara M, 163

G

Gagné I, 82
Gakiopoulou H, 178
Ganesan R, 112
Ganguly A, 114
Garratt J, 15
Gauchotte G, 190
Gavett BE, 219
Gerst SR, 242
Gertler R, 34
Gibson P, 221
Gilks B, 15
Giptner A, 311
Giunti L, 143
Gnepp DR, 186
Goldman R, 124
Goletti D, 298
Gonen M, 242
Gonzalez-Obeso E, 36
Gopaul R, 222
Gorrill TS, 320
Grant-Casey J, 332
Greiner TC, 348
Grimes MM, 5
Grimm KE, 351
Gronowski KS, 275
Grzybicki DM, 3
Guan B, 107
Guy CD, 55

H

Ha KC, 297
Haj-Hassan T, 300

Hall BJ, 234
Hambly NM, 242
Hammond S, 259
Hanna E, 198
Hao S, 110
Harada K, 57
Harris NL, 248
Hassan A, 245
Hasserjian RP, 248
Haug U, 284
Hayward CPM, 338
Heinze G, 109
Henderson P, 295
Hendi A, 80
Hirschowitz L, 105
Hoffman RD, 10
Hol L, 42
Horiuchi Y, 249
Hornick JL, 78
Horsfall LJ, 283
Hoskovec JM, 281
Hosler GA, 345
Hsi ED, 83
Huang J, 86
Huwait HF, 117
Hwang SH, 297

I

Idei M, 249
Idowu MO, 12
Imperiale TF, 33
Ishii K, 333

J

Jack R, 294
Jacobs MA, 80
Jacques SM, 126
Jarell AD, 201
Jenkins J, 179
Jensen JD, 26
Jiang Z, 39
Jimenez RE, 153
Jo VY, 194
Johnson MW, 237
Jones D, 317

K

Kanthan R, 272
Karram S, 141
Kaspirkova-Nemcova J,
    183

Katzenstein A-LA, 89
Kavoura E, 178
Kawamura T, 173
Keller T, 293
Kemetli L, 229
Kerin MJ, 257
Kessler WR, 33
Khanin R, 260
Kidric D, 325
Kim B, 31
Kim CJ, 126
King RL, 261
Kirsch R, 45
Klebanoff MA, 304
Klein RW, 33
Knoop A, 26
Kocerha J, 220
Kocjan G, 240
Kohl SK, 7
Kolker SE, 72
Koni AC, 356
Kouri N, 220
Kraft S, 68
Krag DN, 19
Krogdahl A, 181
Kuffner Akatsu H, 204
Kujala PM, 139
Kung JX, 319
Kurt M, 59

L

Labow DM, 63
Lambert DK, 340
Landau M, 331
Laskin J, 91
La'ulu SL, 292
Laurila M, 139
Law ME, 83, 100
Laxmisan A, 270
Le LP, 74, 263
Leballais L, 336
Ledeboer NA, 308
Leonardi GP, 306
Leung S, 91
Lewis SE, 7
Li B, 350
Li F, 86, 88
Liang J, 63
Likhacheva A, 198
Lima L, 316
Little L, 103
Liu Y, 110
LiVolsi VA, 210
Llombart B, 77

Loh TP, 279
Loos M, 34
Lopez-Beltran A, 153
Lowe AC, 22
Lowe D, 332
Lucarini G, 157
Ludeman L, 112

M

MacGregor MS, 289
Machado I, 77
Mackey A, 115
Magazu LS, 252, 314
Malpica A, 119
Mao T-L, 107
Marberger M, 6
Martignoni G, 166
Martin LJ, 226
Mayall FG, 257
Mbanya D, 336
McCluggage WG, 105, 121
McConnell JD, 6
McDonald AG, 114
McGillicuddy DC, 267
McKee AC, 219
McKenney JK, 135
McLeod RS, 43, 45
McPhail ED, 100
Memeo L, 151
Mendu DR, 288
Mengel M, 170
Merren M, 259
Messenger DE, 43, 45
Methven S, 289
Millar J, 121
Miller JS, 138
Miller K, 121
Miller LJ, 287
Miller N, 257
Mills SE, 194
Minardi D, 157
Misdraji J, 248
Miyamoto H, 138
Miyazaki Y, 173
Moffat KA, 338
Mojtahed A, 71
Montez D, 287
Montironi R, 153
Moog R, 339
Moran CA, 85, 87
Moreira RK, 62
Mounajjed T, 50, 57
Mully TW, 201
Murali R, 65
Murry TC, 72

N

Nadasdy T, 176
Nagar M, 129, 130
Nagaraja HN, 176
Naghashpour M, 261
Nakanuma Y, 57
Nakhleh RE, 12
Nansel TR, 304
Narendra S, 89
Nasr SH, 174
Nassar A, 29
Nese N, 166
Netto GJ, 141
Nielsen TO, 23
Niemeier LA, 204
North JP, 65
Northington FJ, 226
Nugent M, 257

O

Ocque R, 232
Ohori NP, 232, 320
Ohsaka A, 333
Olson JD, 337
Onozato ML, 259
Oschlies I, 250
Oxentenko A, 57
Oxley JD, 17
Ozderin YO, 59

P

Painter MW, 322
Pålsson AS, 305
Paner GP, 135
Panuganti PK, 107
Paraskevakou H, 178
Park DU, 297
Partin A, 159
Paschke R, 238
Pascual M, 171
Perera S, 350
Peter TF, 271
Peters JM, 313
Phadke PA, 74
Philbeck TE, 287
Pieretti B, 307
Pignol JP, 25
Pineda S, 20
Pini B, 307
Powell CB, 115

Powers MLE, 275
Prochazkova-Carlotti M, 66
Pucci R, 22

Q

Qiao W, 317
Quenzel EM, 339
Qureshi F, 126

R

Rabban JT, 115
Raby A, 338
Rait G, 283
Rakheja D, 74
Rakovitch E, 25
Raspollini MR, 143
Recavarren C, 63
Remaley AT, 288
Remotti H, 49
Rialland X, 321
Ricarte-Filho J, 215
Rimondi E, 98
Risio M, 38
Riss P, 109
Rivera M, 215
Roberts WL, 292
Robinson G, 221
Robson A, 75
Rollinger W, 291
Rosai J, 30
Rosenberg N, 331
Rosenthal DI, 198
Ross HM, 47
Rossi G, 98
Roth A, 305
Roth C, 31
Rotz PD, 271
Ruhoy SM, 72
Ryan MS, 3

S

Sahni D, 75
Salomao M, 49
Sanchez LD, 267
Sanders DSA, 14
Sandhaus LM, 325
Sangoi AR, 163
Santos FPS, 317
Sardi I, 143
Satoskar AA, 179

Savage EC, 246
Saw S, 279
Saxe D, 316
Scheding S, 224
Schiess R, 343
Schmidt D, 230
Schmidt RL, 234
Schmitt E, 190
Schork NJ, 349
Schreiber W, 293
Schrijver I, 71
Seethala RR, 186
Sellarés J, 170
Sen C, 17
Senger J-L, 272
Senore C, 38
Shah MA, 260
Shehata F, 123
Shmidt E, 57
Sicilia A, 308
Silva EG, 119
Sima R, 183
Simmons EJV, 14
Sirvent N, 321
Skalova A, 183
Smith LB, 4
Smith M, 268
Smith ML, 3
Smyrk TC, 61
Song C, 204
Souers RJ, 12
Stankovich J, 344
Stanworth SJ, 332
Starikov R, 124
Stein HJ, 34
Stelow EB, 194
Stenson B, 295
Stern RA, 219
Stewart CJR, 103
Stoll LM, 237
Stramer SL, 329
Suciu S, 321
Sun J, 323

T

Tabe Y, 249
Tagny CT, 336

Takeichi H, 69
Tang L, 260
Tao S, 284
Terry J, 91
Therkildsen MH, 181
Thompson LDR, 186
Thompson MJ, 300
Tochigi N, 232
Tolonen TT, 139
Tong G-X, 151
Tong Y, 221
Topol EJ, 349
Traynor JP, 289
Tretiakova M, 53
Trimble S, 335
Trock BJ, 141
Tsitsikotas S, 350
Tsuboi N, 173
Tunnicliffe J, 7
Turhan N, 59
Tuttle RM, 215

V

Valeri AM, 174
van Dekken H, 42
Van Den Bruel A, 300
van Deventer HE, 288
Van Laar RK, 354
Van Overwalle G, 276
van Putten PG, 42
Vanderheyden AD, 246
Vaughan R, 49
Vaughan-Sarrazin M, 270
Veinot JP, 94
Vergier B, 66
Vetto JT, 65
Vivekanandan P, 47
Volz KA, 267
Voss MA, 112

W

Wada DA, 80, 83
Walters K, 283
Walters MP, 100
Walz SE, 268

Wang X, 88
Washington MK, 62
Washington PJ, 345
Watt CD, 261
Weaver DL, 19
Weiss GJ, 347
Weiss LM, 351
Weissferdt A, 85, 87
Welkoborsky H-J, 207
Wend U, 329
West JE, 303
West RB, 163
Westerhoff M, 53
Wicklund CA, 281
Wiklund AE, 305
Wild N, 291
Wild P, 343
Wilkins BS, 253, 254
Wilson AR, 234
Wilson GE, 105
Wood I, 257
Wright TC Jr, 235
Wu T-T, 50

X

Xu H, 88

Y

Yamamoto T, 333
Yang X-J, 224
Yin CC, 323
Youens KE, 345
Young VL, 31
Ypsilantis E, 93
Yu S-P, 224

Z

Zegers I, 293
Zeppieri J, 25
Zhang B, 224
Zhang L, 61, 110
Zhang X, 176
Zimmerman JJ, 294